OXFORD MEDICAL PUBLICATIONS

Fetal Behaviour

The Physical and Developmental Environment
of High-Risk Infant
Division of Child Development
Pediatrics/COM MDC-15
University of South Florida
1 Davis Blvd., Suite 309
Tampa, FL 33606
(813) 272-2755   (813) 272-2793 FAX

Fetal Behaviour

Developmental and Perinatal Aspects

Edited by

JAN G. NIJHUIS

Assistant Professor in Obstetrics and Gynaecology
University Hospital Nijmegen
The Netherlands

OXFORD   NEW YORK   TOKYO
OXFORD UNIVERSITY PRESS
1992

Oxford University Press, Walton Street, Oxford OX2 6DP

Oxford   New York   Toronto
Delhi   Bombay   Calcutta   Madras   Karachi
Petaling Jaya   Singapore   Hong Kong   Tokyo
Nairobi   Dar es Salaam   Cape Town
Melbourne   Auckland

and associated companies in
Berlin   Ibadan

Oxford is a trade mark of Oxford University Press

Published in the United States
by Oxford University Press, New York

© The contributors listed on pp xiii–xiv, 1992

A catalogue record for this book is available from the British Library

Library of Congress Cataloging in Publication Data
(Data available)

ISBN 0 19 262089 4

Set by
Footnote Graphics
Warminster, Wiltshire

Printed in Great Britain
by Bookcraft (Bath) Ltd.
Midsomer Norton, Avon

This book is dedicated to my parents, my wife Marjan Kloen, and my children Tim, Annelijn, and Olivier. Without their stimulating and understanding behaviour (fetal, neonatal, and adult!) this book would not have been written.

Preface

It was not until ultrasonography was introduced into clinical practice that access to the fetus was possible. It rapidly became clear that a fetus was more than a 'positive pregnancy test' or 'audible heart tones'. It became apparent that the fetus exhibits 'behaviour' from seven weeks of gestation (menstrual weeks!) onward, behaviour that is strongly dependent on the gestational age. It is important that clinicians and researchers understand the development of normal fetal behaviour and the concept of behavioural states. Only then can scientific protocols for studying behaviour or behavioural variables be properly written, and only then is an optimal interpretation of the fetal condition possible. Furthermore, the behaviour of the normal fetus must be well understood in order to gain insight into pathological situations and to recognize the abnormal fetus.

This insight into fetal behaviour is also of great importance for those working in the fields of fetal psychology and psychobiology: it is important that they appreciate that a fetus can be observed only within the context of its behaviour and behavioural states. Psychologists have traditionally ignored the fetal period, and a new field of investigation is now opening.

Much basic research has been performed on animals. It is intriguing to see how many behavioural parallels have been drawn during the last decade between several species, especially the chronically instrumented fetal lamb, and man. Animal research has helped a great deal in obtaining insight into fetal behaviour, and human data have also stimulated the physiologists to look to animal models for detailed answers to questions relating to fetal behavioural variables.

It is against this background that this first handbook on fetal behaviour has been written. An overview is given on the subject of fetal behaviour from the very first movements and onward through to neonatal behaviour after birth. The book has four sections. In the first, a description of behaviour in the normal human fetus is given. In the second, chapters are brought together that deal with animal research in relation to fetal behaviour and fetal developmental physiology. The present state of the art is given, and directions are indicated for future research. Attention is also given to medication that may influence behaviour. In the third section two chapters deal with fetal behaviour in relation to fetal psychology and the fetal–maternal axis. All chapters in the fourth and final section have been dedicated to the consequences for clinical practice, fetal monitoring (including biophysical tests and Doppler techniques), and perinatal research.

I hope this book will prove to be of great value for obstetricians, perinatologists, paediatricians, and researchers in the field of perinatal physiology and developmental psychology. Perhaps it will also stimulate students to start to work in these fields, showing possible future directions for their careers.

Nijmegen   J.G.N.
January 1992

Acknowledgements

This seems to be the right place to thank all authors who have—without hesitation—participated in writing this book. All of them are acknowledged leaders in their respective fields, and they have all collaborated with great enthusiasm. This book could not have been published without their efforts.

I would also like to thank Mr Ian Cunningham and my secretary Mrs Leny Aelen for their magnificent help in organizing and editing this book.

Contents

List of contributors   xiii

Introduction   xv
T. K. A. B. Eskes

Part 1   Development of behaviour during normal pregnancy

1   The first trimester   3
J. I. P. de Vries

2   The second trimester   17
G. H. A. Visser

3   The third trimester   26
J. G. Nijhuis

4   Heart-rate patterns and fetal movements   41
E. E. van Woerden and H. P. van Geijn

5   During labour   57
John A. D. Spencer

6   Some remarks on the neonate   65
H. F. R. Prechtl

Part 2   Fetal behaviour in research

7   Development of the central nervous system   75
D. F. Swaab, M. B. O. M. Honnebier, and M. Mirmiran

8   Central nervous control   91
G. S. Dawes

9   Animal investigations   100
P. J. Moore and M. A. Hanson

10   Effects of perinatal medication on the developing brain   112
M. Mirmiran and D. F. Swaab

Part 3   Fetal behaviour and fetal psychology

11   Fetal psychology: an embryonic science   129
     Peter G. Hepper

12   Maternal emotions during pregnancy and
     fetal and neonatal behaviour   157
     B. R. H. van den Bergh

**Part 4   Fetal behaviour and the assessment of
           fetal well-being**

13   Growth retardation   181
     Domenico Arduini, Giuseppe Rizzo, and Carlo Romanini

14   Diabetic pregnancy   193
     E. J. H. Mulder

15   Fetal behaviour in relation to stimulation   209
     Robert Gagnon

16   Doppler flow measurements   227
     J. van Eyck and J. W. Wladimiroff

17   Biophysical profile scoring   241
     F. A. Manning

18   Consequences for fetal monitoring   258
     B. A. P. J. Tas and J. G. Nijhuis

Epilogue: Do we really need the concept of fetal
          behavioural states?   269
     Chester B. Martin Jr

Index   275

Contributors

Domenico Arduini, M.D. *Director of Perinatal Medicine Service, Istituto di Clinica Ostetrica e Ginecologica, Università Cattolica S. Cuore, Rome, Italy.*

B. R. H. van den Bergh, Ph.D. *Psychologist, Pediatric Rehabilitation Centre Pulderbos (affiliated with the University Hospital Gasthuisberg Leuven), 4 Reebergenlaan, 2242 Zandhoven, Belgium.*

G. S. Dawes, C.B.E., D.M., F.R.S. *Professor, Nuffield Department of Obstetrics and Gynaecology, John Radcliffe Hospital, Oxford, UK.*

T. K. A. B. Eskes, M.D., Ph.D., F.R.C.O.G. *Professor of Obstetrics and Gynaecology, Department of Obstetrics and Gynaecology, University Hospital Nijmegen, P.O. Box 9101, 6500 HB Nijmegen, The Netherlands.*

J. van Eyck, M.D., Ph.D. *Department of Perinatal Medicine, Sophia Hospital Zwolle, Dokter Van Heesweg 2, 8025 AB Zwolle, The Netherlands.*

Robert Gagnon, M.D., F.R.C.S. *Assistant Professor of Obstetrics and Gynecology, St. Joseph's Health Centre, 268 Grosvenor Street, London, Ontario, N6A 4V2, Canada.*

H. P. van Geijn, M.D., Ph.D. *Professor in Obstetric Perinatology, Department of Obstetrics and Gynaecology, Free University Hospital, P.O. Box 7057, 1007 MB Amsterdam, The Netherlands.*

M. A. Hanson, M.A., D.Phil. *Department of Obstetrics and Gynaecology, University College and Middlesex School of Medicine, University College London, 86–96 Chenies Mews, London, WC1E 6HX, UK.*

Peter G. Hepper *School of Psychology, The Queen's University of Belfast, Belfast BT7 1NN, N. Ireland.*

M. B. O. M. Honnebier, M.D. *Laboratory for Pregnancy and Newborn Research, NYS College of Veterinary Medicine, Cornell University, Ithaca, New York 14853, USA.*

F. A. Manning, M.D. *Professor and Head, Department of Obstetrics, Gynecology, and Reproductive Sciences, Women's Hospital, 735 Notre Dame Avenue, Winnipeg, Manitoba, R3E 0L8, Canada.*

Chester B. Martin Jr, M.D. *Professor, Department of Obstetrics and Gynecology, University of Wisconsin–Madison, H4/654 Clinical Science Center, 600 Highland Avenue, Madison, Wisconsin 53792, USA.*

M. Mirmiran, M.D., Ph.D. *Netherlands Institute for Brain Research, Meibergdreef 33, 1105 AZ Amsterdam, The Netherlands.*

P. J. Moore, B.Sc., Ph.D. *Department of Obstetrics and Gynaecology, University College and Middlesex School of Medicine, University College London, 86–96 Chenies Mews, London, WC1E 6HX, UK.*

E. J. H. Mulder, M.Sc., Ph.D. *Department of Obstetrics and Gynaecology, University Hospital, Heidelberglaan 100, 3584 CX Utrecht, The Netherlands.*

J. G. Nijhuis, M.D., Ph.D. *Assistant Professor of Obstetrics and Gynaecology, Department of Obstetrics and Gynaecology, University Hospital Nijmegen, P.O. Box 9101, 6500 HB Nijmegen, The Netherlands.*

H. F. R. Prechtl, M.B., D.Phil. *Professor and Head, Department of Developmental Neurology, University of Groningen, Groningen, The Netherlands.*

Giuseppe Rizzo, M.D. *Assistant Professor, Istituto di Clinica Ostetrica e Ginecologica, Università Cattolica S. Cuore, Rome, Italy.*

Carlo Romanini, M.D. *Professor and Chairman, Istituto di Clinica Ostetrica e Ginecologica, Università di Ancona, Ancona, Italy.*

John A. D. Spencer, M.D., B.Sc., M.R.C.O.G. *Senior Clinical Lecturer and Consultant, Department of Obstetrics and Gynaecology, University College and Middlesex School of Medicine, University College London, 86–96 Chenies Mews, London, WC1E 6HX, UK.*

D. F. Swaab, M.D., Ph.D. *Professor of Neurobiology, Director of the Netherlands Institute for Brain Research, Meibergdreef 33, 1105 AZ Amsterdam ZO, The Netherlands.*

B. A. P. J. Tas, M.D. *Department of Obstetrics and Gynaecology, St. Elisabeth Hospital, Leopoldstraat 26, 2000 Antwerpen, Belgium.*

G. H. A. Visser, M.D., Ph.D. *Professor of Obstetrics and Gynaecology, Department of Obstetrics and Gynaecology, University Hospital, Heidelbergliaan 100, 3584 CX Utrecht, The Netherlands.*

J. I. P. de Vries, M.D., Ph.D. *Department of Obstetrics and Gynaecology, Free University Hospital, P.O. Box 7057, 1007 MB Amsterdam, The Netherlands.*

J. W. Wladimiroff, M.D., Ph.D. *Professor, Department of Obstetrics and Gynaecology, Erasmus University Rotterdam, The Netherlands.*

E. E. van Woerden, M.D., Ph.D. *Department of Obstetrics and Gynaecology, Free University Hospital, P.O. Box 7057, 1007 MB Amsterdam, The Netherlands.*

Introduction

T. K. A. B. ESKES

As a clinician with a deep interest in fetal physiology, I was very pleased to be asked to write the Introduction to a book on fetal behaviour. I would like to begin with a little history.

History

Not too long ago the first aim of obstetric care was to prevent maternal death due to tuberculosis, syphilis, difficult deliveries, and haemorrhage. When this battle was won, at least in developed countries, and when perinatal mortality had dropped spectacularly, more time and interest could be focused on the developing fetus.

The history of fetal physiology goes back to the nineteenth century, following an era of anatomical observations (Harvey 1651; Barclay *et al.* 1944). The fascinating work of Sir Joseph Barcroft (1946) also paid tribute to his colleague physiologists in the past and described the numerous animal studies in goats and sheep that contributed so much towards our current understanding of fetal functions.

Techniques to study the fetus

It took some time however, to discover that information obtained from experiments performed under general anaesthesia and/or on the exteriorization of the fetus was rather incomplete. Meschia *et al.* (1965) introduced the technique of chronic fetal catheterization, enabling many researchers to re-write various chapters of fetal physiology (Dawes 1968; Windle *et al.* 1944; Myers 1977).

Research first focused on fetal oxygenation (Hellegers 1970), and later on fetal circulation because of the development of the microsphere technique to measure blood flow accurately (Rudolph and Heymann 1967; Peeters 1978).

Studies in the human started with measurements in cord blood (Walker and Turnbull 1959) leading to concepts like 'Mount Everest in utero' (i.e. low oxygen pressure, similar to living at high altitude) (Eastman 1954). At this time it was thought that almost all neonatal handicaps, especially, cerebral palsy, resulted from hypoxia during labour. Techniques such as measurement of intrauterine pressure (Alvarez and Caldeyro-Barcia 1950), fetal heart-rate recording (Hon 1958), determination of acid–base balance in fetal blood (Saling 1966), ultrasound (Donald *et al.* 1958), and pulsed-wave Doppler ultrasound (Gill 1979) were rapidly introduced into clinical practice. All these efforts led to 'fetal surveillance' in obstetrical practice, using fetal heart-rate tracings (cardiotachograms—CTG) as a screening method. A suspect tracing is now followed by an assessment of the biophysical profile (Manning *et al.* 1980), and sometimes ultrasound Doppler flow studies of fetal vessels. Cordocentesis can now be done to assess acid–base balance of fetal blood (Daffos *et al.* 1983).

As researchers worked with these techniques, and thereby improved their clinical skills, the gap between basic research and clinical obstetrics narrowed.

It is now generally accepted that fetal asphyxia can lead to neuropathology and handicaps. It is also recognized that many infants with asphyxia during delivery can demonstrate normal development thereafter. This indicates that the degree of asphyxia (hypoxia, acidosis), the duration of asphyxia, and the susceptibility and recovery-potential of the individual are major determinants of damage. The fetal response to asphyxia includes a complex sequence of systemic and local reactions. The first fetal response is a cardiovascular one.

Fetal stress/distress

The oxygen consumption of the fetal brain and myocardium can be maintained because of the existence of parallel circulatory channels such as the ductus venosus, foramen ovale, and ductus arteriosus, and is affected by catecholamine production and decreased oxygen requirements due to alterations in the fetus's behavioural state.

Nevertheless, progressive asphyxia can lead to cardiovascular decompensation, and can cause hypotension leading to ischaemia and hypoxia of cerebral tissue. Periventricular leukomalacia and neural necrosis can then lead to neurological malfunction, including cerebral palsy.

Despite the fact that the incidence of birth trauma as a cause of cerebral damage decreased, cerebral palsy, a well-defined cerebral lesion, still occurs.

Cerebral palsy

Illingworth (1979) wrote; 'It is essential to look behind obvious difficulties in labour, such as abnormal presentation or anoxia, to the underlying causes, which are often genetic or social or concern other prenatal factors.'

Nelson and Ellenberg (1986) provided evidence for this statement by demonstrating that in cases of cerebral palsy, although labour accounts for only 3 per cent of cases, in 34 per cent of cases the underlying factors can be found during pregnancy, and in 15 per cent of cases even before conception. This finding led to the insight that techniques now used for fetal surveillance are valid for monitoring and documentation of events not only during labour, but also (and this may be quantitatively more important) during pregnancy. The implication of all this is that fetal asphyxia can be detected early, allowing adequate and timely intervention to avoid definite damage.

Ultrasound

The introduction of real-time ultrasound imaging enabled the examination of the human fetus in the intra-uterine environment in a non-invasive manner.

De Vries *et al.* (1982) studied the emergence of spontaneous fetal motility during the first 20 weeks of gestation. The first movements were observed at 7.5 weeks post-menstrual age. All types of movements that develop later on, such as startles, general movements, hiccups, and breathing, were present at 15 weeks. After the fifteenth week, developmental processes such as neuronal proliferation, migration, and organization continue (Volpe 1987).

Despite the fact that studies in animals from the early 1950s onwards described the development of behavioural states such as sleep states (Dawes *et al.* 1970; van der Wildt 1982), it took much longer to discover the same in the human fetus.

Cyclic changes in fetal activity accompanied by changes in the fetal heart variability were first described at the end of the 1970s (Junge 1979; Timor-Tritsch *et al.* 1978), but the work of Prechtl and Beintema (1964) on neonates was not linked with these findings.

Fetal behaviour

Prechtl's description of the behaviour of the neonate and his classic work with Beintema on the neurological examination of the neonate (Prechtl and Beintema 1964) clearly touched upon the sleep–wake states of neonates, and their classification of five behavioural states in the neonate gained wide acceptance. The variables describing behavioural states in the neonate were, however, not easy to assess in the human fetus. Further progress was hampered by the fact that the presence of behavioural states *in utero* could not be definitely proved. Although electrodes could easily be attached to fetal lambs to record electrical cortical activity and eye movements, these techniques were clearly not applicable in the human fetus.

Bots *et al*. (1981) and Birnholz (1981) described eye movements in the human fetus by means of real-time ultrasound scanning. Since the presence or absence and the type of eye movements are related to sleep and behavioural states, this raised the possibility of distinguishing between REM and non-REM sleep.

Nijhuis and coworkers (1982) took advantage of this finding to study fetal behavioural states. They were able to detect and define four states analogous to four of the five states described in neonates (Prechtl 1974). These behavioural states were present only after 36 weeks of pregnancy. Before this, the variables appeared to cycle relatively independently of one another and no distinct states could be recognized.

It is now clear that from fetal heart-rate tracings alone, several fetal conditions can be recognized (de Haan *et al*. 1971; Timor-Tritsch *et al*. 1978; Jongsma *et al*. 1978; Junge 1979; Arduini *et al*. 1986; van Geijn *et al*. 1980; Patrick *et al*. 1982; Nijhuis *et al*. 1990). Among the conditions that are now known to influence heart-rate variability are age, circadian and ultradian rhythms, stress, hypoxia, brain damage, diabetes mellitus, and drugs.

Our understanding of the relationship between fetal behaviour and the structure of the central nervous system is limited to a few studies in which observed behaviour and morphology, as obtained by autopsy, are correlated (Birnholtz *et al*. 1978; Hooker 1952; Humphrey 1978; Ianniruberto and Tajani 1981; Minkowski 1928).

Further studies are urgently needed to be able to assess fetal condition in relation to fetal age (Prechtl 1990). This is necessary not only for the mature or postmature fetus, but also for the various periods in the immature and premature period of fetal development.

Fetal biophysical profile

In the fetal biophysical profile, fetal heart-rate, fetal movements, fetal breathing movements, and fetal tone can be regarded as 'markers', which may indicate acute fetal distress, whereas the volume of amniotic fluid is more sensitive as a marker of chronic deprivation or malfunction of the fetal–placental unit.

Much more understanding of basic fetal physiology and endocrinology is needed to understand the chain of events in fetal hypoxaemia/hypoxia. Vintzileos *et al*. (1983) presented data suggesting that the biophysical profile could accurately identify hypoxia. The fetal tone centre (cortex–subcortical area), which is the earliest to function during intrauterine life at 7.5–8.5 weeks (Humphrey 1978), seems to be the last to disappear during asphyxia. The fetal movement centre (cortex–nuclei) starts functioning at 9 weeks (Ianniruberto and Tajani 1981) and accordingly appears to be more sensitive to hypoxia than the fetal tone centre. Regular fetal breathing does not occur until 20–21 weeks (Ianniruberto and Tajani 1981) when the fetal breathing movement centre (ventral surface of the fourth ventricle) is fully developed and functioning. The fetal heart-rate centre—located in the posterior hypothalamus, thalamus, and medulla—starts operating by the end of the second trimester and is most sensitive to hypoxia. This hypothesis (Vintzileos *et al.* 1983) seems to contrast with the serial observations on adaptation in the growth-retarded human fetus (Visser and Bekedam 1990).

Conclusion

From the above mentioned issues it will be clear that, although the field is wide open for further research, the time has come to bring together the knowledge that has already been gained.

This book should therefore be warmly welcomed. Its multidisciplinary approach should guarantee progress in our understanding of what I consider the most difficult subject to study: human life from conception to birth.

References

Alvarez, H. and Caldeyro-Barcia, R. (1950). Contractility of the human uterus recorded by new methods. *Surgery Gynecology Obstetrics* **91**, 1.

Arduini, D., Rizzo, G., Parlati, E. *et al.* (1986). Modifications of ultradian and circadian rhythms of fetal heart rate after fetal-maternal adrenal gland suppression: A double blind study. *Prenatal Diagnosis* **6**, 409–17.

Barclay, A. E., Franklin, K. J., and Prichard, M. L. (1944). *The foetal circulation and cardiovascular system and the changes that they undergo at birth*. Blackwell Scientific Publications, Oxford.

Barcroft, J. (1946). *Researches on prenatal life*. Blackwell Scientific Publications, Oxford.

Birnholz, J. C., Stephens, J. C., and Faria, M. (1978). Fetal movement patterns: a possible means of defining neurologic developmental milestones in utero. *American Journal of Roentgenology* **130**, 537–40.

Birnholz, J. C. (1981). The development of human fetal eye movement patterns. *Science* **213**, 679–81.

Bots, R. S. G. M., Nijhuis, J. G., Martin Jr, C. B., and Prechtl, H. F. R. (1981).

Human fetal eye movements: detection in utero by ultrasonography. *Early Human Development* **5**, 87–94.

Daffos, F., Capella-Pavlovsky, M., and Forestier, F. (1983). Fetal blood sampling via the umbilical cord using a needle guided by ultrasound. Report of 66 cases. *Prenatal Diagnosis* **3**, 271–7.

Dawes, G. S. (1968). *Fetal and neonatal physiology*. Year Book Medical Publishers, Chicago, Illinois.

Dawes, G. S., Fox, H. E., Leduc, B. M., Liggins, G. C., and Richards, R. T. (1970). Respiratory movements and paradoxical sleep in fetal lamb. *Journal of Physiology* **210**, 47–8.

Donald, I., MacVicar, J., and Brown, T. G. (1958). Investigations of abdominal masses by pulsed ultrasound. *Lancet* **i**, 1188–94.

Eastman, N. J. (1954). Mount Everest in utero. *American Journal of Obstetrics and Gynecology* **67**, 701–11.

Geijn, H. P. van, Jongsma, H. W., Haan, J. de, Eskes, T. K. A. B., and Prechtl, H. F. R. (1980). Heart rate as an indicator of the behavioural state: studies in the newborn infant and prospects for fetal heart rate monitoring. *American Journal of Obstetrics and Gynecology* **136**, 1061–6.

Gill, R. W. (1979). Doppler with B-mode imaging for quantitative blood flow measurement. *Ultrasound Medical Biology* **5**, 222–35.

Haan, J. de, Bemmel, J. H. van, Stolte, L. A. M., Janssens, J., Eskes, T. K. A. B., Versteeg, B., Veth, A. F. L., and Braaksma, J. T. (1971). Quantitative evaluation of fetal heart rate patterns II. The significance of the fixed heart rate during pregnancy and labor. *European Journal of Obstetrics and Gynecology* **3**, 103–10.

Harvey, W. (1651). *Excertilationes de generatione animatium*. Pulleyn, London.

Hellegers, A. E. (1970). Developments in opinions about the placenta as a barrier to oxygen. *Yale Journal of Biologic Medicine* **42**, 180–90.

Hon, E. W. (1958). The electronic evaluation of the fetal heart rate. Preliminary report. *American Journal of Obstetrics and Gynecology* **75**, 1215–30.

Hooker, D. (1952). *The prenatal origin of behaviour*. University of Kansas Press, Lawrence, Kansas.

Humphrey, T. (1978). Function of the nervous system during prenatal life. In: *Perinatal Physiology*, 2nd edn (ed. U. Stave), pp. 651–83. Plenum, New York.

Ianniruberto, A. and Tajani, E. (1981). Ultrasonographic study of fetal movements. *Seminar Perinatology* **5**, 175–81.

Illingworth, R. S. (1979). Why blame the obstetrician? A review. *British Medical Journal* **1**, 797–801.

Jongsma, H. W., Geijn, H. P. van, and Haan, J. de (1978). The analysis of heart rate variability in the perinatal period. In *Computerdiagnostik in der Geburtsmedizin* (ed. W. Krause), p. 249. Friedrich Schiller Universität, Jena.

Junge, H. D. (1979). Behavioral states and state related heart rate and motor activity patterns in the newborn infant and the fetus antepartum. A comparative study. I. Technique, illustration of recordings and general results. *Journal of Perinatal Medicine* **7**, 85–107.

Manning, F. A., Platt, L. D., and Sipos, L. (1980). Antepartum fetal biophysical profile score. *American Journal of Obstetrics and Gynecology* **136**, 787–95.

Meschia, G., Cotter, J. R., Breathnach, C. S., and Barron, D. H. (1965). The hemoglobin, oxygen, carbon dioxide and hydrogen ion concentration in the umbilical bloods of sheep and goats as sampled via indwelling catheters. *Quarterly Journal Experimental Physiology* **50,** 185–95.

Minkowski, M. (1928). Neurobiologische Studien am menschlichen Foetus. In: Handbuch der Biologischen Arbeitsmethoden (ed. E. Abderhalden), Abt. V, Teil 5 B, Heft 5, Leif 253, pp 511–618.

Myers, R. E. (1977). Experimental models of perinatal brain damage: relevance to human pathology. In: *Intrauterine asphyxia and the developing brain* (ed. L. Gluck), pp. 37–99, Year Book Medical Publishers, Chicago, Illinois.

Nelson, K. B. and Ellenberg, J. H. (1986). Antecedents of cerebral palsy, multivariate analysis of risk. *New England Journal of Medicine* **315,** 81–6.

Nijhuis, J. G., Prechtl, H. F. R., Martin Jr, C. B., and Bots, R. S. G. M. (1982). Are there behavioural states in the human fetus. *Early Human Development* **6,** 177–95.

Nijhuis, J. G., Crevels, A. J., and van Dongen, P. W. J. (1990). Fetal brain death: The definition of a fetal heart rate pattern and its clinical consequences. *Obstetrical and Gynecological Survey* **45,** 229–32.

Patrick, J., Campbell, K., Carmichael, L. *et al* (1982). Influence of maternal heart rate and gross body movements on the daily pattern of fetal heart rate near term. *American Journal of Obstetrics and Gynecology* **144,** 533–8.

Peeters, L. H. (1978). Fetal blood flow at various levels of oxygen—A study in a chronic sheep preparation with radioactive microspheres. Ph.D. Thesis, University of Nijmegen, The Netherlands.

Prechtl, H. F. R. (1974). The behavioural states of the newborn infant (a review). *Brain Research* **76,** 185–212.

Prechtl, H. F. R. (1990). Special issue: New studies on movement assessment in fetuses and preterm infants. *Early Human Development* **23,** 151–246.

Prechtl, H. F. R. and Beintema, D. J. (1964). The neurological examination of the full term newborn infant. *Clinics in developmental medicine*, Vol. 12. Heinemann, London.

Rudolph, A. M. and Heymann, M. A. (1967). The circulation of the fetus in utero. *Circulation Research* **21,** 163–84.

Saling, E. (1966). *Das Kind im Bereich der Geburtshilfe*. Thieme, Stuttgart.

Timor-Tritsch, I. E., Dierker, L. J., Hertz, R. H. *et al.* (1978). Studies of antepartum behavioural state in the human fetus at term. *American Journal of Obstetrics and Gynecology* **132,** 524–8.

Vintzileos, A. M., Campbell, W. A., Ingardia, Ch. J., and Nochimson, D. J. (1983). The fetal biophysical profile and its predictive value. *Obstetrics and Gynecology* **62,** 271–87.

Visser, G. H. A. and Bekedam, D. J. (1990). Serial observations on adaptation in the human fetus. In: *Fetal autonomy and adaptation* (ed. G. S. Dawes, A. Zacutti, F. Borruto, and A. Zacutti Jr), pp. 67–80. Wiley, New York.

Volpe, J. (1987). *Neurology of the newborn*, 2nd edn. W. B. Saunders, Philadelphia, Pennsylvania.

Vries, J. I. P. de, Visser, G. H. A., and Prechtl, H. F. R. (1982). The emergence of fetal behaviour. *Early Human Development* **7,** 301–22.

Walker, J. and Turnbull, A. C. (ed.) (1959). *Oxygen supply to the human fetus.* Blackwell Scientific Publications, Oxford.

Wildt, B. van der (1982). Heart rate, breathing movements and brain activity in fetal lambs. Ph.D. Thesis, University of Nijmegen, The Netherlands.

Windle, W. F., Beeker, R. F., and Weil, A. (1944). Alterations in brain structure after asphyxiation birth. *Journal of Neuropathology* **3,** 224.

Part 1

Development of behaviour during
normal pregnancy

1
The first trimester
J. I. P. DE VRIES

Introduction

The aim of this chapter is to describe the development of embryonic and fetal motility during the first trimester in uncomplicated pregnancies. The latter has the restriction that in the human, it has been possible to study motility *in utero* only since the early 1970s, when real-time ultrasound imaging was introduced.

It has long been known that motility in early gestation is present in many organisms. In the seventeenth century, van Leeuwenhoek (1695) described spontaneous movements in a mussel embryo, and some 40 years later Swammerdam (1739) saw through a home-made microscope those of a snake embryo. Despite these historical roots, there is still a lack of knowledge about the neural substrates underlying prenatal movements and what functions they may serve. Nevertheless it seems evident that movements of the embryo and fetus are a fundamental expression of early neural activity. In this respect, however, marked differences of opinion have arisen with regard to the human fetus. The elaborate studies of Minkowski (1928), Hooker (1952), and Humphrey (1978) on exteriorized fetuses led to the conclusion that early fetal behaviour consists merely of reflexes rather than spontaneously generated movement patterns. It was Reinold (1976), the first observer of the fetus to use ultrasound, who stressed that the fetus of 8–10 weeks postmenstrual age moves spontaneously *in utero* under normal circumstances. He and others provided descriptions of the variety of movement patterns they observed in early pregnancy. Their respective descriptions markedly contrasted with each other. This situation has led to the need for an unambiguous classification of the various movements that is applicable throughout gestation. Once a thorough knowledge of normal development has been achieved by this means, the assessment of the fetal neurological condition *in utero* may become a practical procedure for clinical purposes.

Classification of movement patterns

In three ultrasound studies, attempts were made to develop a classification of various movement patterns. Birnholz *et al.* (1978) based their classification on the reflex patterns reported by Hooker (1952). Ianniruberto and Tajani (1981) resorted to the motoscopy of Milani-Comparetti and Gidoni (1967). In both investigations, straightforward categories were not used but, especially in the latter, categories were used in which interpretations were made about what the fetus might actually be doing. In contrast the study by de Vries *et al.* (1982) attempted to describe not only which parts of the body were actually involved in a particular movement but also how the movement was performed in terms of speed, amplitude, and force. In addition, their classification was based on movements that had been noted previously in low-risk preterm and fullterm infants (Prechtl 1977; Prechtl *et al.* 1979).

In this study, fetuses of 12 healthy nulliparous women were investigated from 7 to 40 weeks gestation. All recordings were performed between 1600 and 1800 hours. To ensure an adequate analysis of fetal motility, a sufficiently long observation period was deemed necessary (60 minutes duration from 7 to 15 weeks weekly, and every two weeks up to 25 weeks, and 60–120 minutes every four weeks thereafter). Such durations do not involve any hazardous or harmful side-effects in humans in the low-MHz frequency, using the low-intensity exposures of diagnostic ultrasound (AIUM 1976 and 1983). Furthermore, the previously held view that ultrasound itself can induce fetal activity has proved to be untrue (Hertz *et al.* 1979; Powell-Phillips and Towell 1979).

The various movement patterns are specific from their very onset (de Vries *et al.* 1982). In the following sections, their descriptions are given together with the ages at which a pattern occurred for the first time (Table 1.1) p. 5.

Just-discernible movements, 7 weeks

The contour of the embryo shows small and short-lasting changes (1–2 seconds). Lateral flexion of head and rump are likely to occur. However, the small size of the embryo and the limited resolution of the available equipment prevents more detailed analyses. Van Dongen and Goudie (1980) and Ianniruberto and Tajani (1981) described the same type of movements as rippling and vermicular movements, respectively.

Startle, 8 weeks

Abrupt flexion and/or extension of both arms and legs at the same time. The amplitude of the movement is mostly large but can also be small, and even just discernible.

Table 1.1 First appearance of movement patterns during the first trimester in 12 fetuses (de Vries *et al.* 1985)

Movement patterns	First appearance: range in weeks postmenstrual age
Just-discernible movements	7.5–8.5
Startle	8.0–9.5
General movements	8.5–9.5
Stretch	10.0–15.5
Rotation of the fetus	10.0
Hiccups	8.5–10.5
Breathing movements	10.0–11.5
Isolated arm/leg movements	9.0–10.5
twitches	10.0–12.5
cloni	13.0
Finger movements	12.0
Isolated head movements	
backward	9.5–12.5
rotation	9.5–12.5
forward	10.5–14.5
Jaw opening	10.5–12.5
Sucking and swallowing	12.5–14.5
Tongue movements	11.0
Hand-face contact	10.0–12.5
Yawn	11.5–15.5
Eye movements*	
slow	16.0
rapid	23.0

* Birnholz *et al.* (1981).

General movements, 8–9 weeks

Head, trunk, and/or extremities participate in a variable sequence. The speed and amplitude of the displacements vary considerably. However, the movements always remain graceful in character. Frequent changes in fetal position occur from 10 to 12 weeks onwards during such movements.

Stretch, 10 weeks

A movement with a clear sequence that is always performed at a slow speed: head backwards, followed by trunk arching and arms lifting.

Hiccups, 8–9 weeks

Abrupt displacements of the diaphragm, thorax, and abdomen. They may occur as a single event but are frequently seen at regular intervals of 2–3 seconds.

Breathing movements, 10 weeks

These fluent movements are paradoxical in nature, involving simultaneous movements of the diaphragm (downwards), thorax (inwards), and abdomen (outwards). They may occur in regular and irregular intervals or as a single event. A single large displacement of the diaphragm may resemble a sigh.

Isolated arm/leg movements, 9 weeks

Movements in one extremity only, without other parts moving, mostly performed slowly with varying speed and amplitude. They can also occur abruptly as an isolated (twitch, 10 weeks) or repetitive event (clonus, 13 weeks).

Finger movements, 12 weeks

Flexion and extension of one or more fingers are seen from 12 weeks onwards.

Isolated head movements, 9–10 weeks

These movements also occur as an isolated event. Mostly they are performed slowly but sometimes involve twitches. The displacement can be small or large. Backward movements are present earliest (9 weeks) and can last for 1 second to more than 1 minute. Head rotation emerges at 9–10 weeks and thereafter the head can be seen bending forwards (10 weeks)

Jaw opening, 10–11 weeks

This movement occurs as a single or repetitive event and may be either slow or quick. The extent of opening varies. The duration can be from less than 1 second to 5 seconds.

Sucking and swallowing, 12 weeks

Regular opening and closing of the jaw at a rate of about one per second, followed by displacement of tongue and fluid in larynx.

Tongue movements, 11 weeks

These movements occur during sucking and swallowing and also as an isolated event. Tongue protrusions can be seen.

Hand–face contact, 10 weeks

Insertion of fingers into mouth can be seen but are frequently missed because of the two-dimensional images. The movement occurs isolated or as a part of a general movement.

Yawn, 11 weeks

This movement occurs as a single event: prolonged wide opening of the jaws followed by quick closure, head backwards, and often elevation of the arms.

Eye movements, 16–23 weeks

Slow eye movements at 16 weeks and rapid eye movements at 23 weeks (Birnholz *et al*. 1981).

Rotation of the fetus, 10 weeks

Displacements around the longitudinal or transversal axis of the fetus can be achieved by alternating leg extensions, hip rotation, and/or rotation of head and trunk within as little as 2 seconds, but often take longer.

Development of specific movement patterns

All fetuses follow a specific sequence in which the different movement patterns are rank-ordered according to the first age of their appearance. These ages have a scatter of about two weeks. The scatter is partly due to the one-week interval between the observations. A wider scatter is found for movements with an infrequent occurrence (e.g., yawn, stretch, head bending forwards, isolated leg movements, and sucking–swallowing).

All the movement patterns appear for the first time between 8 to 16 weeks and remain recognizable throughout gestation and after birth. One exception is the 'just-discernible movement', which is present only between 7–8 weeks. Slight changes in appearance can be seen in general movements, isolated movements of the arms, and jaw opening (e.g. at 20

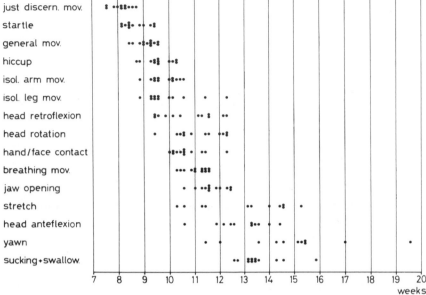

Fig. 1.1. First occurrence of specific fetal movement patterns. Each dot represents an individual. Ages at observations are given in full weeks and days. (Reproduced with permission from de Vries *et al.* 1984.)

weeks of gestation the movements of the extremities and head appear to be more brisk during general movements).

Once a particular movement pattern has appeared, it is unpredictable as to what the next one will be at any one age, as illustrated in the actogram at 13 weeks.

All movement patterns vary in amplitude, speed, and force. They are not jerky in character but co-ordinated and graceful. Exceptions are startles, hiccups, twitches, and cloni.

Inter-observer training was carried out until a high degree of agreement was reached in recognizing the various movement patterns (above 90 per cent).

Quantitative aspects

Attempts have been made to quantify the amplitude and/or speed of a single movement (Henner *et al.* 1975). Experienced observers of the fetus, however, claim that the judgement of these parameters by means of gestalt

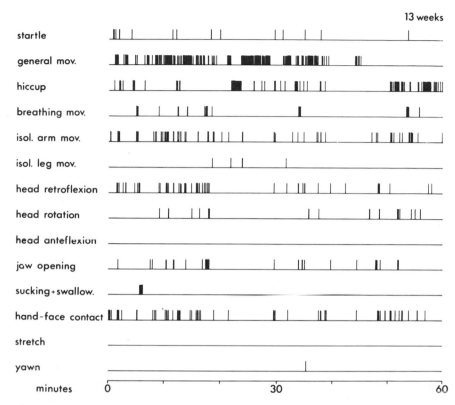

Fig. 1.2. Compiled actogram of one-hour observation of one fetus from 1600–1700 hours at 13 weeks.

perception gives more information than quantification of the movements (in a two-dimensional image in which it is not possible to follow all complete fetal parts continuously).

Aspects of fetal motility that can be quantified are the rate of occurrence of the specific movements and the duration of periods without fetal activity. The specific movement patterns vary considerably in incidence per week. For most patterns, however, a particular trend could be distinguished (de Vries *et al.* 1985). They consisted of a gradual increase in incidence with age (breathing movements, head rotation, jaw openings, sucking, and swallowing), an increase in incidence followed by a decrease (startles, hand–face contacts, head bending forwards), or an increase in incidence until a plateau is reached (general movements, isolated arm movements). Other less-frequently occurring movements showed no such discernible trends.

Table 1.2 Longest period of total quiescence and longest pause
between general movements observed in 12 fetuses from 7 to 19
weeks (from de Vries *et al.* 1985)

Week	Longest period (s) of quiescence		Longest pause (s) between general movements	
	Median	Range	Median	Range
7	—	417–1468	0	0–1468
8	260	108–780	294	226–939
9	226	125–298	250	284–334
10	292	225–447	340	338–595
11	298	159–544	463	304–925
12	380	167–715	466	337–721
13	206	127–399	374	100–449
14	144	68–368	359	208–767
15	121	62–446	300	142–613
17	144	48–328	272	188–449
19	127	77–306	329	141–505

Number of observations at 7 weeks is two.

Total fetal activity, defined as the sum of the duration of all movement
patterns, attained a strikingly high value by 11 weeks (de Vries *et al.* 1988).
By this age a plateau was reached, with median values of 21 to 30 per cent
of the recording time. Fetuses were found to be active for at least 14 per
cent of the observation time. During the first trimester, periods without
fetal movements were short-lasting (median values 2–6 minutes), with a
maximum of 13 minutes (de Vries *et al.* 1985). Between 14–19 weeks
gestational age, median values of the longest periods without activity were
more or less stable: 2 minutes without any activity; 5–6 minutes without
general movements (Table 1.2); 15 minutes without breathing movements;
20–25 minutes without hiccups (Table 1.3). However, breathing movement and hiccups can be absent for nearly an hour. The chance that during
an ultrasound examination the fetus has a long period of inactivity is so
small that adequate studies on responses to stimulation are difficult to
obtain in the young fetus, unless of course one gets a significant reduction
in activity.

Individual differences

It should be emphasized that the appearance of the various movements is

Table 1.3 Longest period between breathing movements and hiccups observed in 12 fetuses from 7 to 19 weeks

Week	Longest period (s) between breathing movements		Longest period (s) between hiccups	
	Median	Range	Median	Range
8			3600	1510–3600
9	3600	1267–3600	1660	551–3600
10	3600	984–3600	660	406–2147
11	1517	965–3600	1160	504–2644
12	1289	823–3600	1267	825–2078
13	1103	612–3324	1226	610–2431
14	898	603–2255	1416	707–2132
15	608	334–1358	1161	371–2801
17	899	359–2017	1432	927–3307
19	922	584–2409	1580	719–3600

strikingly similar from one fetus to another in terms of smoothness and variability in amplitude, speed and force. Considerable inter-individual differences, however, exist in their quantitative expression. For each of the twelve fetuses, there was to some degree a week to week consistency in total motor activity and general movements during the first trimester (de Vries *et al.* 1988). For general movements even a slight tendency in intrafetal consistency was seen throughout gestation. Inter-individually, however, large differences were found in the quantity of the various movements.

The different movement patterns were rank ordered according to incidence per week. The twelve fetuses showed a strikingly similar trend in their development. General movements are always seen most frequently, followed by hiccups at 8–13 weeks. Thereafter hiccups are replaced by breathing movements.

The movement patterns showed no quantitative differences between the six female and six male fetuses. In the second half of gestation no sex differences were found for general movements.

All infants were appropriately grown at birth. All subjects had a neurological examination at 4–6 days after birth, at 6 weeks after birth, and at 1.5 years. No abnormalities were found.

What is normal fetal motility?

Is it possible to recognize and judge the motility of any fetus as being normal? The 12 fetuses of the longitudinal study reached full term without complications and were found to have a normal neurological development up to 1.5 years of age. These fetuses showed movements which were so specific and contained so many recognizable aspects that their motility can be claimed to be normal. The characteristics of normal motility are as follows.

1. All movements have to be recognized as described for the normal population.
2. All movements emerge at the same age as those seen in the normal population.
3. All movements vary in amplitude, speed, and force. They are not jerky in character but are co-ordinated and graceful. Exceptions are startles, hiccups, twitches, and cloni.
4. Once a particular movement has appeared it is unpredictable as to what the next movement pattern will be at any one age.
5. The incidences of movement patterns show certain age-dependent changes but fluctuate considerably from week to week for each fetus.
6. The presence and rank ordering of the incidence of the various types of movements is age dependent.
7. The periods without fetal motility are relatively short during the first trimester. The longest period of inactivity ever observed lasted 13 minutes.

In conclusion, it should be stressed that normal fetal motility can not be recognized by a single movement, but through variations in speed, amplitude, and force of the various movement patterns. Such knowledge might prevent inappropriate interpretation of the movement repertoire. For example a change in motility has been reported from 'rather jerky' around 12 weeks to 'slow and harmonious' at 17 to 19 weeks (Boué *et al.* 1982). As we now know, it is not the movement patterns, but their incidence that changes. The 'jerky' movements, hiccups and startles, are only superseded in frequency by general movements until 12 weeks, but are far less numerous at 17 to 19 weeks (de Vries *et al.* 1988, p. 97). It has to be stressed that the individual movement patterns and not a specific aspect over a short period of time should be judged. The individual pattern hardly changes in appearance from its emergence until full term.

Milestones in motility and anatomy

Motor patterns are specific and recognizable from their onset at a very early gestational age. These movements are not preceded by other movements, which are amorphous at random. Neuroanatomical evidence suggests that motility starts as soon as neural and muscular structures are present (de Vries *et al*. 1982). It supports the view that neural connectivity mediating motor activity is established correctly from the beginning of its formations (Bekoff 1981; Landmesser 1980). The earliest activity seen is not myogenic in origin as it is not restricted to one body part. This point is illustrated by the category of 'just-discernible movements', in which there are both cranial and caudal movements.

Between 9.5 and 10.5 weeks the first rapid increase in axodendritic and axosomatic synapses occurs (Okado 1980). This change facilitates an increase in the number of signals which have to be transmitted. In this period all movements differentiate rapidly while the general movements have already reached a plateau in terms of the percentage of recording time they are present. Okado and Kojima (1984) describe a striking increase in the number of axosomatic synapses between 13 and 15.5 weeks. During this period the differentiation of motility is complete and the rate of occurrence becomes stable (de Vries *et al*. 1988).

The movements differentiate quickly, are age-related, and show a distinct developmental course, suggesting that a variety of endogenous generators are involved and that they are not elicited exogenously. The generation of spontaneous motility has been found *in vitro*. Droge *et al*. (1986) and Stafström *et al*. (1980) found that when a degree of connectivity had been achieved in embryonic tissues, neurons fired spontaneously. This activity was even organized into a number of recognizable patterns. 'So in early life movements need only a few motor neurones to emerge, but an intact, although poorly developed, nervous system to executed normally' (Visser *et al*. 1985).

More details on the relationship between fetal behaviour and central nervous system activity can be found in Chapter, 3.

Functional significance of fetal motility

In all species that have been studied, embryonic and fetal motility is found and can be considered to be a fundamental property of the developing nervous system. Such motility may involve other functional properties. The frequent changes in position during general movements, head rotations followed by rump rotations, alternating extension of legs, and long-lasting bending of the head backwards, may prevent adhesions and local stasis of the circulation in the skin. Such movements can therefore be considered as specific adaptations to the intrauterine environment. Another example of such adaptation is swallowing, which regulates the amount of amniotic fluid. Movements which do not have a clear function prenatally may constitute the earliest stages of postnatal functions (e.g. rotation of the head, eye movements, yawns, stretches, hand–face contact, and breathing movements). It is now known that fetal breathing movements influence the maturation of lung tissue to a certain extent before birth. In animal studies it has been shown that a high spinal cord transection causes cessation of breathing resulting in lung hypoplasia (Liggings *et al.* 1981; Wigglesworth and Desai 1979). Three human fetuses have been described with anencephaly and lung hypoplasia: in one case breathing movements were present in 2 per cent of the recording time (Visser *et al.* 1985).

The data on fetal motility presented in this chapter illustrate the normal course of fetal motor development and are the first step in the creation of a prenatal neurology.

Assessment of motility reveals the condition of the fetal nervous system. Observations of fetuses in sub-optimal intrauterine circumstances show changes in the qualitative rather than the quantitative aspects of the movements. This finding implies that in order to recognize abnormal motility the fetal observer needs to be thoroughly conversant with normal motility at the various ages.

References

American Institute of Ultrasound in Medicine (1976). Report: biological effects of ultrasonic energy in living animals. *Ultrasound in Medicine and Biology* **2**, 351.

American Institute of Ultrasound in Medicine (1983). Safety Statements. *Journal of Ultrasound in Medicine* **2**, (Suppl.), 1–49.

Bekoff, A. (1981). In: *Studies in developmental neurobiology: Essays in Honor of Viktor Hamburger* (ed. W. M. Cowan), pp. 134–70. Oxford University Press.

Birnholz, J. C. (1981). The development of human fetal eye movement patterns. *Science* **213**, 679–81.

Birnholz, J. C., Stephens, J. C., and Faria, M. (1978). Fetal movement patterns: a possible means of defining neurologic developmental milestones *in utero*. *American Journal of Roentgenology* **130**, 537–40.

Boué. J., Vignal, P., Aubry, J. P., Aubry, M. C., and Aleese, J. M. (1982). Ultrasound movement patterns of fetuses with chromosome anomalies. *Prenatal Diagnosis* **2**, 61–5.

Dongen, L. G. R. van and Goudie, E, G. (1980). Fetal movement patterns in the first trimester of pregnancy. *British Journal of Obstetrics and Gynaecology* **87**, 191–3.

Droge, M. H., Gross, G. W., Hightower, M. H., and Czisny, L. E. (1986). Multi-electrode analysis of coordinated, multiside, rhythmic bursting in cultured CNS monolayer networks. *Journal of Neuroscience* **6**, 1583–92.

Henner, H., Haller, U., Wolf-Zimper, O., Lorenz, W. J., Bader R., Müller, B., and Kubli, F. (1975). Quantification of fetal movement in normal and pathologic pregnancy. *Excerpta Medica International Congress Series* **363**, 316–19.

Hertz, R. H., Timor-Tritsch, I. E., Dierker, L. J., Chik, L., and Rosen, M. G. (1979). Continuous ultrasound and fetal movement. *American Journal of Obstetrics and Gynecology* **135**, 152–4.

Hooker, D. (1952). *The prenatal origin of behaviour*. University of Kansas Press, Lawrence, Kansas.

Humphrey, T. (1978). Function of the nervous system during prenatal life. In: *Perinatal physiology* (ed. U. Stave), pp. 651–83. Plenum, New York.

Ianniruberto, A. and Tajani, E. (1981). Ultrasonographic study of fetal movements. *Seminars in Perinatology* **5**, 175–81.

Landmesser, L. T. (1980). The generation of neuromuscular specificity. *Annual Review of Neuroscience* **3**, 279–302.

Leeuwenhoek, A. Van (1695). *Briefe über die enthüllten Geheimnisse der Natur*.

Liggins, G. C., Vilos, G. A., Kitterman, J. A., and Lee, C. H. (1981). The effect of spinal cord transection on lung development in the fetal sheep. *Journal of Developmental Physiology*, **3**, 267–74.

Milani-Comparetti, A. and Gidoni, E. A. (1967). Pattern analysis of motor development and its disorders. *Developmental Medicine in Child Neurology* **9**, 625–30.

Minkowski, M. (1928). Neurobiologische Studien am menschlichen Foetus. *Handbuch der Biologischen Arbeitsmethode*, Abt. v, Teil 5B, 511–618.

Okado, N. (1980). Development of the human cervical spinal cord with reference to synapse formation in the motor nucleus. *The Journal of Comparative Neurology* **191**, 495–513.

Okado, N. and Kojima, T. (1984). Ontogeny of the central nervous system: Neurogenesis, fibre connection, synaptogenesis and myelination in the spinal cord. In: Continuity of neural functions from prenatal to postnatal life. *Clinics in Developmental Medicine* (ed. H. F. R. Prechtl), Vol. 94, pp. 46–64. Blackwell Scientific Publications, Oxford.

Powell-Phillips, W. D. and Towell, M. E. (1979). Doppler ultrasound and subjective assessment of fetal action. *British Medical Journal* **2**, 101–2.

Prechtl, H. F. R. (1977). The neurological examination of the full-term newborn infant, second revised and enlarged edition. In: *Clinics in Developmental Medicine*, Vol. 63, pp. 65. Heinemann, London.

Prechtl, H. F. R., Fargel, J. W., Weinmann, H. M., and Bakker, H. H. (1979). Posture, motility and respiration in low-risk preterm infants. *Developmental Medicine in Child Neurology* **21**, 3–27.

Reinold, E. (1976). Ultrasonics in early pregnancy. Diagnostic scanning and fetal motor activity. *Contributions to Gynaecology and Obstetrics* **1**, 148.

Stafström, C. E., Johnston, D., Wehner, J. M., and Sheppard, J. R. (1980). Spontaneous neural activity in fetal brain reaggregate cultures. *Neuroscience* **5**, 1681–90.

Swammerdam, J. (1739). *Bibliae Naturae*. Leiden. (Published by H. Boerhaave 59 years after Swammerdam's death).

Vries, J. I. P. de, Visser, G. H. A., and Prechtl, H. F. R. (1982). The emergence of fetal behaviour. I. Qualitative aspects. *Early Human Development* **7**, 301–22.

Vries, J. I. P. de, Visser, G. H. A. de, and Prechtl H. F. R. (1984). Fetal mortality in the first half of pregnancy. In: Continuity of neural functions from prenatal to postnatal life (ed. H. F. R. Prechtl), Vol. 94, pp. 46–64, *Clinics in Developmental Medicine*, Blackwell Scientific Publications, Oxford.

Vries, J. I. P. de, Visser, G. H. A., and Prechtl, H. F. R. (1985). The emergence of fetal behaviour. II. Quantitative aspects. *Early Human Development* **12**, 99–120.

Vries, J. I. P. de, Visser, G. H. A., and Prechtl, H. F. R. (1988). The emergence of fetal behaviour. III. Individual differences and consistencies. *Early Human Development* **16**, 85–103.

Visser, G. H. A., Laurini, R. N., Vries, J. I. P. de, Bekedam, D. J., and Prechtl, H. F. R. (1985). Abnormal motor behaviour in anencephalic fetuses. *Early Human Development* **12**, 173–82.

Wigglesworth, J. S. and Desai, R. (1979). Effects of lung growth on cervical cord section in the rabbit fetus. *Early Human Development* **3**, 51–65.

2
The second trimester
G. H. A. VISSER

Introduction

Embryonic and fetal movements emerge during the first trimester of pregnancy, and almost all the movement patterns that can be recognized during the remainder of pregnancy and the neonatal period are present as early as 16 weeks (see Chapter 1). Initially, movements appear scattered in a random order, but progressive clustering occurs in the second trimester with discernible relative rest and activity cycles. Later on, during the third trimester, this results in the development of fetal behavioural states (see Chapter 3). During the second trimester, considerable changes also occur in the rate of occurrence of movement patterns. This chapter reviews the clustering of fetal movement patterns and the changes in their incidence in normal pregnancy between 16 and 32 weeks.

Individual movement patterns

During the second trimester there are no real changes in the quality of motor patterns, thus the execution of individual movement patterns remains similar to that described for the first trimester of pregnancy (de Vries et al. 1982; Roodenburg et al. 1991). There are, however, considerable changes in incidence of most of the movements. Data from the literature on the incidence (percentage of recording time) of the two most frequent motor patterns, generalized body movements and breathing movements, are summarized in Figs 2.1 and 2.2.

Generalized movements

Generalized movements decrease in number per hour (Natale et al. 1985; Roodenburg et al. 1991) and in percentage of time present (de Vries et al. 1988), during the second trimester (Fig. 2.1). The data of two of the studies are compatible; but Roodenburg et al. (1991) found a considerably higher incidence of movements between 20 and 28 weeks, and a fall in incidence only after this age. They attribute their different results to the fact that two

Fetal behaviour

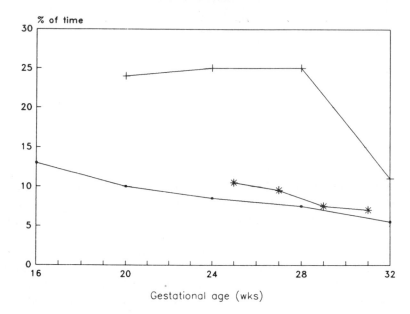

Fig. 2.1. Median incidence of general movements between 16 and 32 weeks, according to the studies of de Vries *et al.* 1985 and 1987 (●——●), Natale *et al.* 1985 (*——*), and Roodenburg *et al.* 1991 (⊦——⊦).

scanners were used instead of one. It is, however, unlikely that the use of two scanners would have a major impact at 20 weeks of gestation, when one scanner with a large probe is still capable of visualizing most of the fetus.

The lowest incidence of general movements in normal pregnancies between 20 and 30 weeks of gestation was 2.5 per cent of time, according to the data of de Vries *et al.* (1988), and about 4 per cent of recording time according to Roodenburg *et al.* (1991). In 33 cases that we studied for one hour between 28 and 31 weeks, the lowest incidence was 3.0 per cent, with a tenth centile of 3.6 per cent of recording time (Ribbert, unpublished observations).

At 20 to 22 weeks of gestation there are already diurnal variations in general movements, with peak values at night (de Vries *et al.* 1987). These diurnal changes become more pronounced during the third trimester (Patrick *et al.* 1982).

Breathing movements

Breathing movements increase during the second trimester from less than 5 per cent to about 30 per cent of recording time (Fig. 2.2). The data from

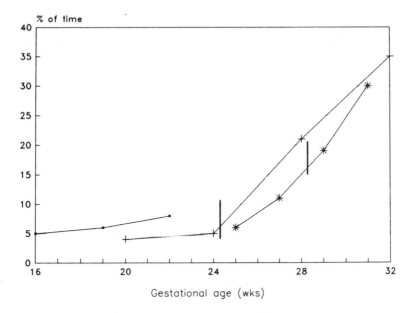

% of time

Gestational age (wks)

Fig. 2.2. Median incidence of fetal breathing movements between 16 and 32 weeks, according to the studies of de Vries *et al*. 1985 and 1987 (●——●), Natale *et al*. (*——*) and Roodenburg *et al*. 1991 (⊦——⊦). The vertical bars at 24 and 28 weeks indicate the breathing incidence during placebo- (lower end) or glucose-infusion (top) as found in a controlled study by Nijhuis *et al*. 1986.

the literature are quite consistent, despite differences in study design (time of day, relation to maternal meals). The mean breath-to-breath interval decreases from 1 to 2 seconds at 16 weeks to less than 1 second at 19 weeks (de Vries *et al*. 1985). From 30 weeks onwards an increase in breath-to-breath interval from 1 to 1.3 seconds has been reported (Trudinger *et al*. 1980). Thus in the course of gestation, the intervals initially decrease (increasing breathing rate), and then increase between 20 and 30 weeks.

It is likely that during the second trimester breathing already increases following a meal or glucose intake, though such an effect could be demonstrated in only two of four studies. De Vries *et al*. (1987) found a significantly higher incidence of breathing during the second hour after breakfast or lunch than during the third hour at 20 to 22 weeks of gestation. Others could demonstrate such an effect only from 30 weeks onwards (Natale *et al*. 1985). Following administration of glucose to the mother, Nijhuis *et al*. (1986) observed a significant increase in breathing compared with that observed after administration of a placebo, both at 24 and 28 weeks. Such an increase was not found by others (Meis *et al*. 1985). The early emergence of breathing movements in embryos of women with type 1 diabetes mellitus and the high incidence of breathing movements in these embryos and fetuses, suggests that glucose affects breathing activity from its emergence (see Chapter 14). During the third trimester there are also diurnal changes in fetal breathing which are unrelated to maternal meals. Breathing tends to decrease during the day and the lowest incidence occurs between 1900 and 2400 hours; between 0400 and 0700 hours breathing increases again (Patrick *et al.* 1980). At 20 to 22 weeks breathing activity follows a different pattern over the day, with the lowest values in the morning and higher values in the afternoon and evening (de Vries *et al.* 1987).

Other movements

Second trimester data on other movement patterns are largely restricted to the studies of de Vries *et al.* (1985, 1987) (below 22 weeks) and Roodenburg *et al.* (1991) (from 20 weeks onwards). In summary there is a decrease in the incidence of hiccups, startles, and stretches. Before 20 weeks hiccups are present during every one hour recording, but between 20 and 30 weeks they are noted in one out of two recordings, and after 30 weeks only two to four episodes occur per 24 hours (Patrick *et al.* 1980).

Fetal eye movements have been observed as early as 16 to 18 weeks of gestation (Birnholz 1981). Three different eye movement patterns can be distinguished: a slow and rolling movement; a more rapid and regular movement; and occasionally a nystagmoid movement. During the second trimester eye movements gradually increase in incidence, and at 30 weeks approximately 75 such movements can be observed per hour (Inoue *et al.* 1986; Roodenburg *et al.* 1991).

Movement patterns that do not show clear changes during the second trimester are jaw movements (isolated, sucking, swallowing, yawn), hand–face contacts, head rotations and ante- and retroflexion of the head. Their incidences may vary considerably and at 28 weeks the following ranges and median values have been reported from one-hour observations: jaw movements 60–460, median 300; hand–face contacts 30–190, median 95; head rotations 20–125, median 37; head retroflexions 4–29, median 12 (Roodenburg *et al.* 1991).

Development of rest–activity cycles

In the fetus the periodicity of the different movements undergoes several changes in the course of gestation. General movements, for example, are scattered over the record at 8 weeks, whereas they become grouped into bursts during the following weeks. After 14 weeks these bursts are replaced by much longer periods of fluctuating activity (de Vries *et al.* 1982). In early gestation, periods without any detectable movement are usually short. De Vries *et al.* (1985), studying 12 fetuses at 19 weeks, reported that the longest period without movements ranged from 1.3 to 5.1 minutes (median 2.1 minutes) in one-hour recordings. At 20 weeks Swartjes *et al.* (1990) observed an absence of movements lasting longer than 3 minutes in 55 per cent of one-hour recordings; as random scattering of movements on a time axis could not imitate these results, they concluded that clustering already exists at 20 weeks of gestation. Between 20 and 30 weeks the clustering of movements in rest–activity cycles becomes more and more evident and using 2 tocodynanometers Soronkin *et al.* (1982) could demonstrate such cycles in only 2 of 10 recordings made at 20 to 22 weeks, and in 8 of 10 recordings made at 28 to 30 weeks. The duration of episodes without movements also increases. According to Natale *et al.* (1985) the longest interval without general movements is, in 95 per cent of cases, less than 6 minutes at 24 to 28 weeks, and less than or equal to 10 minutes at 28 to 32 weeks. At 25 to 30 weeks Drogtrop *et al.* (1990) also found that 95 per cent of episodes without general movements lasted 10 minutes or less, with the longest interval between movements of 16 minutes. Drogtrop *et al.* concluded that when assessing fetal condition in early gestation, different criteria of normality should be used from those applied later in pregnancy. For instance, using the biophysical profile score, three or more fetal body movements per 30 minutes is considered optimal. Thus a fetus of less than 30 weeks gestation that starts to move after a period of 20 minutes would obtain an optimal score, although at this age absence of body movements for 20 minutes or longer is probably abnormal.

Using fetal heart-rate (FHR) variation (bandwidth), general movements, and eye movements as state variables, it has been shown that the fetus has fully-developed behavioural states from about 36 weeks of gestation onwards (see Chapter 3). These behavioural states—with relatively stable periods in which particular combinations of the variables are displayed and changes of the characteristics occur more or less simultaneously at transitions—gradually develop from about 28 weeks.

An association between the rest–activity cycles (absence or presence of general movements) and FHR pattern, and between eye movements and heart rate has been found from about 28 weeks onwards (Visser *et al.* 1981; Drogtrop *et al.* 1990). Eye movement and general movement patterns are linked from 30 weeks onwards (Awoust and Levi 1984; Visser *et al.* 1987). At this age co-ordination is, however, far from perfect and a significant correlation between incidence of eye movements and body movements was demonstrated in only 7 of 11 fetuses at 30 to 32 weeks (Visser *et al.* 1987). Moreover, changes in the state variables seldom occur at exactly the same time, and during coincidence 1 F (*see also* Chapter 3) neither body move-

ments nor eye movements disappear completely (Fig. 2.3). These data are
consistent with observations of premature infants. 'Quiet'-sleep (similar to
'non-REM-sleep' or state 1), with atypical components, may be recognized
as early as 31 weeks (Dreyfus-Brisac 1970) and differentiation between
active and quiet sleep using electroencephalography and rapid eye movement criteria appears to be possible from the same age onwards (Karch *et
al.* 1982; Curzi-Dascalova *et al.* 1983). In addition, from 30 weeks onwards
movements predominate in active sleep compared to quiet sleep (Curzi-
Dascalova *et al.* 1985).

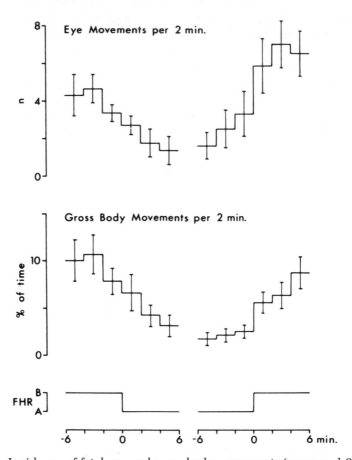

Fig. 2.3. Incidence of fetal eye and gross body movements (mean and SEM) of
10 fetuses at 30 to 32 weeks of gestation during the 6 minutes preceding and
following a change in fetal heart-rate (FHR) pattern. During episodes of low
heart-rate variation (FHR-A) eye and body movements are reduced but not
absent. (Reproduced with permission from Visser *et al.* 1987.)

At 32 weeks of gestation the length of a complete rest–activity cycle is about 50 to 70 minutes (Hoppenbrouwers *et al.* 1981; Dierker *et al.* 1982; Visser *et al.* 1982). This is considerably shorter than the average cycle length of 80 to 100 minutes observed in term fetuses.

Conclusion

During the second trimester of pregnancy the incidence of generalized body movements gradually decreases, whereas that of breathing movements increases considerably. Breathing movements become the most frequent of all fetal movement patterns and by this time their incidence appears to be related to maternal meals. Eye movements emerge early during the second trimester and increase gradually. The incidence of hiccups, startles, and stretches decreases, whereas other movement patterns (jaw movements, hand–face contacts, head movements) show no clear developmental changes.

At all ages there are large inter-fetal differences in the incidence of the different movement patterns. The large variety in motor repertoire, with continuous changes between large generalized movements and movements of specific parts of the body, can be considered as an expression of normality of the developing central nervous system.

Fetal rest–activity cycles and subsequent behavioural states develop gradually during the second trimester, though co-ordination between the state variables still remains far from perfect. These developments imply that with increasing age longer periods without general movements, or with a flat (non-reactive) FHR pattern have to be considered as signs of normality. The duration of such episodes is, however, shorter than during the third trimester when other criteria of normality have to be used to assess the fetal condition.

References

Awoust, J. and Levi, S. (1984). New aspects of fetal dynamics with a special emphasis on eye movements. *Ultrasound in Medicine and Biology* **10**, 107–16.

Birnholz, J. C. (1981). The development of human fetal eye movement patterns. *Science* **213**, 679 81.

Curzi-Dascalova, L., Lebrun, F., and Korn, G. (1983). Respiratory frequency according to sleep states, and age in normal premature infants. *Pediatrics research* **17**, 152–6.

Curzi-Dascalova, L., Peirano, P., and Vicente, G. (1985). Body motility according to sleep states in normal newborn infants: a preliminary study. In: *The physiological development of the fetus, and newborn* (ed. C. T. Jones and P. N. Nathanielsz), pp. 817–20. Academic Press, London.

Dierker, L. J., Pillay, S., Soronkin, Y., and Rosen, M. G. (1982). The change in fetal activity periods in diabetic, and nondiabetic pregnancies. *American Journal of Obstetrics and Gynecology* **143**, 181–5.

Dreyfus-Brisac, C. (1970). Ontogenesis of sleep in human prematures after 32 weeks of conceptional age. *Developmental Psychobiology* **3**, 91–121.

Drogtrop, A. P., Ubels, R., and Nijhuis, J. G. (1990). The association between fetal body movements, eye movements, and heart rate patterns between 25, and 30 weeks of gestation. *Early Human Development* **23**, 67–73.

Hoppenbrouwers, T., Combs, D., Ugartechea, J. C., Hodgman, J., Sterman, M. B., and Harper, R. M. (1981). Fetal heart rate during maternal wakefulness, and sleep. *Obstetrics and Gynecology* **57**, 301–9

Inoue, M., Koyanagi, T., Nakahara, H., Hara, K., Hori, E., and Nakano, H. (1986). Functional development of human eye movement in utero assessed quantitatively with real-time ultrasound. *American Journal of Obstetrics and Gynecology* **155**, 170–4.

Karch, D., Rothe, R, Jurich, R., Heldt-Hildebrandt, R., Lübbesmeier, A., and Lemburg, P. (1982). Behavioural changes, and bioelectric brain maturation of preterm, and full term newborn infants: a polygraphic study. *Developmental Medicine and Child Neurology* **24**, 30–47.

Meis, P. J., Rose, J. C., Swain, M., and Nelson, L. H. (1985). Gestational age alters fetal breathing response to intravenous insulin, and intravenous glucose administration. *American Journal of Obstetrics and Gynecology* **151**, 438–40.

Natale, R., Nassello-Paterson, C., and Turlink, R. (1985). Longitudinal measurements of fetal breathing, body movements, and heart rate accelerations, and decelerations at 24 and 32 weeks of gestation. *American Journal of Obstetrics and Gynecology* **151**, 256–63.

Nijhuis, J. G., Jongsma, H. W., Crijns, I. J. M. J., de Valk, I. M. G. M., and van der Velden, J. W. H. J. (1986). Effects of maternal glucose ingestion on human fetal breathing movements at weeks 24, and 28 of gestation. *Early Human Development* **13**, 183–8.

Patrick, J., Campbell, K., Carmichael, L., Natale, R., and Richardson, B. (1980). Patterns of human fetal breathing during the last 10 weeks of pregnancy. *Obstetrics and Gynecology* **56**, 24–30.

Patrick, J., Campbell, K. Carmichael, L., Natale, R., and Richardson, B. (1982). Patterns of gross fetal body movements over 24 hours observation intervals during the last 10 weeks of pregnancy. *American Journal of Obstetrics and Gynecology* **136**, 471–7.

Roodenburg, P. J., Wladimiroff, J. W., van Es, A., and Prechtl, H. F. R. (1991). Classification, and quantitative aspects of fetal movements during the second half of normal pregnancy. *Early Human Development* **25**, 19–36.

Soronkin, Y., Bottoms, S. F., Dierker, L. J., and Rosen, M. G. (1982). The clustering of fetal heart rate changes, and fetal movements in pregnancies between 20, and 30 weeks of gestation. *American Journal of Obstetrics and Gynecology* **143**, 952–7.

Swartjes, J. M., van Geijn, H. P., Mantel, R., van Woerden, E. E., and Schoemaker, H. C. (1990). Coincidence of behavioural state parameters in the human fetus at three gestational ages. *Early Human Development* **23**, 75–83.

Trudinger, B. J., Aust, F., and Knight, P. C. (1980). Fetal age and patterns of human fetal breathing. *American Journal of Obstetrics and Gynecology* **137**, 724–8.

Visser, G. H. A., Dawes, G. S., and Redman, C. W. G. (1981). Numerical analysis of the normal human antenatal fetal heart rate. *British Journal of Obstretrics and Gynaecology* **88,** 792–802.

Visser, G. H. A., Goodman, J. D. S., Levine, D. H., and Dawes, G. S. (1982). Diurnal, and other cyclic variations in human fetal heart rate near term. *American Journal of Obstetrics and Gynecology* **142,** 535–44.

Visser, G. H. A., Poelmann-Weesjes, G., Cohen, T. M. N., and Bekedam, D. J. (1987). Fetal behaviour at 30 to 32 weeks of gestation. *Pediatrics Research* **22,** 655–8.

Vries, J. I. P. de, Visser G. H., A., and Prechtl, H. F. R. (1982). The emergence of fetal behaviour I. Qualitative aspects. *Early Human Development* **7,** 301–22.

Vries, J. I. P. de, Visser, G. H. A., and Prechtl, H. F. R. (1985). The emergence of fetal behaviour II. Quantitative aspects. *Early Human Development* **12,** 99–120.

Vries, J. I. P. de, Visser, G. H. A., Mulder, E. J. H., and Prechtl, H. F. R. (1987). Diurnal, and other variations in fetal movement, and heart rate patterns at 20 to 22 weeks. *Early Human Development* **15,** 333–48.

Vries, J. I. P. de, Visser, G. H. A., and Prechtl, H. F. R. (1988). The emergence of fetal behaviour III. Individual differences, and consistencies. *Early Human Development* **16,** 85–103.

3
The third trimester
J. G. NIJHUIS

Introduction

During the last weeks of the third trimester of human pregnancy, fetal behaviour can be almost totally explained in terms of 'behavioural states', that is as a concept of a recognizable and well-defined association of variables which are stable over time, with clear state transitions in between.

This concept may seem difficult to understand. However, fetal behaviour is very similar to neonatal behaviour, and those dealing with neonates use the concept in daily practice. For example, if one looks at a neonate in its crib, who has its eyes closed and breathes regularly, then everyone would accept a diagnosis of a quiet state (state 1, non-REM sleep). Nobody would, in order to differentiate this state from coma, shake the crib or the neonate, and I have never seen a mother applying a vibro-acoustic stimulus to the neonatal head! The most obvious thing to do is to wait for the baby to move to a more active state (state 2, REM-sleep). If this did not happen spontaneously, then there would be reason for concern, and other actions could be considered. We are, therefore, used to the concept of states that are stable over time and that change spontaneously into other states. Another aspect to consider is the age. Nobody would expect this baby to walk or talk when it is awake. However, if the same child did not talk or walk during wakefulness at an age of three years, then this would be considered very abnormal. So, the absence of speech may be physiological at one age, but pathological at another. The same holds for the fetus: one needs to realize what behaviour can be expected at what ages, and what one may expect to see in an older fetus.

Definition of behavioural states

Behavioural states are defined as combinations of physiological and behavioural variables (e.g., eyes closed, no body movements, and regular respiration), which are stable over time and recur repeatedly, not only in the same infant, but also in similar forms in all infants (modified from Prechtl et al. 1969).

The concept of behavioural states has been used as a descriptive categorization of behaviour, and also as an explanatory concept in which states are considered to reflect particular forms of response-modifying nervous activity in the infant (Prechtl 1974).

The behavioural characteristics used to describe and define a behavioural state are called state-criteria (e.g. eyes open, regular breathing). Other phenomena which are state-related but not always present (e.g. regular mouthing movements, regularity of fetal breathing) are referred to as state-concomitants.

Assessment of behavioural states in the human fetus

Although descriptions of behavioural states in the neonate are in part based on variables that cannot be assessed in the human fetus, several investigators have postulated the existence of behavioural states in the human fetus. De Haan et al. (1977) found that 'quiet' and 'active' states in the neonate could be distinguished only by heart-rate analysis, both heart rate and heart-rate variability being significantly higher during the active state than during the quiet state. Using polygraphic recordings in neonates, Van Geijn et al. (1980) also found that heart-rate indices (long-term irregularity or LTI index; RR-interval index; interval difference or ID index) were closely related to neonatal behavioural states. Both groups extrapolated from these recordings that fetal behavioural states may also be recognized from fetal heart-rate (FHR) recordings.

Timor-Tritsch and coworkers (1978) claimed to identify fetal behavioural states by visual analysis of FHR base-line and variability in relation to fetal movements in 16 fetuses of 38 to 40 weeks' gestation. They distinguished 'quiet', 'active', and 'intermediate' states. The mean duration of a complete cycle consisting of these three states was 62.3 minutes. The mean duration of the quiet states was 22.8 minutes, and of the non-quiet states, 39.5 minutes. In a subsequent investigation, they included another variable, fetal breathing movements, as recorded by external tocodynamometers, and showed that breathing movements are significantly more regular during the quiet state than during a non-quiet state (Timor-Tritsch et al. 1980). They thus provided additional evidence that a state resembling quiet sleep might exist in the term fetus; however, since fetal breathing movements are not continually present, the evidence remained inconclusive.

Junge (1979) recorded FHR and fetal movements of near-term and post-term fetuses during 8-hour sessions and compared these recordings with those obtained from neonates. He applied Prechtl's state classification (Prechtl 1969), but combined state 3, 4, and 5 into one category. In 10 near term fetuses the FHR resembled that recorded from neonates in states 1 and 2 during 97.6 per cent of the recording time. A pattern corresponding to wakefulness (states 3 to 5) in the neonate was seen in only 1.2 per cent of the recording time. In 26.3 per cent of 'total sleeping time' a state 1 FHR pattern was found. In the post-term fetuses the FHR pattern resembled that of the neonate during wakefulness for 21.5 per cent of the recording time. This increase came at the expense of state 2, since the relative duration of the assumed state 1 FHR pattern remained nearly constant, being evident for 22.6 per cent of the recording time. The distribution of time among the assumed behavioural states in the post-term fetuses was similar to that found in the neonates. However, since both FHR and FHR variability are affected by fetal motility (John 1967; Wheeler and Guerard 1974), it was possible that 'states' defined on the basis of FHR and movement patterns represent only cycles in fetal activity and not true behavioural states. These studies did not therefore provide conclusive evidence of the presence of behavioural states and their development during the fetal period in man.

An important step forward was the demonstration that fetal eye movements could be visualized using real-time ultrasound (Bots *et al.* 1981; Birnholz 1981). Thus another independent behavioural variable became available for the description of fetal behaviour; this prompted many researchers to study the existence and development of fetal behavioural states.

Monitoring fetal behaviour

To assess fetal behaviour it is necessary to record fetal body movements, FHR, and fetal eye movements simultaneously (Nijhuis *et al.* 1982). Therefore two real-time ultrasound scanners are needed. One transducer can be oriented to give an oblique sagittal section through the fetal face, including the orbit and mouth, and the second transducer can be placed transversely just below the level of the fetal diaphragm. With the first transducer it is then possible to visualize head and facial (including mouth) movements, as well as eye movements. Also, a hand and forearm can often be seen. With the second transducer fetal breathing movements, movements of the trunk and usually movements of one or more extremities can be detected. Images from the first scanner (head and face) can be recorded on videotape for subsequent analysis, whereas fetal somatic and breathing movements can be recorded verbally by the observer on the audio-channel of the videorecorder. A clinical cardiotocograph (CTG) can be used to record the FHR.

Synchronization of the FHR recording on paper with the videotape is the next important step. This may be achieved by repeated marking with the event marker of the CTG which also produces an audible signal on the videotape. For standardization it is important to make all recordings at about the same time of the day. In order to record at least one complete activity cycle the minimum duration of a recording should be at least 1 hour, but preferably 2 (Timor-Tritsch *et al.* 1978; Junge 1979; Visser *et al.* 1981*a*).

Analysis of the fetal movement data (audio and video) can subsequently be carried out off-line using a multiple push-button event marker connected to the uterine activity channel of the CTG. The two records (FHR and motility) can be aligned by using the previously recorded synchronization signals. In this way a graphic display of fetal behaviour during the entire observation period can be obtained. Segments of such behavioural records are shown in Figs 3.1, 3.2, and 3.3.

Certain FHR patterns, the presence or absence of various kinds of fetal body movements, and the presence or absence of eye movements can be recognized and meet the criteria of stability, simultaneity of change, and

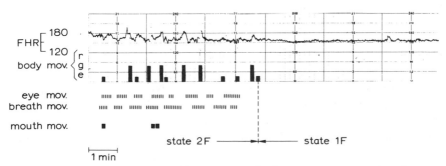

Fig 3.1. Graphic display of fetal behaviour. The first 7 minutes consist of a state 2F, followed by a transition to state 1F. (r, rotation; g, general movement; e, extremity movement). (From Nijhuis and Tas 1991).

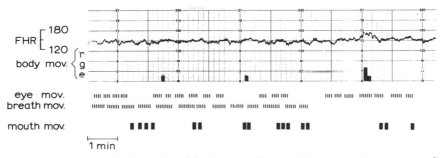

Fig. 3.2. Graphic display of fetal behavioural state 3F. (r, rotation; g, general movement; e, extremity movement).

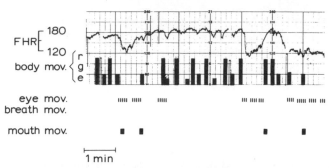

Fig. 3.3. Graphic display of fetal behavioural state 4F. (r, rotation; g, general movement; e, extremity movement).

recurrence needed to prove the presence of states. A similar method has been described by Arduini *et al.* (1985), Caron *et al.* (1986), Rizzo *et al.* (1988), and Shinozuka *et al.* (1989) who use a computer programme for on-line analysis of fetal behaviour.

Definition of fetal behavioural states

We have defined four fetal behavioural states (Nijhuis *et al.* 1982), which resemble the neonatal behavioural states 1 (quiet sleep), 2 (active sleep), 3 (quiet awake), and 4 (active awake) outlined by Prechtl *et al.* (1969). To indicate that we did not use the same criteria the suffix 'F' (for fetal) was added.

1. State 1F (see Fig. 3.1) is quiescence, which can be regularly interrupted by brief gross body movements, mostly startles. Eye movements are absent. The FHR is stable, with a narrow oscillation bandwidth. Isolated accelerations occur, strictly related to movements. This FHR pattern is called FHR pattern A.

2. State 2F (see Fig. 3.1) comprises frequent and periodic gross body movements, mostly stretches and retroflexions, and movements of the extremities. Eye movements are continually present. The FHR (pattern B) shows a wider oscillation bandwidth than pattern A. Frequent accelerations occur in association with movements.

3. State 3F (see Fig. 3.2) is characterized by the absence of gross body movements, but eye movements are continually present. The FHR (pattern C) is stable, but exhibits a wider oscillation bandwidth than pattern A and a more regular oscillation frequency than pattern B. There are no accelerations.

4. State 4F (Fig. 3.3) is vigorous, continual activity, including many trunk
   rotations. Eye movements are present (when observable). The FHR
   (pattern D) is unstable, showing large and long-lasting accelerations,
   which are often fused into sustained tachycardia.

'It should be emphasized that, with respect to heart-rate patterns, each
fetus shows small but distinct individual characteristics. The observer is
therefore advised to obtain a global impression of the spectrum of patterns
exhibited in a total registration, before the definitive assignment of episodes
of heart-rate patterns A to D, respectively, is attempted' (Nijhuis *et al.*
1984).
   In the neonate a state 5 (crying) has been defined and states 3, 4, and 5
are awake states. Although the definitions of the fetal and neonatal states
are similar, it is not thought that the fetus is awake in the uterus. At
present there is no substantial evidence for intrauterine wakefulness or
crying.

Coincidence and behavioural states

The development of behavioural states in the human fetus has been investigated in both healthy multigravidae and nulligravidae (Nijhuis *et al.* 1982;
van Vliet *et al.* 1985*a*; Arduini *et al.* 1986). These studies all described the
existence of behavioural states from 36 to 38 weeks onwards.
   By definition, behavioural states are present if specific combinations of
parameters are present, if the combination is stable over time (at least 3
minutes), and if there are state transitions shorter than 3 minutes.
   Before about 36 weeks of gestation there is a cyclic alternation of the
parameters of the variables, but these combinations are not stable, and
synchronized transitions can not be detected (Drogtrop *et al.* 1990; Swartjes
et al. 1990). These specific combinations are therefore called periods of
'coincidence' and not states (Fig. 3.4). Thus the concept of coincidence
emphasizes that certain combinations of parameters may occur by chance
in the absence of the two other criteria used to prove the presence of a
behavioural state.

Quantitative analysis of fetal behaviour

The behavioural records were analysed by the moving window technique.
This is a smoothing technique that emphasizes stable properties and elim-
inates short-lasting or isolated events. The actual effect of this technique
depends on the duration of the window. After window durations of 1, 2,

Fetal behaviour

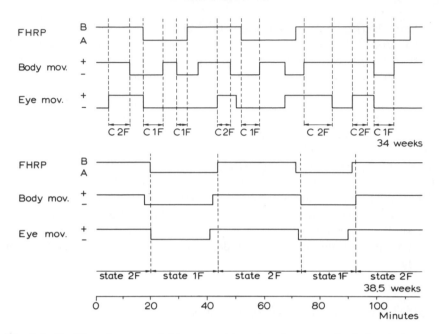

Fig. 3.4. Profiles of state variables at 34 (above) and 38.5 weeks (below). At 38.5 weeks, but not at 34 weeks, the variables are linked to form behavioural states. (C1F and C2F, coincidence 1F and coincidence 2F.) (From Nijhuis and Tas 1991.)

and 3 minutes were tested, a 3-minute window appeared to be the most suitable (Nijhuis *et al.* 1984). The technique is fairly simple. A rectangular hole is made in the centre of an A4-sheet of paper. The length of the rectangle should correspond with 3 minutes and thus depends on the paper-speed used during the recording (e.g. 9 cm long if the paper-speed is 3 cm/min). This window is now shifted over each of the state variables to identify their parameters. For example, body movements are scored as present as long as movements are visible in the window. The first complete window without a movement identifies a period of absence of body movements lasting for more than 3 minutes. Periods are approximated to the nearest 30 seconds.

In this way a profile of the behavioural variables is created and periods of coincidence, state transitions or states can be identified (see Fig. 3.4). The incidence and duration of periods of coincidence and of states are summarized in Tables 3.1 and 3.2.

Table 3.1 Distribution of the percentage (median, quartiles, and range) of coincidence and no coincidence per recording in relation to gestational age in low risk fetuses. (From Nijhuis *et al.* 1982; van Vliet *et al.* 1985*a*)

	Gestational age (weeks)				
	32 (n = 19)	34 (n = 26)	36 (n = 27)	38 (n = 27)	40 (n = 16)
Coincidence 1F					
Median	7	18.5	15	25	36
Q1–Q3	2.5–16	12–26	9–25	15.5–37	22–42.5
Range	0–25	0–29	0–42	7–49	21–51
Coincidence 2F					
Median	49	53	47.5	52	47.5
Q1–Q3	41–63	45–65	31–60	39–64	39.5–56
Range	24–76	23–66	17–65	23–74	23–80
Coincidence 3F					
Median			5 values	2 values	(2.5; 5.5; 5.5)
Q1–Q3				(6.5; 8)	
Range			3–6		
Coincidence 4F					
Median	9 values	10 values	6	0.3	0.4
Q1–Q3			0–46	0–15	0–12
Range	2.5–41.5	3–36	0–100	0–19	0–76
No coincidence					
Median	29	20.5	19.5	15	5.5
Q1–Q3	22.5–37	11–26	16–28	10–19.5	2.5–14
Range	13–63	6–49	0–53	1–54	0–26

State concomitants and behavioural states

Fetal breathing movements

As mentioned on p. 27 Timor-Tritsch *et al.* (1980) observed regular breathing during 'quiet' periods and irregular breathing during 'active' periods. Nijhuis *et al.* (1983) analysed M-mode recordings of fetal breathing movements during states 1F and 2F, and demonstrated that breathing is indeed much more regular during state 1F than during state 2F. Furthermore, it was demonstrated that the incidence of fetal breathing movements is much higher during state 2F than during 1F (mean 73 per cent *vs* 36 per cent) (van Vliet *et al.* 1985*b*). A similar relationship between the incidence of

Table 3.2 Distribution of the percentage and duration (median, quartiles, and range) of states 1F to 4F, and no state identified in low risk fetuses. (From Nijhuis *et al.* 1982; van Vliet *et al.* 1985*a*)

	Percentages 38 (n = 19)	Gestational age (weeks) 40 (n = 15)	38 (n = 19)	Durations 40 (n = 15)
State 1F				
Median	29	39	21	26
Q1–Q3	19–39	27–45	13–26.5	22–30
Range	9–54	29–52	8.5–37.5	12.5–30.5
State 2F				
Median	50	47	20	11.5
Q1–Q3	34–64	41–57	10–26	4–42.5
Range	23–76	24–80	4.5–82	4–54.5
State 3F				
Median	2 values	3 values		7
Q1–Q3	(6; 8)	(2; 6; 6)	2 periods	5.5–14
Range			(3; 6)	3.5–20
State 4F				
Median	2.4	21.5		8
Q1–Q3	0–18.5	0–10	4 periods	6–20.5
Range	0–25	0–76	(3; 3; 4; 6; 5)	5–38
No state identified				
Median	9	3		
Q1–Q3	4–14.5	0–8		
Range	0–53	0–26.5		

fetal breathing movements and behavioural states 1F and 2F has been reported by Arduini *et al.* (1986).

Fetal micturition

Visser *et al.* (1981*b*) studied fetal micturition in relation to FHR patterns. In 95 per cent of their observations of fetuses of 37 to 39 weeks' gestation, voiding occurred within 30 minutes of a transition from a low to a high FHR variation. At this age FHR pattern A is almost entirely confined to periods of absent eye and body movements, whereas FHR pattern B is strongly associated with the criteria of state 2F. Fetal voiding may therefore be inhibited during state 1F, or initiated or facilitated by a change to state 2F. These findings were confirmed by Arduini *et al.* (1986).

Regular mouthing movements

In the neonate, bursts of rhythmic mouthing movements occur at a frequency of 2–3 Hz during states 1 and 2 (Prechtl *et al.* 1986). We have observed similar bursts of regular mouthing in many fetuses; however, these movements occurred only during 1F periods (Nijhuis 1986). Fetal regular mouthing movements may therefore also be a state 1F concomitant. These behavioural phenomena are more extensively discussed in Chapter 4.

Behavioural states in pathological pregnancies

Using the methodology discussed on p. 28, the development of behavioural states has been studied in growth-retarded fetuses (van Vliet *et al.* 1985c; Arduini see Chapter 13) in fetuses of epileptic women (van Geijn *et al.* 1986) and in fetuses of women with type 1 diabetes mellitus (Mulder *et al.* 1987, see Chapter 14), and the findings from these studies are discussed in Section IV.

The first data on cocaine exposure *in utero* and fetal behaviour in relation to neonatal outcome have been published by Hume *et al.* (1989). Archie *et al.* (1989) reported decreased body movements and heart-rate accelerations in narcotic-addicted women who were treated with methadone, but they did not look at fetal eye movements.

Discussion

The study of fetal behavioural states is time-consuming; the minimum duration of a recording is 60 minutes and its analysis may take even more time. Furthermore, the duration and incidence of states is so variable that in most cases no conclusion can be drawn from a single recording. Of course, in healthy fetuses, the coincidence of variables is such that protocols using only two variables will yield similar results (Arabin *et al.* 1988; Weiner *et al.* 1990).

It is important to be aware of the existence of fetal behavioural states when the fetal condition is assessed. It is clear that the biophysical profile (Manning *et al.* 1980) scores are completely different in states 1F and 2F. Several pulsatility indices of the fetal circulation are also state-dependent (see Chapter 16).

Recordings should be made at about the same time of the day because fetal behaviour shows a diurnal variation, which may be related to circulating maternal adrenal hormones (Visser *et al.* 1982; Arduini *et al.* 1986).

Table 3.3 Comparison of behavioural states in the human neonate, the human fetus, and the fetal lamb. Fetal lamb body movements refer mainly to neck muscle activity, as not much is known about general body movements in the fetal lamb. (From Nijhuis and Tas 1991)

	Behavioural state 1(F)			Behavioural state 2(F)		
	Human neonate	Human fetus	Fetal lamb	Human neonate	Human fetus	Fetal lamb
Electrocorticogram	HV (High voltage)	—	HV (High voltage)	LV (Low voltage)	—	LV (Low voltage)
Heart-rate pattern	Stable	Stable pattern A	—	Unstable	Unstable pattern B	—
Average variability	Decreased	Decreased	Increased	Increased	Increased	Decreased
Eye movements	Absent	Absent	Absent	Present	Present	Present
Body movements	Isolated	Isolated	Frequent	Frequent	Frequent	—
Breathing movements	Regular	Regular (if present)	Absent (isolated deep breaths may occur)	Irregular	Irregular (if present)	Irregular (if present)

Clearly the simultaneous recording of three or more variables provides more information about the output of the fetal nervous system. Arduini *et al.* (1986) suggested that in some cases it may be easier to focus on the transitions (see Chapter 13). In individual cases it is sometimes possible to use behavioural observations to discriminate between hypoxia, anomalies, etc. (Pillai *et al.* 1991; see Chapter 18).

In conclusion, it is now clear that fetal behavioural states do exist. These stable constellations are an expression of the activity of the fetal nervous system. Therefore, disturbances in the development of behavioural states near term in growth-retarded fetuses and in fetuses of diabetic women may indicate a disturbance in the development of the central nervous system activity.

Knowledge of the existence of fetal behavioural states is required for adequate interpretation of FHR recordings. This is also the case during labour (Spencer *et al.* 1986; see Chapter 5). Fetal micturition, fetal mouthing movements, and fetal breathing movements, in both regularity and incidence, are state concomitants. Studies involving fetal breathing or other phenomena should therefore always be standardized for behavioural states. The importance of behavioural states for other aspects of fetal surveillance will be dealt with in Sections 2 and 4. The recognition of such states has also had consequences for animal research (see Section 2). In the chronically instrumented fetal lamb for example, two states have been defined, based merely on the recording of the electrocorticogram; these are high-voltage (HV) and low-voltage (LV), respectively. These states show some similarities with the behavioural states in the human neonate and fetus (Table 3.3).

Further human and animal research is necessary to discover which changes in fetal behavioural variables, or combinations of variables (e.g. disturbances of transitions) are the best indicators for the assessment of the integrity and disturbances of the fetal central nervous system.

References

Arabin, B., Riedewald, S., Zacharias, C., and Saling, E. (1988). Quantitative analysis of fetal behavioural patterns with real-time sonography and the acto-cardiograph. *Gynecologic and Obstetrics Investigation* **26**, 211–18.

Archie, C. L., Milton, I. G., Sokol, R. J., and Norman, G. (1989). The effects of methadone treatment on the reactivity of the nonstress test. *Obstetrics and Gynecology* **74**, 254–5.

Arduini, D., Rizzo, G., Giorlandino, C., Vizzone, A., Nava, S., Dell'Acqua, S. *et al.* (1985). The fetal behavioural states: an ultrasonic study. *Prenatal Diagnosis* **5**, 269–76.

Arduini, D., Rizzo, G., Parlati, E., Giorlandino, C., Valensise, H., Dell'Acqua, S., and Romanini, C. (1986). Modifications of ultradian and circadian rhythms of fetal heart rate after fetal–maternal adrenal gland suppression: a double blind study. *Prenatal Diagnosis* **6**, 409–17.

Birnholz, J. C. (1981). The development of human fetal eye movement patterns. *Science* **213**, 679–81.

Bots, R. S. G. M., Nijhuis, J. G., Martin, C. B. Jr., and Prechtl, H. F. R. (1981). Human fetal eye movements: detection *in utero* by ultrasonography. *Early Human Development* **5**, 87–94.

Caron, F. J. M., Geyn, H. P. van, Woerden, E. E. van, and Swartjes, J. M. (1986). Processing of fetal behavioural state patterns. In: *Computers in obstetrics and gynaecology* (ed. K. J. Dalton and R. D. S. Fawdrey), pp. 179–86. IRL Press, Oxford.

Drogtrop, A. P., Ubels, R., and Nijhuis, J. G. (1990). The association between fetal body movements, eye movements and heart rate patterns in pregnancies between 25 and 30 weeks of gestation. *Early Human Development* **23**, 67–73.

Dierker, L. J. Jr., Pillay. S., Sorokin. Y., and Rosen, M. G. (1982). The change in fetal activity periods in diabetic and nondiabetic pregnancies. *American Journal of Obstetrics and Gynecology* **143**, 181–5.

Eyck, J. van, (1987). Blood flow and behavioural states in the human fetus. *Thesis*, Rotterdam.

Geijn, H. P. van, Jongsma, H. W., Haan, J. de, Eskes, T. K. A. B., and Prechtl, H. F. R. (1980). Heart rate as an indicator of the behavioral state: studies in the newborn infant and prospects for fetal heart rate monitoring. *American Journal of Obstetrics and Gynecology* **136**, 1061–6.

Geijn, H. P. van, Swartjes, J. M., Woerden, E. E. van, Caron, F. J. M., Brons, J. T. J., and Arts, N. F. T. (1986). Fetal behavioural states in epileptic pregnancies. *European Journal of Obstetrics and Gynecology and Reproductive Biology* **21**, 309–14.

Haan, R. de, Patrick, J., Chess, J. F., and Jaco, M. T. (1977). Definition of sleep state in the newborn infant by heart rate analysis. *American Journal of Obstetrics and Gynecology* **127**, 753–8.

Hume, R. F. Jr., O'Donnell, K. J., Stanger, C. L., Killam A. P., and Gingras, L. (1989). *In utero* cocaine exposure: Observations of fetal behavioral state may predict neonatal outcome. *American Journal of Obstetrics and Gynecology* **161**, (3), 685–90.

John, A. H. (1967), Effect of fetal movements on the fetal heart rate. *Journal of Obstetrics and Gynaecology of the British Commonwealth* **74**, 60–3.

Junge, H. D. (1979). Behavioral states and related heart rate and motor activity patterns in the newborn infant and the fetus antepartum–A comparative study. I. Technique, illustration of recordings and general results. *Journal of Perinatal Medicine* **7**, 85–103.

Manning, F. A., Platt, L. D., and Sipos, L. (1980). Antepartum fetal evaluation: Development of a fetal biophysical profile. *American Journal of Obstetrics and Gynecology* **136**, 787–95.

Mulder, E. J. H., Visser, G. H. A., Bekedam, D. J., and Prechtl, H. F. R. (1987). Emergence of behavioural states in fetuses of type-1-diabetic women. *Early Human Development* **15**, 231–51.

Nijhuis, J. G. (1986). Behavioural states: concomitants, clinical implications and the assessment of the condition of the nervous system. *European Journal of Obstetrics and Gynecology and Reproductive Biology* **21**, 301–8.

Nijhuis, J. G. and Tas, B. A. P. J. (1991). Physiological and clinical aspects of the development of fetal behaviour. In: *The fetal and neonatal brainstem* (ed. M. A. Hanson), pp. 268–80. Cambridge University Press, Cambridge.

Nijhuis, J. G., Prechtl, H. F. R., Martin, C. B. Jr., and Bots, R. S. G. M. (1982). Are there behavioural states in the human fetus? *Early Human Development* **6**, 177–95.

Nijhuis, J. G., Martin, C. B. Jr., Gommers, S., Bouws, P., Bots, R. S. G. M., and Jongsma, H. W. (1983). The rhythmicity of fetal breathing varies with behavioural state in the human fetus. *Early Human Development* **9**, 1–7.

Nijhuis, J. G., Martin, C. B. Jr. and Prechtl, H. F. R. (1984). Behavioural states of the human fetus. In: Continuity of neural functions from prenatal to postnatal life. *Clinics in Developmental Medicine* (ed. H. F. R. Prechtl), **94**, 65–79. Blackwell Scientific Publications, Oxford.

Pillai, M., Garrett, C., and James, D. (1991). Bizarre fetal behaviour associated with lethal congenital anomalies. *European Journal of Obstetrics and Gynecology and Reproductive Biology* **39**, (3), 215–8.

Prechtl, H. F. R. (1974). The behavioural states of the newborn infant (a review). *Brian Research* **76**, 185–212.

Prechtl, H. F. R., Akiyama, Y., Zinkin, P., and Kerr Grant, D. (1986). Polygraphic studies of the full-term newborn: I. Technical aspects and qualitative analysis. In: Studies in infancy. *Clinics in Developmental Medicine* (ed. R. MacKeith and M. Box), **27**, 1–21. London SIMP with Heinemann Medical.

Prechtl, H. F. R., Weinmann, H. M., and Akiyama, Y. (1969). Organization of physiological parameters in normal and neurologically abnormal infants. *Neuropädiatrie* **1**, 101–29.

Rizzo, G., Arduini, D., Mancuso, S., and Romanini, C. (1988). Computer-assisted analysis of fetal behavioural states. *Prenatal Diagnosis* **8**, 479–84.

Shinozuka, N., Masuda, H., Okai, T., Kuwabara, Y., and Mizuno, M. (1989). Computer-assisted analysis of fetal behavior in fetal abnormalities. *Fetal Therapy* **4**, 97–109.

Spencer, J. A. D. and Johnson, P. (1986). Fetal heart rate variability changes and fetal behavioural cycles during labour. *British Journal of Obstetrics and Gynaecology* **93**, 314–21.

Swartjes, J. M., van Geijn, H. P., Mantel, R., van Woerden, E. E., and Schoemaker, H. C. (1990). Coincidence of behavioural state parameters in the human fetus at three gestational ages. *Early Human Development* **23**, 75–83.

Timor-Tritsch, I. E., Dierker, L. J., Hertz, R. H., Deagan, C., and Rosen, M. G. (1978). Studies of antepartum behavioral states in the human fetus at term *American Journal of Obstetrics and Gynecology* **132**, 524–8.

Timor-Tritsch, I. E., Dierker, L. J., Hertz, R. H., Chik, L., and Rosen M. G. (1980). Regular and irregular human fetal respiratory movements. *Early Human Development* **4**, 315–24.

Visser, G. H. A., Dawes, G. S., and Redman, C. W. G. (1981*a*). Numerical analysis of the normal human fetal heart rate. *British Journal of Obstetrics and Gynaecology* **87**, 792–802.

Visser, G. H. A., Goodman, J. D. S., Levine, D. H., and Dawes, G. S. (1981*b*).

Micturition and the heart rate period cycle in the human fetus. *British Journal of Obstetrics and Gynaecology* **88,** 803–5.

Visser, G. H. A., Goodman, J. D. S., Levine, D. H., and Dawes, G. S. (1982). Diurnal and other cyclic variations in the human fetal heart rate near term. *American Journal of Obstetrics and Gynecology* **142,** 535–44.

Vliet, M. A. T. van, Martin, C. B. Jr., Nijhuis, J. G., and Prechtl, H. F. R. (1985*a*). Behavioural states in the fetuses of nulliparous women. *Early Human Development* **12,** 121–35.

Vliet, M. A. T. van, Martin, C. B. Jr., Nijhuis, J. G., and Prechtl, H. F. R. (1985*b*). The relationship between fetal activity and behavioural states and fetal breathing movements in normal and growth-retarded fetuses. *American Journal of Obstetrics and Gynecology* **153,** (5), 582–8.

Vliet, M. A. T. van, Martin, C. B. Jr., Nijhuis, J. G., and Prechtl, H. F. R. (1985*c*) Behavioural states in the growth-retarded human fetuses. *Early Human Development* **12,** 183–97.

Wheeler, T. and Guerard, P. (1974). Fetal heart rate during late pregnancy. *Journal of Obstetrics and Gynaecology of the British Commonwealth* **81,** 348–56.

Weiner, E., Serr, D. M., and Shalev, E. (1990). Human fetal behavioral state at term. *Gynecologic and Obstetrics Investigation* **29,** 37–40.

4

Heart-rate patterns and fetal movements

E. E. VAN WOERDEN and H. P. VAN GEIJN

The recording of fetal heart-rate (FHR) both antenatally and during labour has become an indispensable part of fetal surveillance. Features of interest in the FHR pattern are the base-line frequency and variability, and the presence or absence of FHR accelerations and decelerations. A base-line variability of more than 10 beats per minute and the presence of accelerations in relation to fetal movements (the so-called reactive or normal FHR pattern) is regarded as a sign of fetal well-being by many authors (Gultekin-Zootsman 1975; Zuspan *et al.* 1979). Another reassuring sign is the presence of normal fetal movements, using maternal perception, the real-time ultrasound imaging, or phonosignals.

FHR accelerations are known to be related to fetal movements, especially gross fetal body movements. This relationship has been studied by many investigators (Timor-Tritsch *et al.* 1978; Dawes *et al.* 1981; Schmidt *et al.* 1983; Patrick *et al.* 1984; Natale *et al.* 1984). At term and in healthy human fetuses, a wide range of heart-rate patterns can be observed as well as a large variety of movements. This chapter focuses on these heart-rate patterns and their relationship with specific movements within particular fetal behavioural states.

In Chapter 3 the concept of fetal behavioural states is described. In this chapter fetal behavioural states are assessed applying the criteria described by Nijhuis *et al.* (1982) (Table 4.1). Because the term human fetus spends

Table 4.1 Fetal behavioural state parameters (from Nijhuis *et al.* 1982)

Fetal state	Eye movements	Body movements	Heart-rate pattern
1F	—	—	A
2F	+	+	B
3F	+	—	C
4F	+	+	D

more than 95 per cent of its time in behavioural states 1F and 2F (van
Woerden *et al.* 1989*a*), we will focus on these two sleep states.

One parameter of state is the FHR rhythm. Figure 4.1 shows the four
FHR patterns that coincide with the fetal behavioural states 1F to 4F.
During state 1F, the FHR pattern has a rather small bandwidth, and
accelerations occur only sporadically. During state 2F on the other hand,
the bandwidth becomes larger, and accelerations are common.

Most of the information given in this chapter is derived from a study

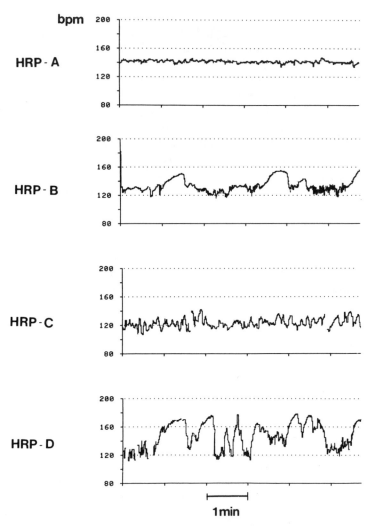

Fig. 4.1. The four fetal heart-rate (FHR) patterns A, B, C, and D, which occur
during behavioural states 1F, 2F, 3F, and 4F, respectively.

using real-time ultrasound to detect fetal movements in 36 term human fetuses (van Woerden 1989*b*). Only healthy pregnant women with uncomplicated pregnancies participated. The mean pH of the umbilical artery of the neonates was 7.27 ± 0.06. The Apgar score was 8.7 ± 1.1 at 1 minute and 10 at 5 minutes. The mean birth-weight was 3.44 ± 0.46 kilograms. All birth-weights were above the 25th centile for parity, gestational age, and sex. The infants were examined neurologically according to Prechtl and Beintema (1977), and were found to be normal. The recording technique which we used to study fetal behaviour is similar to that described in Chapter 3. Some modifications, however, have been made. The FHR is obtained by abdominal electrocardiography (Hewlett-Packard 8030), or by using wide-range Doppler ultrasound (Hewlett-Packard 8040), and each observer uses a set of coded push-buttons. A button is pressed when a movement starts and not released until the movement has finished. Control devices are used to indicate visibility of the fetal orbit and the fetal trunk to provide optimal information on fetal movements. The marking of the visibility of the fetal orbit is an essential part of the recording technique since it enables discrimination between real absence of eye movements and 'pseudo-absence' caused by a temporary loss of visualization.

The FHR and information on fetal movements are stored on-line. With the use of an automated procedure behavioural states are determined, and movements and heart rate are analysed within these states. Detailed information on the technical aspects of the recording method has been published elsewhere (van Woerden *et al.* 1989*a*).

Behavioural state 1F (quiet sleep state)

For approximately 25 per cent of recording time behavioural state 1F can be recognized, with a mean duration of 17 ± 8 minutes. In the FHR tracings of these periods of 1F different types of heart rhythm can be recognized and relate to the presence or absence of fetal movements specific to the 1F state. For approximately 6 per cent of time the fetus does not move at all (Fig. 4.2), and during these periods the bandwidth of the FHR has the lowest value (7.0 ± 0.5 beats). There is little variation in the FHR frequency, and it may be mistaken for a 'silent pattern', which is an ominous sign, indicating deteriorating fetal condition, especially when combined with the occurrence of so-called late decelerations. In such cases the bandwidth is almost uniformly less than 5 beats.

Regular mouthing

A typical feature of the behavioural state 1F is the presence of so-called

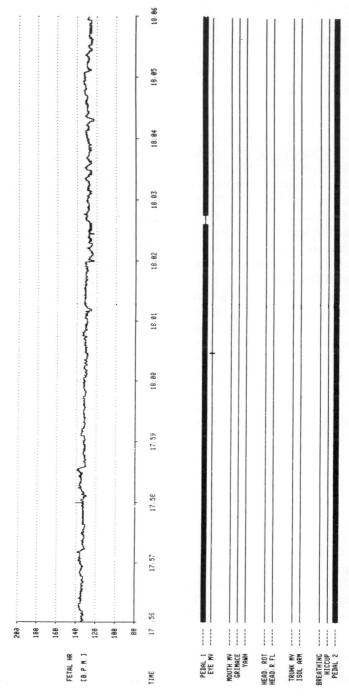

Fig. 4.2. Recording of fetal heart-rate (FHR) and fetal movements showing 10 minutes of state 1F without fetal body movements. Pedal 1 indicates visibility of the fetal orbit, while pedal 2 indicates visibility of the fetal trunk (control devices). Each bar represents a movement or a cluster of movements, the length of the bar indicating the length of the movement or cluster.

regular mouthing (Fig. 4.3). This movement pattern consists of small movements of the mouth or chin in clusters of 5 to 14 movements. The clusters are present in a regular pattern. The average frequency of the clusters is 3 per minute, while the average frequency of the mouth movements within a cluster is 2.5 per second. Regular mouthing is present for 75–93 per cent of the time of behavioural state 1F (van Woerden *et al.* 1988*a*; Pillai and Janes 1990). The latter investigators also noted an absence of regular mouthing movements in cases of fetal compromise of different aetiologies. In state 2F this movement pattern is present sporadically while other mouth movements such as mouth opening, tongue protrusion, and yawning are common.

During periods of regular mouthing the FHR shows a typical oscillatory pattern, with the oscillation frequency relating closely to the cluster frequency of the mouthing movements. In the lower spectrum of the FHR recorded during regular mouthing, there is a dominant peak at the frequency of 60 mHz, which is the frequency of the clusters of regular mouthing (van Woerden *et al.* 1990).

Breathing

Another commonly observed movement in state 1F is fetal breathing (Fig. 4.4). The fetal chest moves in and out in a repetitive fashion. Fetal breathing can also be observed during behavioural state 2F, but the fetal thoracic movements are generally much more irregular (Nijhuis *et al.* 1983). The bandwidth of the FHR in state 1F increases in the presence of breathing movements to 11 ± 2 beats, and has been observed by several investigators (Nijhuis *et al.* 1983; Timor-Tritsch *et al.* 1977; Wheeler *et al.* 1979). In adults many different mechanisms have been proposed to explain this so-called respiratory sinus arrhythmia, such as parasympathetic modulation and intrathoracic pressure changes. For the fetus this phenomenon has not yet been fully explained. Beretska *et al.* (1989) observed a sinusoidal fetal heart-rate in combination with fetal breathing. However the authors suggest that other fetal movements such as mouthing and sucking could also be involved.

Sucking

Sometimes, during a period of fetal rest, fetal sucking movements can be recognized by large and regular movements of the buccal region and the larynx (Fig. 4.5). The movements also have a typical cluster pattern. The characteristics of the two fetal mouth movement patterns, regular mouthing and sucking, are summarized in Table 4.2. The differences are statistically significant (van Woerden *et al.* 1988*a*). During sucking the heart

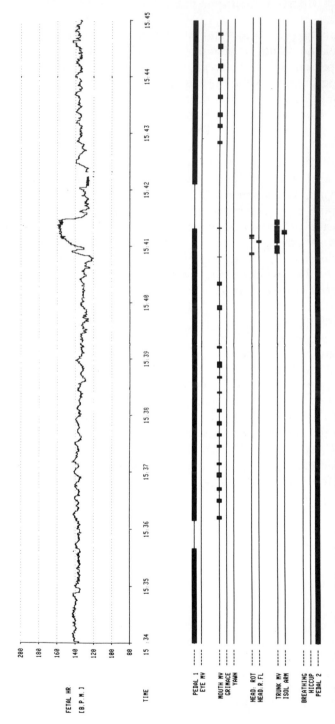

Fig. 4.3. Recording of fetal heart-rate (FHR) and movements showing two periods of state 1F with regular mouthing interrupted by a cluster of body movements. Note the concurrence of the clusters of mouthing movements with the oscillations in the FHR.

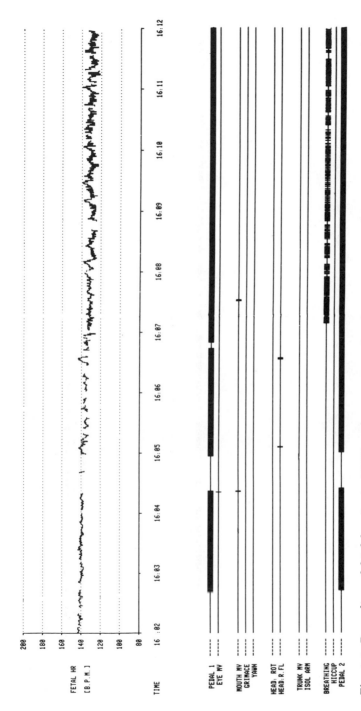

Fig. 4.4. Recording of fetal heart-rate (FHR) and movements showing 10 minutes of state 1F with the presence of fetal breathing movements from 5 minutes into the recording time. Note the increase in the bandwidth of the FHR at the start of the breathing movements.

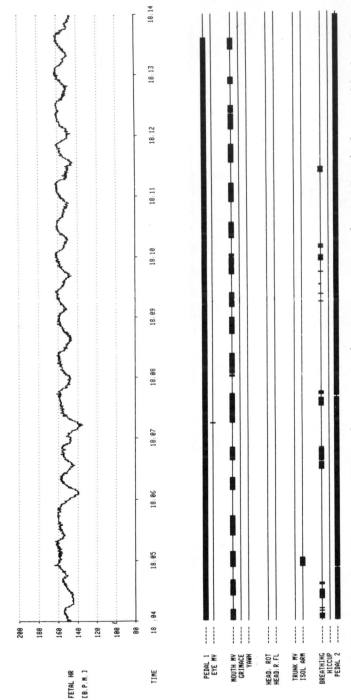

Fig. 4.5. Recording of fetal heart-rate (FHR) and movements showing 10 minutes of state 1F with clusters of fetal sucking movements. Each cluster of sucking coincides with a smooth acceleration in the FHR, resulting in a sinusoidal-like pattern.

Table 4.2 Data on the clusters of regular mouthing and sucking
(From van Woerden *et al.* 1988*a*)

Cluster characteristics	Regular mouthing	Sucking
Onset-to-onset interval between clusters (s)	21 ± 5	28 ± 5
Cluster duration (s)	3 ± 2	14 ± 2
Number of movements per cluster	7 ± 5	20 ± 11
Frequency of movements within clusters/sec	2.5 ± 0.2	1.4 ± 0.2

rhythm shows an oscillatory pattern (sinusoidal-like), with a larger amplitude and a lower frequency than during regular mouthing. These oscillations coincide with the clusters of fetal sucking movements (van Woerden *et al.* 1988*b*). It can be mistaken for a sinusoidal heart rhythm (Nijhuis *et al.* 1984). In contrast to the true sinusoidal pattern, which is associated with severe fetal distress, particularly in cases of severe fetal anaemia (Modanlou and Freeman 1982), the sinusoidal-like rhythm is not symmetrical. In the sinusoidal-like pattern occurring with fetal sucking, an accelerative (sympathetic) and a decelerative (parasympathetic) phase can be recognized.

Behavioural state 2F (active sleep)

Behavioural state 2F can be recognized by the presence of eye movements, body movements, and FHR pattern B (Fig. 4.1). It is present for 60–70 per cent of the time. The mean duration of state 2F is 34 ± 6 minutes, but there is wide variation (10 to 75 minutes, van Woerden *et al.* 1989*a*). The observed movements are single movements of the head, limbs, or trunk, and combinations of these movements.

Most body movements, especially the combinations of movements, coincide with accelerations in the FHR, which are defined as a rise in frequency of at least 10 beats and lasting for 10 seconds or more. It appears that single head, arm, or trunk movements lasting less than 4 seconds are not usually accompanied by accelerations. On the other hand, single movements lasting more than 10 seconds and combinations of movements with trunk movements nearly always coincide with accelerations (van Woerden *et al.* 1991). The duration of movements correlates with the duration of the simultaneously occurring acceleration ($r = 0.75$ for single movements, and $r = 0.9$ for compilations of movements).

The amplitude of all changes in the FHR frequency, such as oscillations during regular mouthing and sucking, appears to be related to the type of movement. In Table 4.3 a summary of the various types of movements is given, together with the concomitant increase in FHR from the base-line frequency. Regular mouthing, a delicate movement type, is accompanied by a small increase in FHR, while combinations of body movements coincide with large accelerations.

The relationship between movements and accelerations has been analysed in detail. Analogous to the distinction between single movements and combinations of movements, one can differentiate single and more complex accelerations. The complex accelerations have one or more notches. In the combinations of movements short-lasting pauses can be present. It appears that in 77 per cent the number of notches in the accelerations correlates with the number of pauses lasting 5 to 10 seconds. In the majority of cases in which there is a discrepancy between the number of notches and the number of pauses there has been a superimposed short-lasting single head or arm movement. Even mouth movements can play a role in this respect (van Woerden *et al.* 1991). This phenomenon is shown in Fig. 4.6. When all observed fetal movements are ordered sequentially and accumulated when they occur simultaneously the compilation of the movements resembles the shape of the acceleration.

Hiccups

Fetal hiccups can also be related to the FHR (Fig. 4.7). Fetal hiccups are frequently noted by the pregnant woman during the second half of pregnancy (Swann 1978). It can be perceived as a jerky movement with a typical and repetitive character, and has been observed with real-time ultrasound from nine weeks of gestation onwards (de Vries *et al.* 1982).

At term, the incidence of hiccups is low, and they occur for 1–2 per cent of the time. Hiccupping frequency varies from 10 to 21 per minute with a

Table 4.3 Increase in fetal heart-rate (FHR) during fetal movements

Fetal movement	Increase in FHR (beats/min; mean ± SD)
Regular mouthing	9 ± 2
Head movements	15 ± 4
Arm movements	16 ± 3
Trunk movements	18 ± 6
Sucking	16 ± 4
Compilations of movements	22 ± 8

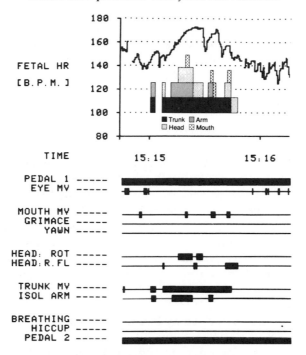

Fig. 4.6. Timing of movements and shape of the acceleration. Below the fetal heart-rate (FHR) pattern is a compilation of the movements in sequential order. Note the resemblance in shape of the acceleration and the compilation of movements. (From van Woerden *et al.*, 1991.)

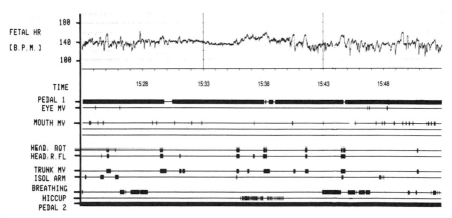

Fig. 4.7. Recording of fetal heart-rate (FHR) and movements. For four minutes a period of fetal hiccuping is present, and coincides with an increase in the FHR.

mean of 15. The movement occurs in both states 1F and 2F. In both states the hiccupping is accompanied by an increase in the base-line FHR of approximately five beats. When body movements are present at the same time, accelerations are superimposed. When hiccupping has finished, the base-line frequency returns to its original level (van Woerden *et al.* 1989*b*).

Implications for fetal heart-rate monitoring

The FHR is an easily and continuously available parameter of fetal condition. The interpretation of the FHR pattern is, however, less easy, especially in pathological conditions. Presence of base-line FHR variability and accelerations is regarded as a sign of fetal well-being. Decelerations are usually not present antenatally in healthy fetuses. In the past, scoring systems were developed to classify FHR tracings as normal, suspicious, or ominous (Hammacher *et al.* 1974; Fischer *et al.* 1976). Following these scoring systems, guidelines were supplied for obstetric management. The criteria for the classification of the FHR patterns were however based mainly upon empiricism.

The scoring system described by Fischer *et al.* (1976) is shown in Table 4.4. A score of 8 to 10 points is regarded as normal, while 5 to 7 points arouses suspicion of a deterioration of the fetal condition, and 0 to 5 points is an ominous sign. Most of the criteria scoring 1 point are within the physiological range. An amplitude of variability (bandwidth) of 5 to 10 beats can be present in periods of behavioural state 1F in the absence of fetal movements, or when there is regular mouthing. A frequency of variability

Table 4.4 Scoring system for antenatal cardiotocography according to Fischer *et al.* (1976)

| | Score | | |
	0	1	2
Basal fetal heart-rate	<100 >180	100–120 160–180	120–160
Amplitude of variability	<5	5–10 >30	10–30
Frequency of variability (number/min)	<2	2–6	>6
Accelerations	none late	sporadic	periodic
Decelerations	profound variable	variable	none

(oscillations in the heart rhythm) of 2 to 6 per minute can be observed during regular mouthing in normal physiological conditions. Sporadic accelerations are common in behavioural state 1F in the healthy human fetus. Thus based on this scoring system a substantial number of physiological FHR patterns are unjustly classified as suspicious. Obstetricians should be aware of the limited value of these scoring criteria. A physiological basis for scoring the FHR patterns as published by Fischer and others is lacking.

This chapter demonstrates that the fetal heart rhythm is closely related to the presence or absence of fetal movements. In the absence of any fetal movement, the FHR pattern is stable and has a bandwidth of 7 ± 0.5 beats per minute. The moment the fetus exhibits movements, the heart rhythm alters. All observed fetal movements, even small movements like breathing and regular mouthing, are accompanied by particular FHR patterns. In periods of fetal activity even small fetal movements can contribute to the final fetal heart rhythm.

In the relationship between FHR patterns and fetal movements a number of associations can be distinguished. The bandwidth of the FHR and the amplitude of oscillations and accelerations is predominantly related to the type of movement (see Table 4.3). The duration of accelerations in the FHR is highly correlated with the duration of the (compilations of) fetal body movements. The shape of the fetal heart rhythm appears to be determined not only by the type of movement, but also by the timing of events. Fetal trunk and extremity movements are of interest in this respect, but fetal mouth movements can also play a role (see Fig. 4.6).

No clear correlation exists between the amplitude of accelerations and the duration of movements. Particular movement patterns, such as regular mouthing and sucking, relate to specific changes in the FHR. Regular mouthing is associated with a smaller rise in heart-rate than fetal sucking and body movements. In the latter two types of movements a larger muscular mass is involved, which is probably associated with a more intense stimulation of the sympathetic system (increase in FHR), followed by a rapid return to the base-line level through parasympathetic control.

It is usually stated that there is a causal relationship between fetal movements and accelerations in the FHR. In 1985 Clewlow and Dawes, and Bocking *et al.* denied this causal relationship. After administration of gallamine to sheep, which acts as a neuromuscular blocking agent, fetal movements were abolished, but accelerations in the fetal heart-rate continued to be present. It was concluded that the majority of accelerations occurred as a result of central neuronal output rather than as a consequence of the fetal movement itself (Bocking *et al.* 1985). A link between motor activity and cardiac acceleration through activation of the reticular formation was suggested (Clewlow and Dawes 1985). In a fetus with Duchenne muscular dystrophy we noticed accelerations in the FHR, while fetal movements were absent (unpublished observation), which also suggests central regulation of heart-rate accelerations.

In our opinion, fetal movements and FHR, though closely related, are both expressions of the functioning central nervous system. Further evidence is needed to support initial observations that in the jeopardized fetus, not only are the patterns of movements and FHR altered, but the normal close association between heart rhythm and movements can be severely disturbed.

References

Beretska, J. S., Johnson, T. R. B., and Hrushesky, W. J. M. (1989). Sinusoidal fetal heart rate pattern during breathing is related to the respiratory sinus arrhythmia; A case report. *American Journal of Obstetrics and Gynecology* **160**, 690.

Bocking, A. D., Harding, R., and Wickham, J. D. (1985). Relationship between accelerations and decelerations in heart rate and skeletal muscle activity in fetal sheep. *Journal of Developmental Physiology* **7**, 47.

Clewlow, F. and Dawes, G. S. (1985). The association between fetal movements and cardiac accelerations in fetal sheep. *Journal of Developmental Physiology* **7**, 281.

Dawes, G. S., Visser, G. H. A., Goodman, J. D. S., and Levine, L. H. (1981). Numerical analysis of the human fetal heart rate. Modulation by breathing and movements. *American Journal of Obstetrics and Gynecology* **14**, 535.

Fischer, W. M., Stude, L., and Brandt, H. (1976). Ein Vorschlag zur Beurteilung des antepartualen Kardiotokogramm. *Zeitschrift zur Geburtshilfe und Perinatologie* **180**, 117.

Gultekin-Zootsman, B. (1975). The history of monitoring the human fetus. *Journal of Perinatal Medicine* **3**, 135.

Hammacher, K., Brun Del Re, R., Gaudenz, R., Degrandi, P., and Richter, R. (1974). Kardiotoko-graphischer Nachweis einer fetalen Gefährdung mit einem CTG-score. *Gynaecologisches Rundschrift Supplement* **1**, 61.

Modanlou, H. D. and Freeman, R. K. (1982). Sinusoidal fetal heart rate pattern: its definition and clinical significance. *American Journal of Obstetrics and Gynecology* **142**, 1033.

Natale, R., Nasello, C., and Turliuk, R. (1984). The relationship between movements and accelerations in the heart rate at 24 to 32 weeks' gestation. *American Journal of Obstetrics and Gynecology* **148**, 591.

Nijhuis, J. G., Prechtl, H. F. R., Martin, Jr. C. B., and Bots R. S. G. M. (1982). Are there behavioural states in the human fetus? *Early Human Development* **6**, 177–95.

Nijhuis, J. G., Martin, C. B., Gommers, S., Bouws, P., Bots, R. S. G. M., and Jongsma, H. W. (1983). The rhythmicity of fetal breathing varies with behavioural state in the human fetus. *Early Human Development* **9**, 1–7.

Nijhuis, J. G., Staisch, K. J., Martin, C. B. Jr., and Prechtl, H. F. R. (1984). A sinusoidal-like fetal heart rate pattern in association with fetal sucking. Report of two cases. *European Journal of Obstetrics and Gynecology and Reproductive Biology* **16**, 353.

Patrick, J. P., Carmichael, L., Chess, L., and Staples, C. (1984). Accelerations of the human fetal heart rate at 38 to 40 weeks gestational age. *American Journal of Obstetrics and Gynecology* **148**, 35.

Pillai, M. and James, D. (1990). Human fetal mouthing movements: a potential biophysical variable for distinguishing state 1F from abnormal fetal behaviour; report of 4 cases. *European Journal of Obstetrics and Gynecology and Reproductive Biology* **38**, 151.

Prechtl, H. F. R. and Beintema, D. J. (1977). The neurological examination of the full-term newborn infant. In: *Clinics in developmental medicine*, p. 63. Heinemann, London.

Schmidt, W., Hara, K., and Cseh, I. (1983). Fetale Bewegungsaktivitat und Akzelerationen im CTG. *Zeitschrift Geburtshilfe und Frauenheilkunde* **43**, 548.

Swann, I. (1978). Intrauterine hiccup (letter). *British Medical Journal*, 1497.

Timor-Tritsch, I. E., Zador, I., Herz, R. H., and Rosen, M. G. (1977). Human fetal respiratory arrhythmia. *American Journal of Obstetrics and Gynecology* **127**, 662.

Timor-Tritsch, I. E., Dierker, L. J., Zador, I., Hertz, R. H., and Rosen, M. G. (1978). Fetal movements associated with fetal heart rate accelerations and decelerations. *American Journal of Obstetrics and Gynecology* **131**, 276.

Vries, J. I. P. de, Visser, G. H. A., and Prechtl, H. F. R. (1982). The emergence of fetal behaviour 1. Qualitative aspects. *Early Human Development* **7**, 301.

Wheeler, T., Gennser, G., Lindvall, R., and Murrills, A. F. (1979). Changes in fetal heart rate associated with fetal breathing and fetal movements. *British Journal of Obstetrics and Gynecology* **87**, 1068.

Woerden E. E. van. (1989). Fetal movements and heart rate: their relationship within behavioural states 1F and 2F. Thesis, Vrije Universiteit Amsterdam.

Woerden, E. E. van, Geijn, H. P. van, Caron, F. J. M., Valk A. W. van der, Swartjes, J. M., and Arts N.F.Th. (1988*a*). Fetal mouth movements during behavioural states 1F and 2F. *European Journal of Obstetrics and Gynecology and Reproductive Biology* **29**, 97.

Woerden, E. E. van, Geijn, H. P. van, Swartjes, J. M., Caron, F. J. M., Brons, J. T. J., and Arts N.F.Th. (1988*b*). Fetal heart rhythms during behavioral state 1F. *European Journal of Obstetrics and Gynecology and Reproductive Biology* **28**, 29–38.

Woerden, E. E. van, Geijn, H. P. van, Caron, F. J. M., Swartjes, J. M., Mantel, R., and Arts N.F.Th. (1989*a*). Automated assignment of fetal behavioural states near term. *Early Human Development* **19**, 137–46.

Woerden E. E. van, Geijn, H. P. van, Caron, F. J. M., Mantel, R., Swartjes, J. M., and Arts N. F. Th. (1989*b*). Fetal hiccups; characteristics and relation to the fetal heart rate. *European Journal of Obstetrics and Gynecology and Reproductive Biology* **30**, 209–16.

Woerden, E. E. van, Geijn, H. P. van, Caron, F. J. M., and Mantel, R. (1990). Spectral analysis of fetal heart rhythm in relation to fetal regular mouthing. *International Journal of Biomedical Computing* **25**, 253.

Woerden E. E. van, Geijn, H. P. van, Mantel, R., and Swartjes, J. M. (1991)

Amplitude and shape of accelerations in relation to fetal body movements in behavioural state 2F. *Journal of Perinatal Medicine* **19**, 73–80.

Zuspan, E. P., Quilligan, E. J., Iams, J. D., and Geijn, H. P. van. (1979). NICHD Consensus Development Task Force Report. Predictors of intrapartum fetal distress; the role of electronic fetal heart rate monitoring. *American Journal of Obstetrics and Gynecology* **135**, 287–91.

5

During labour

JOHN A. D. SPENCER

Introduction

During late pregnancy the fetus exhibits behavioural characteristics that resemble aspects of neonatal behaviour (Nijhuis *et al.* 1982). These features may also be seen during labour (Griffin *et al.* 1985). This chapter will describe the effect of labour on fetal activity and fetal breathing movements, and will emphasize the influence of fetal behaviour state changes on the fetal heart-rate (FHR) during labour.

Fetal movements and the FHR

FHR accelerations associated with fetal activity are the basis of a 'reactive' FHR record (non-stress test) and are a reliable indicator of fetal well-being (Lee *et al.* 1975). However, the suggested optimum number of accelerations required in a 20 or 30 minute recording period has varied between one and five (Spencer 1990). The fetal rest–activity cycle has a profound effect on the FHR (Timor-Tritsch *et al.* 1978; Wheeler and Murrills 1978; Junge 1979; Dawes *et al.* 1982). Fetal quiescence, associated with a non-reactive FHR, may be observed until spontaneous transition from quiet to active state (Brown and Patrick 1981), or be terminated by vibro-acoustic stimulation of the fetus (Divon *et al.* 1987). The fetal response to vibro-acoustic stimulation is characterized by an increase in fetal movements and a transient tachycardia, irrespective of the preceding state; this probably represents an abrupt change to wakefulness although subsequent behavioural cycles, as indicated by alternating episodes of high and low FHR variability, are normal (Spencer *et al.* 1991).

Fetal movements, as perceived by the mother (Nyholm *et al.* 1983) and as seen by ultrasound (Carmichael *et al.* 1984), continue during labour. Most fetal movements during labour are associated with uterine contractions and account for the majority of FHR accelerations in labour (Wittmann *et al.* 1979; Sadovsky *et al.* 1984; Zimmer *et al.* 1987). FHR accelerations contribute to the effect of rest–activity cycles on the FHR during labour (Spencer and Johnson 1986).

Prognostic value of FHR accelerations in labour

FHR accelerations during labour are known to be associated with fetal well-being (Powell et al. 1979; Nyholm et al. 1983). Many early studies of continuous FHR monitoring and fetal acid-base measurement showed that accelerations were the only pattern to consistently predict a normal fetal pH (Kubli et al. 1969; Tejani et al. 1975). There has been recent interest in the FHR response to stimulation during labour. FHR accelerations that occur at the time of fetal blood sampling (Clark et al. 1982; Rice and Benedetti 1986; Spencer 1991), in response to scalp stimulation (Clark et al. 1984; Zimmer and Vadasz 1989), and in response to vibro-acoustic stimulation (Edersheim et al. 1987; Divon et al. 1987) suggest fetal well-being as indicated by a fetal scalp pH above 7.20, and a healthy neonate at delivery. However, the absence of FHR accelerations during labour is not predictive of fetal compromise, although it is associated with twice the risk of caesarean section (Spencer 1991). The value of a provoked FHR acceleration in response to stimulation during labour has yet to be compared with fetal blood sampling in a prospective, randomized study. Fetal stimulation in labour may have a role in screening high-risk pregnancies at the onset of labour (Ingemarsson et al. 1988; Sarno et al. 1990), and in the evaluation of episodes of reduced FHR variability during labour (Spencer and Johnson 1986; Divon et al. 1987), particularly following analgesia (Zimmer et al. 1990).

Effect of fetal behaviour on the fetal heart-rate in labour

Decreased FHR variability during labour has been attributed to 'fetal sleep' for many years. Intermittent episodes of increased fetal movements and FHR variability continue during labour (Richardson et al. 1979; Greene et al. 1980), and the presence of behavioural state changes during labour has been demonstrated by ultrasound (Griffin et al. 1985). Alternating episodes of high and low FHR variability during labour were used to examine the influence of fetal behaviour on the FHR during labour (Spencer and Johnson 1986).

In a study of 301 term labours that had a continuous FHR record for at least six hours duration, agreement between two observers regarding visual recognition of FHR variability cycles was 89 per cent (Spencer and Johnson 1986). Nearly 60 per cent of FHR records showed at least two complete cycles of consecutive episodes of high and low FHR variability and such cycles were almost twice as common in induced labours (Fig. 5.1) compared with spontaneous labours (p < 0.0001). Table 5.1 shows the mean durations of these episodes, which are remarkably similar to the durations

Table 5.1 Fetal heart-rate (FHR) variability cycles during labour

FHR characteristic	Duration (mins) Mean (SD)	Range
Low FHR variability (fetal quiescence)	25 (11)	12–93
High FHR variability (fetal activity)	66 (31)	22–180
Complete cycle	92 (32)	47–202

of such episodes reported during late pregnancy (Timor-Tritsch *et al.* 1978; Wheeler and Murrills 1978) and in neonates (Junge 1979). The only obvious difference was that the duration of low variability episodes during labour extended to 90 minutes, compared with 40 minutes during pregnancy. However, only 5 per cent of these episodes during labour extended beyond 46 minutes. When labours with cycles were compared to those without, there was no effect of time of day, or difference in incidence of labour factors, such as use of uterine stimulation, artificial rupture of membranes, type of analgesia, or mode of delivery.

The amplitude of FHR variability during quiet (low variability) episodes was less than 5 beats per minute in nearly half the cases (Spencer and Johnson 1986). All labours ended with delivery of a healthy neonate, and reduced variability was observed in 26 of the 52 labours in which fetal blood sampling was performed. Variability above 5 beats per minute was 93 per cent predictive of a scalp pH > 7.25, whereas low variability was only 32 per cent predictive of a low pH. Eighteen per cent of labours that did not show cycles had long-term FHR variability which was mainly less than 5 beats per minute in amplitude. Thus, loss of FHR variability alone does not seem to indicate fetal distress during labour.

The absence of FHR changes suggestive of fetal behavioural cycles in more than half of the spontaneous labours, all of which resulted in a healthy neonate, indicates that the process of efficient labour may transiently inhibit such activity (Spencer and Johnson 1986). FHR records from induced labours longer than 12 hours' duration were nearly three times more likely to show FHR variability cycles, compared with those of 6 to 9 hours' duration, but this may have been due to commencing the FHR record earlier during the labour, possibly even during the latent phase. Labours with cycles continued to show evidence of behavioural state changes until a mean of 3 hours prior to delivery. Thus, there was no evidence that cycles of FHR variability disappear as labour progresses, or even during the transition from latent to active phase of labour. This agrees with the report by Richardson *et al.* (1979), which also described the continuation of intermittent episodes of increased body movement and

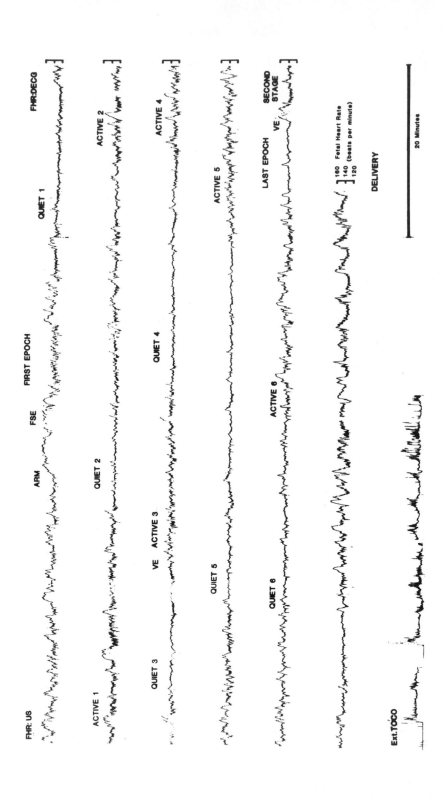

FHR: US

FIRST EPOCH

ARM   FSE

QUIET 1

FHR:DECG

ACTIVE 1

QUIET 2

ACTIVE 2

QUIET 3

VE   ACTIVE 3

QUIET 4

ACTIVE 4

QUIET 5

ACTIVE 5

ACTIVE 6

LAST EPOCH

QUIET 6

SECOND
STAGE

VE

180   Fetal Heart Rate
140   (beats per minute)
120

DELIVERY

Ext.TOCO

20 Minutes

Fig. 5.1. The complete FHR record from an induced labour illustrating the presence of six complete cycles of consecutive episodes of low and high FHR variability, consistent with alternating periods of quiet and active fetal behaviour. Behavioural changes still occurred in the second stage of labour. Note that accelerations were larger, and more prominent during fetal activity. The transient tachycardia ('prolonged accelerations') at the time of artificial rupture of the membranes (ARM), and application of the fetal scalp electrode (FSE), is an example of a FHR response to fetal scalp stimulation. FHR:US, fetal heart-rate recorded by ultrasound; FHR: DECG, fetal heart-rate recorded by Direct ElectroCardioGraphy; VE, vaginal examination; Ext. TOCO, external tocography. (From Spencer and Johnson 1986, reproduced with permission from *British Journal of Obstetrics and Gynaecology*.)

FHR variability during labour, despite the cessation of fetal breathing movements. Greene *et al.* (1980) suggested that the episodic pattern of FHR variability is not the result of breathing and body movements during labour even though the continuation of body movements may modulate the FHR. The implications of the presence or absence of FHR variability cycles, indicative of fetal rest–activity cycles, during labour, remains far from clear.

Fetal breathing and behavioural states

Although the incidence of fetal breathing activity is higher during active states than during quiet states (Junge and Walter 1980; Van Vliet *et al.* 1985), it is not a state criterion, but a state concomitant (Nijhuis 1986). Fetal breathing movements are reduced in active labour (Richardson *et al.* 1979; Boylan 1980), presumably due to a rise in prostaglandins (Kitterman *et al.* 1983), and have been shown to decline over the last three days of pregnancy prior to spontaneous labour (Carmichael *et al.* 1984). Artificial rupture of the membranes also results in an abrupt diminution in fetal breathing, whereas fetal movements continue (Boylan *et al.* 1980; Greene *et al.* 1980). The clinical use of estimates of fetal breathing movements are confined to the biophysical profile (Manning 1991), and to the prediction of preterm labour in women with preterm uterine activity and intact membranes (Castle and Turnbull 1983; Besinger *et al.* 1987).

Summary

Fetal movements with their associated FHR accelerations, as well as the cyclic alternation between episodes of low and high FHR variability, particularly in late pregnancy, give a clear indication of the fetal rest–activity cycle. FHR variability changes during labour indicate that the rest–activity cycle continues, even though perceived movements may diminish and fetal breathing may stop. Fetal behavioural states, known to be present by term, and characterized by the concordant association of fetal movements, FHR changes, and fetal eye movements, have also been shown to continue during labour. However, not all labours show evidence of fetal behaviour despite a normal outcome, and the significance of this remains unknown. Recognition of the influence of fetal behaviour is essential for appropriate interpretation of the FHR during labour.

References

Besinger, R. E., Compton, A. A., and Hayashi, R. H. (1987). The presence or absence of fetal breathing movements as a predictor of outcome in preterm labour. *American Journal of Obstetrics and Gynecology* **157,** 753–7.

Boylan, P. and Lewis, P. J. (1980). Fetal breathing in labor. *Obstetrics and Gynecology* **56,** 35–8.

Brown, R. and Patrick, J. (1981). The nonstress test: How long is enough? *American Journal of Obstetrics and Gynecology* **141,** 646–51.

Carmichael, L., Campbell, K., and Patrick, J. (1984). Fetal breathing, gross fetal body movements, and maternal and fetal heart rates before spontaneous labor at term. *American Journal of Obstetrics and Gynecology* **148,** 675–9.

Castle, B. M. and Turnbull, A. C. (1983). The presence or absence of fetal breathing movements predicts the outcome of preterm labour. *Lancet* **ii,** 471–3.

Clark, S. L., Gimovsky, M. L., and Miller, F. C. (1982). Fetal heart rate response to scalp blood sampling. *American Journal of Obstetrics and Gynecology* **144,** 706–8.

Clark, S. L., Gimovsky, M. L., and Miller, F. C. (1984). The scalp stimulation test: a clinical alternative to fetal scalp blood sampling. *American Journal of Obstetrics and Gynecology* **148,** 274–7.

Dawes, G. S., Houghton, C. R. S., Redman, C. W. G., and Visser, G. H. A. (1982). Pattern of the normal human fetal heart rate. *British Journal of Obstetrics and Gynaecology* **89,** 276–84.

Divon, M. Y., Braverman, J. J., Guidetti, D. A., Langer, O., and Merkatz, I. R. (1987). Intrapartum vibratory acoustic stimulation of the human fetus during episodes of decreased heart rate variability. *American Journal of Obstetrics and Gynecology* **157,** 1355–8.

Edersheim, T. G., Huston, J. M., Druzin, M. L., and Kogut, E. A. (1987). Fetal heart rate response to vibratory acoustic stimulation predicts fetal pH in labor. *American Journal of Obstetrics and Gynecology* **157,** 1557–60.

Greene, K. R., Natale, R., and Harrison, C. Y. (1980). Heart period variation and gross body and breathing movements after amniotomy in the human fetus. In: *Fetal and neonatal physiological measurements* (ed. P. Rolfe), pp. 250–5. Pitman Medical Limited, London.

Griffin, R. L., Caron, F. J. M., and van Geijn, H. P. (1985). Behavioral states in the human fetus during labour. *American Journal of Obstetrics and Gynecology* **152,** 828–33.

Ingemarsson, I., Arulkumaran, S., Paul, R. H., Ingemarsson, E., Tambyraja, R. L., and Ratnam, S. S. (1988). Fetal acoustic stimulation in early labor in patients screened with the admission test. *American Journal of Obstetrics and Gynecology* **158**, 70–4.

Junge, H. D. (1979). Behavioural states and state related heart rate and motor activity patterns in the newborn infant and the fetus antepartum. A comparative study. II Computer analysis of the state related heart rate baseline and macrofluctuation patterns. *Journal of Perinatal Medicine* **7**, 134–48.

Junge, H. D. and Walter, H. (1980). Behavioral states and breathing activity in the fetus near term. *Journal of Perinatal Medicine* **8**, 150–7.

Kitterman, J. A., Liggins, G. C., Fewell, J. E., and Tooley, W. H. (1983). Inhibition of breathing movements in fetal sheep by prostaglandins. *Journal of Applied Physiology* **54**, 687–92.

Kubli, F. W., Hon, E. H., Khazin, A. F., and Takemura, H. (1969). Observations on heart rate and pH in the human fetus during labor. *American Journal of Obstetrics and Gynecology* **104**, 1190–206.

Lee, C. Y., Di Loreto, P. C., and O'Lane, J. M. (1975). A study of fetal heart rate acceleration patterns. *Obstetrics and Gynecology* **45**, 142–6.

Manning, F. A. (1991). The biophysical profile. In: *Fetal monitoring* (ed. J. A. D. Spencer), pp. 73–7. Oxford University Press, Oxford.

Nijhuis, J. G. (1986). Behavioural states: concomitants, clinical implications and the assessment of the condition of the nervous system. *European Journal of Obstetrics and Gynecology and Reproductive Biology* **21**, 301–8.

Nijhuis, J. G., Prechtl, H. F. R., Martin Jr, C. B., and Bots, R. S. G. M. (1982). Are there behavioural states in the human fetus? *Early Human Development* **6**, 177–95.

Nyholm, H. C., Hansen, T., and Neldam, S. (1983). Fetal activity acceleration during early labour. *Acta Obstetricia et Gynecologica Scandinavica* **62**, 131–3.

Powell, O. H., Melville, A., and MacKenna, J. (1979). Fetal heart rate acceleration in labor: excellent prognostic indicator. *American Journal of Obstetrics and Gynecology* **134**, 36–8.

Rice, P. E. and Benedetti, T. J. (1986). Fetal heart rate acceleration with fetal blood sampling. *Obstetrics and Gynecology* **68**, 469–72.

Richardson, B., Natale, R., and Patrick, J. (1979). Human fetal breathing activity during electively induced labor at term. *American Journal of Obstetrics and Gynecology* **133**, 247–55.

Sadovsky, E., Rabinowitz, R., Freeman, A., and Yarkoni, S. (1984). The relationship between fetal heart rate accelerations, fetal movements, and uterine contractions. *American Journal of Obstetrics and Gynecology* **149**, 187–9.

Sarno, A. P., Ahn, M. O., Phelan, J. P., and Paul, R. H. (1990). Fetal acoustic stimulation in the early intrapartum period as a predictor of subsequent fetal condition. *American Journal of Obstetrics and Gynecology* **162**, 762–7.

Spencer, J. A. D. (1990). Antepartum cardiotocography. In: *Modern antenatal care of the fetus* (ed. G. Chamberlain), pp. 163–88. Blackwell Scientific Publications, Oxford.

Spencer, J. A. D. (1991). Predictive value of a fetal heart rate acceleration at the time of fetal blood sampling in labour. *Journal of Perinatal Medicine.* **19**, 207–15.

Spencer, J. A. D. and Johnson, P. (1986). Fetal heart rate variability changes and fetal behavioural cycles during labour. *British Journal of Obstetrics and Gynaecology* **93**, 314–21.

Spencer, J. A. D., Deans, A., Nicolaidis, P., and Arulkumaran, S. (1991). Fetal heart rate response to vibratory-acoustic stimulation during high and low heart rate variability episodes in late pregnancy. *American Journal of Obstetrics and Gynecology* **165**, 86–96.

Tejani, N., Mann, L. I., Bhakthavathsalan, A., and Weiss, R. R. (1975). Correlation of fetal heart rate–uterine contraction patterns with fetal scalp blood pH. *Obstetrics and Gynecology* **46**, 392–6.

Timor-Tritsch, I. E., Dierker, L. J., Hertz, R. H., Deagan, N. C., and Rosen, M. G. (1978). Studies of antepartum behavioral state in the human fetus at term. *American Journal of Obstetrics and Gynecology* **132**, 524–8.

Vliet, M. A. T. van, Martin, C. B., Nijhuis, J. G., and Prechtl, H. F. R. (1985). The relationship between fetal activity and behavioural state and fetal breathing movements in normal and growth-retarded fetuses. *American Journal of Obstetrics and Gynecology* **153**, 582–8.

Wheeler, T., and Murrills, A. (1978). Patterns of fetal heart rate during normal pregnancy. *British Journal of Obstetrics and Gynaecology* **85**, 18–27.

Wittmann, B. K., Davison, B. M., Lyons, E., Frohlich, J., and Towell, M. E. (1979). Real-time ultrasound observation of fetal activity in labour. *British Journal of Obstetrics and Gynaecology* **86**, 278–81.

Zimmer, E. Z., Divon, M. Y., and Vadasz, A. (1987). The relationship between uterine contractions, fetal movements and fetal heart rate patterns in the active phase of labor. *European Journal of Obstetrics and Gynecology and Reproductive Biology* **25**, 89–95.

Zimmer, E. Z. and Vadasz, A. (1989). Influence of the fetal scalp electrode stimulation test on fetal heart rate and body movements in quiet and active behavioral states during labor. *American Journal of Perinatology* **6**, 24–9.

Zimmer, E. Z., Vadasz, A., and Reem, Z. (1990). Intrapartum fetal vibratory acoustic stimulation during spontaneous and induced states of low activity and low heart rate variability. *Journal of Reproductive Medicine* **35**, 250–5.

6

Some remarks on the neonate

H. F. R. PRECHTL

Introduction

The previous five chapters have dealt with behaviour of the fetus from the embryonic stage up to term. It is of special interest to consider the behaviour of the full-term infant from the point of view of the prenatal development of behaviour. Extensive knowledge of the neonate has long existed, but a meaningful comparison of fetal behaviour with that of the neonate has become possible only recently. The last ten years have seen systematic and longitudinal ultrasound studies of fetal behaviour, but it was essential that these investigations were carried out within the theoretical framework of developmental neurology. These studies have provided a wealth of data and have outdated the previously available fragmentary observations of fetal behaviour *in utero* (see Chapter 1 and Roodenburg *et al.* 1991). The other source of knowledge, the stimulation experiments by Hooker and Humphrey on exteriorized fetuses (Humphrey 1978), unfortunately completely neglected any kind of spontaneous motility, and focused exclusively on artificially elicited reflexes.

Neural mechanisms of fetal movements

The new ultrasound observations of fetal motility have substantiated the view of an endogenous generation of fetal movements. Hence, the overwhelming majority of these movements are not reflexes or responses elicited by external stimuli. Recent studies of neural tissue cultures have revealed patterns of neurone activity as soon as inter-neuronal connections are made, and transmitter substances are formed (Droge *et al.* 1986), and showed that co-ordinated endogenous activity is a primary property of the (young) nervous system.

Perhaps a more surprising aspect is the early differentiation of fetal movement patterns. I personally have been struck by the fact that all fetal movements I have ever observed are similar to motor patterns occurring postnatally, and are easily recognized by an observer who is familiar with the motor repertoire of preterm and full-term infants. It was not difficult to classify the various fetal movements (de Vries *et al.* 1982; see Chapter 1) as such a classification already existed from an investigation of low-risk preterm infants (Prechtl *et al.* 1979), which was explicitly intended to be a pilot study for later fetal observations. Moreover, the old concept of an undifferentiated, amorphic, and random pattern from which later specific and distinct movement patterns differentiate is not valid for the human embryo and fetus. On the contrary, early motor patterns are fully patterned and co-ordinated, and—most remarkably—do not change in form once emerged. Thus, the pattern of yawns and stretches that is evident from the first trimester of pregnancy remains unchanged throughout life. Other movements disappear in early infancy, and are specific only for the early life period. It is incredible that firstly the enormous changes in the physical environment occurring at the transition from the intrauterine to the extra-uterine environment have so little influence on the movements, and secondly that these co-ordinating neural circuitries are independent of the profound structural changes occurring in the nervous system during the fetal and infancy period. Such early pattern-generators must be considered as rather independent modules, not influenced by the development and remodelling of the rest of the nervous system.

Fetal and neonatal behavioural states

Although scientific interest in the sleep of the young infant has been documented since the beginning of the twentieth century, a real break-through was only achieved with the introduction of the concept of be-havioural states (Prechtl and O'Brien 1982). Our systematic investigations of the input–output relation of stimulus–response patterns to different sensory modalities have revealed that states are not only an arbitrary classification of many types of behaviours, but 'are distinct and mutually exclusive conditions, each having its specific properties and reflecting a particular mode of nervous function' (Prechtl 1974). This explains why not only certain responses or reflexes, but also certain spontaneous move-ments, can only be obtained in one, but not in other states. Moreover, this concept refutes earlier ideas of a continuum of arousal or vigilance, and of depth of sleep, which are still held among some developmental psycho-logists (e.g. in the Brazelton test).

There are two ways of monitoring behavioural states in the neonate: these are firstly by direct observation, and secondly, by non-invasive electronic recording of certain physiological variables. The first way is required in all those situations that require knowledge of the on-going state, without manipulating or restraining the infant in any way. Such a technique was for example, needed for the standardization of a neurological examination (Prechtl 1977). Based on similar observations by Wolff (1959) and Prechtl (1958), a categorization was introduced that avoided interpretative terms by numbering the various conditions as states 1 to 5 (Prechtl and Beintema 1964). It has gained wide acceptance, and is defined as follows:

(1) state 1—eyes closed, regular respiration, no movements (except startles, and exceptionally general movements);

(2) state 2—eyes closed, irregular respiration, some small twitches in the limbs, and at 2 to 3 minute intervals, a general movement;

(3) state 3—eyes open, no gross movements;

(4) state 4—eyes open, continual gross movements;

(5) state 5—eyes open or closed, crying or fussing.

These state variables can be easily and reliably observed. There are several other events linked with these states and we have called them 'state concomitants'. Included in this group are slow and rapid eye movements, mouthing (rhythmical small jaw movements at a rate of 1.5 to 2 per second), and a number of movement patterns, mentioned above in the list of criteria.

By definition, states are stable conditions over time and not point events. Therefore it is necessary to decide on a minimum duration. We have chosen 3 minutes as a limit, and did this on empirical grounds. The great advantage is that 'indeterminate states' or, even the more illogical 'transitional states', are avoided.

The second technique of studying states of the neonate are polygraphic recordings. The pioneer work in this field has been carried out in Paris by Delange *et al.* (1962), Monod and Pajot (1965), and Eliet-Flescher and Dreyfus-Brisac (1966). The simultaneous electronic recording of a whole set of physiological variables, such as electroencephalogram, electrooculogram, electromyogram of various trunk and limb muscles, respiration and cardiotachogram, not only on paper, but also on magnetic tape, provided the opportunity for extensive and complex computer analysis of the signals (Amemiya *et al.* 1991; Prechtl 1968; Prechtl *et al.* 1968; Prechtl *et al.* 1969; Scholten *et al.* 1985). These studies have provided a certain degree of insight and understanding of state organization, and of the deviations that can occur in the presence of neurological problems. On the other hand it must be admitted that disorganization of state variables is a non-specific abnormality, and does not carry a great deal of prognostic value. The time course of transitions from state 1 into state 2 and vice versa, as well as from state 1 into state 5 and back, are more useful prognostic indicators. Prolonged transitions (considerably longer than 3 minutes) indicated defects in the switching mechanisms from one state into the other. Other transitions (e.g. 1 into 5) are extremely rare in normal neonates and indicate, when repeatedly present, some abnormality of neural functioning.

Moreover it became evident that in quantitative studies of behavioural states, the awake states must be included, as restriction to sleep states can easily lead to erroneous conclusions (Prechtl *et al*. 1973). Sleep research in young infants may easily produce artifacts.

The repertoire of behavioural states in the full-term neonate must have a developmental history. The formation and organization of states at an earlier age during prenatal development was to be expected. It had been suspected from studies on preterm infants that this might happen at around 36 weeks' post-menstrual age (Parmelee and Stern 1972; Prechtl *et al*. 1979). The first comprehensive and detailed study of fetal behavioural states and their precursors was carried out by Nijhuis *et al*. 1982). For this study it was necessary to adapt the neonatal state criteria to possible measurements in the fetus, and the distinction of four behavioural states was introduced (see Chapter 3). A crucial progress was made by the introduction of the concept of 'coincidence', which covers all those periods of recordings in which the different state variables fit together as during a behavioural state, but without synchronization of changes in the variables. Coincidences are thus the ontogenetic precursors of real states.

A comparison of the quantitative distributions of behavioural states in near-term fetuses with those of neonates showed close similarity (Prechtl 1988). Pillai and James (1990) recorded states in the same individuals before and after birth, and confirmed this close quantitative relationship. As for motor behaviour, behavioural states also show a continuum from pre- to postnatal life.

New requirements after birth

There can be no doubt that the neonate is equipped with neural functions that during a long prenatal period anticipate their adaptive role, which occurs only after birth. This endogenously generated repertoire of specific movement patterns must, after birth, adapt the neonate to his new environment, with its many new requirements. One of the main problems in this situation is to trigger specific behaviour patterns at the right time so that they can fulfil their functional task. For example, sucking movements in the fetus lead to ingestion of amniotic fluid whenever they occur, but in the neonate, sucking is only functional if it is triggered when the mouth of the infant has contact with the nipple. Hence, sucking, like many other fetal patterns, must come under an afferent trigger control to be elicited when needed.

The vestibular system is a special case. We have been unable to elicit vestibular responses in fetuses, even at an age when they are clearly present in the preterm infant. This is a meaningful biological adaptation as it prevents motor responses of the fetus to every brisk movement and turning of the mother. The switch-on of the vestibular system after birth seems to be related to the rise of oxygen tension above a critical value with the onset of lung ventilation. This can be concluded from animal experiments (Schwartze and Schwartze 1977).

The human neonate is immature

As a whole the behavioural equipment of the human neonate is surprisingly limited. This view is very much in contrast to statements made nowadays by many developmental psychologists, who claim a high degree of behavioural competence for the young infant. This is true in a historical perspective, as some 60 years ago, neonates were believed to be blind and deaf. On the other hand, it cannot be denied that social or postural behaviour, for instance, is fragmentary during the first weeks of human life (Prechtl 1989; Van Wulfften-Palthe 1990). This becomes strikingly evident if the repertoire is seen in a biological and evolutionary context, by comparing the behavioural repertoire of human neonates with those of newborn apes. The latter are much more advanced developmentally, and many behaviour patterns, which in the human infant only emerge at about the third month of life, are present in newborn apes from the first few days (personal observations). The end of the second month, and the beginning of the third month, is a period of special change of many neural functions, and this change is one of the major functional transformations in early human development (Prechtl 1984).

One may ask why a process of reconstruction and lability takes place in the human extrauterinely, but obviously occurs in other primate species before birth. The answer may be found in the relatively short duration of gestation in the human species. Seen in the light of allometric relationships between body-weight, brain-weight, birth-weight, maximal lifespan, and metabolic rate, the human has a pregnancy which is too short. It is probable that the energy metabolism of the mother is the limiting factor for prolonged growth and development of the fetus. The human fetus is especially 'expensive' for the maternal metabolism because of the relatively large brain of the fetus, and the subcutaneous white fat, which is unique among primates and obviously compensation for the loss of protecting fur (Prechtl 1986). These special fetal demands could only be met by the maternal metabolism if the human mother had a much larger body size, and correspondingly, a larger metabolic reserve. As this did not happen in evolution, the problem was solved by curtailing the increasing duration of pregnancy during the evolution of the hominids. This may be the most likely explanation for the relative immaturity of many neural functions in the neonate. The large increase in intelligence of the human species resulting from encephalization provided a safeguard for survival; mothers had the capacity to learn to compensate for the immaturity of their offspring in their nursing behaviour.

Neurological assessment of fetus and neonate

Full-term and preterm infants can be relatively easily manipulated, observed, and neurologically tested, while the neurological assessment of the fetus is limited to direct observation with ultrasound. The hope to assess the integrity of the fetal nervous system by observing an acoustic startle response to a click (Divon *et al.* 1985) ignores the complexity of the nervous system at this early age. A method which combines a complex functional expression of the nervous system, such as the general movements (Prechtl *et al.* 1979) with a correspondingly complex assessment, such as the visual Gestalt-perception, has been introduced by Prechtl (Prechtl 1990; Prechtl and Nolte 1984). From the replays of video-recordings of fetal movements, or of motor activity of preterm infants in the incubator, it was possible to distinguish between intact nervous systems and those with brain lesions. There was no difference in the amount of general movements between low-risk infants and high-risk infants with documented haemorrhage and/or leucomalacia (Ferrari *et al.* 1990). However, a striking difference existed in the quality of general movements, with abnormal movements lacking fluency, elegance, and complex rotations superimposed on limb movements. Those who might fear that such an assessment might be too subjective can be reassured by the high inter-observer agreement, which was 90 per cent between ten different observers (Prechtl 1990).

A great advantage is that the same method can be applied for the fetus and for the preterm or full-term infant. This gives a high degree of validation, and is a new and reliable way of neurological assessment, which is quickly performed, cheap, and of high predictive value.

References

Amemiya, F., Vos, J. E., and Prechtl, H. F. R. (1991). Effects of prone and supine position on heart rate, respiratory rate and motor activity in fullterm newborn infants. *Brain and Development* **13**, 148–54.

Brazelton, T. B. (1984). Neonatal behavioural assessment scale (2nd edn). *Clinics in Developmental Medicine*, Vol. 88, London, S.I.M.P., Blackwell Scientific; Lippincott, Philadelphia.

Delange, M. M., Castan, Ph., Cadilhac, J., and Passouant, P. (1962). Les divers stades du sommeil chez de nouveau-né et le nourrisson. *Revue Neurologique* **107**, (3), 271–6.

Divon, M. Y., Platt, L. D., Cantrell, C. J., Smith, C. V., Yeh, S.-Y., and Paul, R. H. (1985). Evoked fetal startle response: a possible intrauterine neurological examination. *American Journal of Obstetrics and Gynecology* **153**, 454–6.

Droge. M. H., Gross, G. W., Hightower, M. H., and Czisny, L. E. (1986). Multielectrode analysis of coordinated, multisite, rhythmic bursting in cultured CNS monolayer networks. *Journal of Neuroscience* **6**, 1583–92.

Eliet-Flescher, J. and Dreyfus-Brisac, C. (1966). Le sommeil du nouveau-né et du prématuré. II. Relations entre l'électroencéphalogramme et l'électromyogramme mentionnier au cours de la maturation. *Biologia Neonatorum*, **10**, 316–39.

Ferrari, F., Cioni, G., and Prechtl, H. F. R. (1990). Qualitative changes of general movements in preterm infants with brain lesions. *Early Human Development* **23**, 193–233.

Humphrey, T. (1978). Function of the nervous system during prenatal life. In: *Perinatal physiology* (ed. U. Stave), pp. 651–83. Plenum, New York.

Monod, N. and Pajot, N. (1965). Le sommeil du nouveau-né et du prématuré. *Biologia Neonatorum* **8**, (5–6), 281–307.

Nijhuis, J. G., Prechtl, H. F. R., Martin, C. B. Jr., and Bots, R. S. G. M. (1982). Are there behavioural states in the human fetus? *Early Human Development* **6**, 177–95.

Parmelee, A. H. and Stern, E. (1972). Development of states in infants. In: *Sleep and the maturing nervous system* (ed. C. Clemente, D. Purpura, and F. Meyer), pp. 199–228. Academic Press, New York.

Pillai, M. and James, D. (1990). Are the behavioural states of the newborn comparable to those of the fetus? *Early Human Development* **22**, 39–49.

Prechtl, H. F. R. (1958). The directed head turning response and allied movements of the human baby. *Behaviour* **13**, 212–42.

Prechtl, H. F. R. (1968). Polygraphic studies of the fulterm newborn infant. II. Computer analysis of recorded data. In: 'Studies in infancy'. *Clinics in Developmental Medicine* (ed. M. C. O. Bax and R. C. MacKeith), Vol. 27, pp. 26–40, Heinemann, London.

Prechtl, H. F. R. (1974). The behavioural states of the newborn infant (a review). *Brain Research* **76**, 185-212.

Prechtl, H. F. R. (1977). The neurological examination of the full-term newborn infant, second revised and enlarged edition. In: *Clinics in Developmental Medicine*, Vol. 63, p. 65. Heinemann, London.

Prechtl, H. F. R. (1984). Continuity of neural functions from prenatal to postnatal life. *Clinics in Developmental Medicine*, Vol. 94, p. 255. Blackwell Scientific Publications, Oxford.

Prechtl, H. F. R. (1986). New perspectives in early human development. *European Journal of Obstetrics and Gynecology and Reproductive Biology* **21**, 347–55.

Prechtl, H. F. R. (1988). Developmental neurology of the fetus. In: *Antenatal and perinatal causes of handicap* (ed. N. Patel and F. W. Kubli). *Baillier's Clinical Obstetrics and Gynecology* **2**, 21–36.

Prechtl, H. F. R. (1989). Development of postural control in infancy. In: Neurobiology of early infant behaviour. *Wenner-Gren International Symposium Series* (ed. C. von Euler, H. Forssberg, and H. Lagercrantz), Vol. 55, pp. 59–68. MacMillan Press Ltd, London.

Prechtl, H. F. R. (1990). Qualitative changes of spontaneous movements in fetus and preterm infant are a marker of neurological dysfunction. *Early Human Development* **23**, 151–8.

Prechtl, H. F. R. and Beintema, D. J. (1964). The neurological examination of the full-term newborn infant. In: *Clinics in Developmental Medicine*, Vol. 12, p. 74. Heinemann, London.

Prechtl, H. F. R. and Nolte, R. (1984). Motor-behaviour of preterm infants. In H. F. R. Prechtl (ed.) Continuity of neural functions from prenatal to postnatal life, In: *Clinics in Developmental Medicine*, Vol. 94, pp. 79–92. Blackwell Scientific, Oxford.

Prechtl, H. F. R., and O'Brien, M. J. (1982). Behavioural states of the full-term newborn. The emergence of a concept. In: *Psychobiology of the newborn infant* (ed. P. Stratton), pp. 53–73. J. Wiley & Sons, Chichester.

Prechtl, H. F. R., Akiyama, Y., Zinkin, P., and Kerr Grant, D. (1968). Polygraphic studies of the fullterm newborn infants. I. Technical aspects and qualitative analysis. In: Studies in infancy. *Clinics in Developmental Medicine* (ed. M. C. O. Bax and P. MacKeith), Vol 27, pp. 1–25. Heinemann, London.

Prechtl, H. F. R., Weinmann, H., and Akiyama, Y. (1969). Organization of physiological parameters in normal and neurologically abnormal infants: computer analysis of polygraphic data. *Neuropädiatrie* Vol 1, 101–29.

Prechtl, H. F. R., Theorell, K., and Blair, A. W. (1973). Behavioural state cycles in abnormal infants. *Developmental Medical Child Neurology* Vol. 1, 606–15.

Prechtl, H. F. R., Fargel, J. W., Weinmann, H. M., and Bakker, H. H. (1979). Posture, motility and respiration in low-risk preterm infants. *Developmental Medicine and Child Neurology* **21**, 3–27.

Roodenburg, P. J., Wladimiroff, J. W., Es, A. van, and Prechtl, H. F. R. (1991). Classification and quantitative aspects of fetal movements during the second half of normal pregnancy. *Early Human Development* **25**, 19–36.

Schwartze, H. P. and Schwartze, P. (1977). *Physiologie des Fötal-, Neugeborenen- und Kinderalters*. Akademie Verlag, Berlin.

Scholten, C. A., Vos, J. E., and Prechtl, H. F. R. (1985). Compiled profile of respiration, heart beat and motility in newborn infants: a methodological approach. *Medical and Biological Engineering and Computing* **23**, 15–22.

Vries, J. I. P. de, Visser, G. H. A., and Prechtl, H. F. R. (1982). The emergence of fetal behaviour. I. Qualitative aspects. *Early Human Development* **7**, 301–322.

Wolff, P. H. (1959). Observations on newborn infants. *Psychosomatic Medicine* **221**, 110–18.

Wulfften-Palthe, T. van, Hopkins, B., and Vos, J. E. (1990). Quantitative description of early mother-infant interaction using information theoretical statistics. *Behaviour* **112**, 117–48.

Part 2

Fetal behaviour in research

7

Development of the central nervous system

D. F. SWAAB, M. B. O. M. HONNEBIER, and M. MIRMIRAN

Introduction

It is, at present, very difficult to make a direct connection between a particular function or behaviour and a brain structure that is responsible for it. This holds true for the adult, but even more so in fetal development. One possible exception is the suprachiasmatic nucleus (SCN), a brain structure that generates and co-ordinates circadian rhythms (Moore 1983; Rusak and Zucker 1979; Reppert 1989). The SCN, the biological clock of the hypothalamus, is a small (0.25 mm^3, Swaab et al. 1985) group of neurones located above the optic chiasm. In the human it also contains pacemakers for the generation of circadian rhythms (Schwartz et al. 1986). Under constant conditions the clock is 'free running' with a rhythm of nearly 24 hours. The circadian rhythm of the clock is synchronized (entrained) with the environment by information on the solar cycle of light and dark. This photic information comes directly to the SCN from the optic nerve by way of the retino-hypothalamic tract (RHT) (Sadun et al. 1984), and indirectly by the geniculo-hypothalamic tract (GHT) from the intergeniculate leaflet that contains e.g. neuropeptide-Y fibres (Moore et al. 1989). Although the latter projections may play a role in phase readjustment of circadian rhythms, the RHT is the only visual pathway sufficient for day–night entrainment of the biological clock (Dark and Asdourian 1975).

Predominantly, the ventral subdivision of the SCN receives mainly retinal and geniculate afferents, and contains a large portion of vasoactive intestinal polypeptide (VIP)-producing neurones. The dorsomedial SCN contains a large proportion of vasopressin (VP)-producing neurones. The SCN sends its circadian information to other parts of the brain by VIP- or VP-containing fibres, which terminate on other brain structures, such as the paraventricular nucleus, by means of peptidergic synapses (Kalsbeek et al. 1992; Inenaga and Yamashita 1986).

During human pregnancy, many overt 24-hour rhythms may be observed, both in the mother and in the fetus, for example, rhythms in hormone levels, breathing activity, heart-rate, uterine activity, and fetal behavioural states. Circadian rhythms may be of crucial importance for the onset of labour, and in brain development. This chapter considers whether the fetal SCN is involved in such circadian rhythms, and discusses the strategy to improve understanding of the relationship between developing brain structures and behaviour; this is based on a combination of data from human autopsy material, observations in the human fetus and neonate, and from animal experiments.

Circadian rhythms in the fetus

During human pregnancy 24-hour rhythms have been described for fetal hormones, physiological parameters, and fetal movements, and for uterine activity. Since 90 per cent of estriol (E3) production is derived from fetal adrenal precursors, E3 can be used to monitor fetal adrenal function. Peak values of this hormone are found during periods of darkness in pregnant women (Patrick *et al.* 1979).

A nadir in breathing activity of the human fetus occurring between 1900 and 2400 hours has been observed as early as 20 to 22 weeks of gestational age (de Vries *et al.* 1985). From 38 to 39 weeks of gestational age a clear daily pattern in fetal movements becomes evident (Patrick *et al.* 1982). The mean hourly number, and incidence, of fetal movements, show peak values during maternal sleep with no relation to maternal meals (Patrick *et al.* 1982; Roberts *et al.* 1979). Similar observations have been made using subjective maternal reports of fetal activity (Minors and Waterhouse 1979). A link with the breathing rhythm might exist, since Dawes *et al.* (1981) suggested that episodes of human fetal movement are characterized by reduction or absence of breathing.

Patrick *et al.* (1984) found that by 38 to 40 weeks of gestation there was a peak increase in fetal heart-rate (FHR) accelerations from 2300 to 0200 hours that coincided with gross fetal movements. In addition, both FHR variability and pulse (R–R)—interval variability (that is, accelerations and decelerations) change in the course of the day (Visser *et al.* 1982). The modulation of R–R intervals seems to be mainly attributable to respiratory activity (Timor-Tritsch 1977). Dawes *et al.* (1981) found that any small increase in FHR variability was associated with the presence of fetal breathing.

A 24-hour rhythm of myometrial activity is present in the late gestational rhesus monkey (Ducsay *et al.* 1983; Harbert 1977; Harbert *et al.* 1979; Harbert and Spisso 1980; Taylor *et al.* 1983; Walsh *et al.* 1984). This rhythm seems to be specific for the primate uterus and is postnatally photoperiod-dependent (Figueroa *et al.* 1990). These variations do not require the presence of a live fetus (Honnebier *et al.* 1989*c*). During the night increased maternal plasma oxytocin levels, and a switch from contractures to contractions, was observed in rhesus monkeys. Administration of an oxytocin antagonist inhibits the contractions that emerge with the onset of darkness (Honnebier *et al.* 1989*c*). These observations, and those of an oxytocin challenge test, indicate that the differences in day and night-time myometrial activity in the pregnant monkey are related to an increased sensitivity of the myometrium to oxytocin in the early hours of darkness (Honnebier *et al.* 1989*b*). Since increased nocturnal uterine activity has also been observed in pregnant women (Germain *et al.* 1990), and recent observations indicate that in the same period the human uterus is also more responsive to oxytocin at night (Main *et al.* 1989), similar changes seem to take place in the human myometrium.

Possible functions of circadian rhythms

Circadian rhythms and parturition

The pattern of birth shows a clear 24-hour rhythm in humans. Based upon analysis of 601 222 spontaneous human births in North America and Western Europe published over a period of 100 years, Kaiser and Halberg (1962) found the time distribution of the moment of birth to peak at about 0300 to 0400 hours and to display a nadir at 1700 to 1800 hours.

Although the time of the onset of labour is rather loosely recorded in many hospitals, available data also demonstrate a 24-hour rhythm. According to Charles (1953), in a series of over 16 000 live and stillbirths in Birmingham from 1951 to 1952, the distribution of 'time of onset of labor' showed the greatest difference between night and day if the 12-hour night period from 2100 to 0900 hours is chosen, when 62 per cent of the labours started, in comparison to a day period from 0900 to 2100 hours when only 38 per cent began. Shettles (1960) studied 4154 pregnant women who went into labour spontaneously; this occurred between 2100 and 0900 hours for 65 per cent of the women. The curves for onset of parturition using either painful contractions or spontaneous rupture of the membranes as a criterion bear a close resemblance. Malek (1952) showed that deliveries starting with the passing of amniotic fluid show the same rhythm as those that start with labour pains.

Malek (1952) also found that labours that start during the night tend to be shorter in duration than those beginning at other times of the day. These observations suggest that an endogenous process, subject to circadian control, is operating so that labour takes place during that part of the day when its course tends to be the most rapid. It is interesting, therefore, to relate ultimate outcome in obstetrics to the time of the day that birth took place.

De Porte (1932) showed that the distribution of stillbirths in New York State over the 24-hour day was opposite to that of live births. The maximum number of live births was recorded between 0300 and 0600 hours, exceeding by more than 38 per cent the minimum number between 1200 and 1500 hours. Conversely, the stillbirth rate was 57 per cent higher between 1500 and 1800 hours, than its minimum rate between 0600 and 0900 hours. Yerushalmy (1938) explored this issue further by adding data from Bradford Hill, and found not only was the highest stillbirth rate recorded between 1500 and 1800 hours, but that the neonatal mortality rate also reached its highest value during this period. Furthermore, the distribution of the percentages of necessary operative deliveries followed a very similar pattern.

From the data of Malek (1952) it appears that deliveries beginning between 2400 and 0300 hours proceed most rapidly, whereas those occurring later in the day are associated with an increasing duration of parturition. These data are in agreement with the phase lag of approximately four hours between the 24-hour curve of delivery onset as described by Charles (1953), and the birth curve according to King (1956).

The data of Malek (1952) raised the question of a possible inhibitory effect of light upon the clinical onset of birth. He showed that 1.5 times more deliveries started in darkness (defined as the period between sunset and sunrise) than during the rest of the day, and that this difference was present in all seasons. This confirms previous findings that parturition in humans seems to start preferentially in the course of the evening, and to terminate preferentially in the early morning hours (Guthmann and Bienhüls 1936; Hosemann 1946; Jenny 1933; Kirchhoff 1935). It remains to be determined what the exact contribution of the human fetal and maternal clock is to the circadian rhythms in the process of labour, and to brain development.

Circadian rhythms and maturation of the brain

Roffwarg et al. (1966) proposed two complementary hypotheses to account for the large quantities of rapid eye movement (REM) sleep in infancy. One was a passive hypothesis, based upon the lack of inhibitory control of REM-generator centres by the immature brain. REM diminution, therefore, reflects maturation of this inhibitory system. The second is the active hypothesis, which suggests that REM sleep serves a functional role, namely to stimulate brain maturation. The REM sleep mechanism of the brain stem would constitute a neural self-stimulating system, and be particularly important when the young organism is relatively cut off from environmental stimuli. Since growth and maintenance of neural tissue are enhanced by stimulation, oscillatory (controlled by the circadian system) excitatory activation provided to the brain by REM sleep would stimulate maturation of neuronal structures, and thereby serve a preparatory function for the central nervous system (Roffwarg *et al*. 1966). Observations in human neonates made the later hypothesis plausible, since REM sleep decreases in relation to wakefulness (Dreyfus-Brisac and Monod 1965; Fagioli and Salzarulo 1982; Becker and Thoman 1983; Denenberg and Thoman, 1981; Parmelee *et al*. 1968; Roffwarg *et al*. 1966).

The active hypothesis is of special interest for this chapter. The relatively high amount of REM sleep in the fetus suggests that such a mechanism might already be operational *in utero*. One of the major factors that may influence the prevalence of REM states during prenatal life is the activity of the myometrium. The daily variation in uterine activity (see pp. 76–8) may contribute to REM stimulation of the brain by the entrainment of fetal sleep states (Nathanielsz *et al*. 1984, 1980; Jansen *et al*. 1979). Maternal myometrial activity, either through concomitant vascular partial pressure of oxygen changes, tactile stimulation, or both, may be able to influence fetal behavioural states. It seems of great importance, therefore, to know how the developing brain is affected when these profound circadian variations in the mother, and the concomitant rhythmicity of the behavioural states in the fetus (REM sleep in particular), are disrupted by external factors.

The hypothesis that REM sleep is required for normal brain development has been tested in animals by Mirmiran (1986) Mirmiran *et al*. 1981) and others Davenne and Adrien 1984; Hilakivi *et al*. 1984; Juvancz 1981; Saucier and Astic 1975; Vogel *et al*. 1990). Suppression of REM sleep during early development in either rats or cats leads to permanent structural brain differences, and physiological and behavioural defects, including sleep disturbances later in life.

Suppression of REM sleep by pharmacological interference with monoaminergic neurotransmitters (with drugs such as clonidine or alpha-methyldopamine) during early brain development has proved to interfere with the normal maturation of behaviour and sleep in later life in humans as well. Huisjes *et al*. (1986; Huisjes 1988) reported a clinical study of 22 children who were exposed to clonidine during gestation. The study group showed an excess of hyperactivity and sleep disturbances, for example night awakening phenomena such as night terrors, somnambulism, and nocturnal enuresis. In addition, there seemed to be a dose–effect relationship, especially with respect to sleeping behaviour. Shimohira *et al*. (1986) presented a case report of a 3-year-old boy whose mother had taken alpha-methyldopa throughout pregnancy. Polysomnographic recording indicated that his sleeping behaviour showed an abnormal circadian sleep–wake pattern. Furthermore, in contrast to normal children of comparable age, an increased frequency of gross movements and twitches (mainly during REM) was observed. Others have reported relatively small head circumferences in neonates from alpha-methyldopa—treated mothers compared with those of non-treated hypertensive controls (Moar *et al.* 1978; Ounsted *et al.* 1980). Drugs that affect brain monoamines are prescribed for several indications (for example, depression, hypertension) during pregnancy. Such drugs might suppress REM sleep, and as a result, disturb maturation of the brain. Smaller head circumference, smaller brain, and smaller cortical pyramidal cells with less branching, are among the various drug-induced defects (Mirmiran and Swaab, see Chapter 10; Swaab and Mirmiran 1984).

In conclusion, although experimental data are far from complete, particularly in human and other non-human primates, the existing empirical data suggest that daily variations in maternal rhythms, such as myometrial activity, may be important factors for the maturation of the fetal central nervous system by influencing fetal behavioural states (in particular REM sleep). Furthermore, postnatal development of daily rhythms in the fetus may be affected. This hypothesis seems to be exemplified by premature discontinuation of the intricate mother–fetus relationship (Sander *et al.* 1972). It has often been observed that sleep problems are more common in infants born prematurely than born at full term (Hellbrügge 1974), particularly if these children stay in neonatal units where they are exposed to constant light and noise (Mann *et al.* 1986; Sander *et al.* 1972). Interestingly, it has been found that an artificial daily environment in the nursery has a beneficial effect on the subsequent sleeping behaviour of preterm infants. Not only did these children sleep more than controls, who were exposed to constant light and noise in their neonatal unit, but they fed better and gained more weight; this difference was still present 3 months after the expected day of delivery. For children, in particular those born prematurely, imposed rhythmicity in the form of a strict daily schedule seems to influence food habits and sleep regulation, and, consequently, overall thriving. Studies addressing weight gain of premature neonates and of children after illness point in the same direction (Fagioli *et al.* 1981; Mann *et al.* 1986).

Neonatal circadian rhythms

In late human gestation several daily rhythms are present in the fetal environment, for example, maternal hormones, body temperature, heart rate, and uterine activity; it can therefore be questioned whether fetal rhythms are generated by the fetal SCN. So far, most observations suggest that those diurnal rhythms that can be discerned in the fetus are, to a large extent, driven by the mother. Human neonates were reported to lack all rhythmicity (Junge 1979; Kleitman 1963; Minors and Waterhouse 1979; Parmelee *et al.* 1968; Prechtl 1974). Studies performed on an infant kept in continuous uniform illumination and fed on demand, indicated that an endogenous rhythm in sleep–wakefulness emerged that was out of phase with the world outside, from about 54 days of postnatal ages whereas at 80 days of age the infant could adjust to an imposed environmental cycle (Martin-du-Pan 1970). A major problem in assessing the functioning of an endogenous clock is that different overt rhythms become manifest at different postnatal ages. In children, the plasma serotonin N-acetyl-transferase rhythm (the enzyme that determines the rate of melatonin production) matures early (Attanasio *et al.* 1986), at around 3 months postnatally, whereas the diurnal body temperature rhythm ultimately matures between 5 and 7 years of age (Abe and Fukui 1979; Abe *et al.* 1978). However, data are usually of transversal origin.

Recently, Mirmiran *et al.* (1990) developed a method for long-term continuous recordings of several physiological variables in humans, including body movements, core temperature, heart-rate, and respiratory rate. This method enabled them to study 24-hour rhythms of body temperature and rest–activity in preterm infants. In five of nine infants (recorded at 28 to 34 weeks of conceptional age) 24-hour rhythms were found in body temperature. They concluded that circadian rhythmicity is present during the early neonatal period for certain physiological variables (body temperature), but not others (rest–activity). Unfortunately, fetal body temperature cannot be monitored *in utero* and is, therefore, not available as an indicator for the development of the fetal circadian system.

Relationship between the development of the human SCN and the development of circadian rhythms

The observation that although, generally speaking, human neonates lack all rhythmicity, some circadian rhythms are present in premature children (Mirmiran *et al.* 1990), makes the question of when the human SCN becomes functional of particular interest. This discrepancy was reinforced by the observation that diurnal metabolic changes are present in the fetal SCN in rat and squirrel monkey (Reppert and Schwartz 1983, 1984*a*, 1984*b*). It is difficult, if not impossible, to visualize the human SCN convincingly by conventional histological staining techniques. However, immunocytochemical staining of the SCN with antibodies against arginine-vasopressin (VP) seems to be a good marker for this nucleus in the human brain. Consequently, a morphometric investigation of the human SCN has become feasible (Swaab *et al.* 1985). The moment during development at which VP is expressed in the rat SCN is closely related to the moment that overt rhythms occur (see below). In order to assess the maturity of the human SCN at the moment of birth, the number of neurones expressing VP has been determined in 45 subjects from fetal week 27 to 30 years of age (Swaab *et al.* 1990).

A clear SCN staining was found only from 31 weeks onwards. For five subjects no VP was found in the SCN region; the youngest was a boy of 27 weeks of gestation, and the oldest was a 2-year-old girl (Fig. 7.1). It is not clear why the latter case (urosepsis for 3 days) did not show any VP staining in the SCN, and only very weak staining in the otherwise strongly positive supraoptic and paraventricular nucleus. VP and total cell numbers (Fig. 7.1(a) and (b), respectively) rose rapidly in the neonatal period reaching a peak value around 1 to 1.5 years' postnatally. When the period around birth is considered in detail, it becomes clear that most cells start to express VP only after birth. At term, (between 38 and 42 weeks of gestational age, n = 7), only about 13 per cent of the adult numbers of VP-expressing neurones were present. The developmental course was similar in boys and girls (Swaab *et al.* 1990).

The moment when VP becomes clearly expressed in the SCN neurones in rat is closely related to the moment when the first overt rhythms occur. The rat SCN neurones are formed between gestational days 14 and 16 (Moore *et al.* 1989). The retinohypothalamic tract, which is the primary pathway through which the light stimulus reaches the SCN (Moore and Lenn 1972), starts to penetrate the SCN on postnatal day 3 to 4 (Stanfield and Cowan 1976; Moore *et al.* 1989). From this period onwards, that is from postnatal day 4 to 6, VP-positive neurones were visible in the SCN in all animals, whereas on the seventh postnatal day VP-containing fibres were spread throughout the SCN (de Vries *et al.* 1981). The major increase in synaptic density in the SCN occurs in exactly the same period, that is between postnatal day 4 and 10 (Lenn *et al.* 1977). On postnatal day 6, retina-mediated photic entrainment of circadian rhythms is functional, and capable of overriding any remaining maternal influence (Duncan *et al.* 1986). The rapid maturation of the SCN around postnatal days 4 to 6, as judged from an increase in VP-staining neurones (de Vries *et al.* 1981) is closely related to the appearance of the first overt rhythm, which is that of N-acetyltransferase (NAT) (Ellison *et al.* 1972). A similar relationship is present between the increasing number of human SCN neurones staining for VP in the first postnatal months (see Fig. 7.1(a), and the occurrence of overt rhythms such as NAT (Attanasio *et al.* 1986), cortisol (Price *et al.* 1983), and sleep–wakefulness patterns (Sander and Julia 1966). This shows that like rats, human VP-expression in the SCN coincides with the moment at which some of the first overt rhythms emerge.

On the basis of VP staining, the human SCN at term seems to be

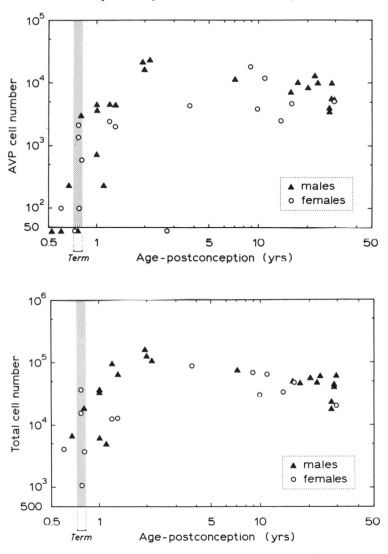

Fig. 7.1. Development of the human suprachiasmatic nucleus (SCN) of the hypothalamus. Term (38 to 42 weeks of gestation) is indicated by the vertical bar. Note that both vasopressin (AVP) and total cell number are low at the moment of birth (13 per cent and 21 per cent respectively of the cell number found in adulthood). There is no difference in the developmental course of the SCN in boys and girls. In the SCN region of five subjects no AVP-expressing neurones were found; these subjects are indicated by symbols below the time axis. Cell numbers around 1 to 15 years postnatally are more than twice the adult cell numbers; thereafter these high levels decrease to adult AVP cell number and total cell number. (Reproduced with permission from Swaab *et al*. 1990.)

comparable to the rat SCN around postnatal day 3, being immature and not capable of regulating most overt rhythms. Our observations consequently reinforce the hypothesis that the human fetal diurnal rhythms are largely driven by the mother. In addition, the 24-hour variation in the timing of birth is probably largely determined by the mother as well (Honnebier *et al.* 1989*a*). On the other hand, SCN neurones seem to be able to express circadian rhythmicity well before this nucleus can co-ordinate overt circadian rhythms; in the rat the rhythm of SCN 2-deoxyglucose-uptake appears on embryonic day 19 (Reppert and Schwartz 1983), a prominent day–night rhythm of VP messenger RNA is evident in the SCN on day 21 of gestation (Reppert and Uhl 1987), and the firing rate of SCN neurons shows a diurnal rhythm on embryonic day 22 (Shibata and Moore 1987). The 2-deoxyglucose rhythm of the fetal SCN depends on the maternal circadian system (Reppert and Schwartz 1983). This means that the SCN neurones express a metabolic rhythm long before they can communicate this rhythm to the rest of the brain. In order to co-ordinate overt rhythms fibre connections with other brain areas need to be developed, and transmitters such as VP have to be expressed.

On the other hand, it should not be forgotten that data relating to the development of the human SCN obtained so far, are based upon the expression of VP in the SCN, whereas VIP expression, according to animal experiments, might appear earlier (Moore *et al.* 1989). Mirmiran's observation on the early development of temperature rhythms might thus be related to such an earlier-developing cell population.

Conclusions

Twenty-four-hour rhythms are present in fetal hormone levels, breathing activity, fetal behaviour, heart-rate, uterine activity, and the onset of birth. The daily variations in rhythm may be important factors for maturation of the fetal central nervous system. An artificial day–night rhythm in the nursery has a beneficial effect on the sleeping behaviour and growth of prematurely born children.

Generally speaking, fetal rhythms such as sleep–wakefulness do not continue after birth. The recently observed exception to this rule, the presence of temperature rhythms in some premature neonates can not unfortunately be monitored *in utero*.

The fetal SCN, the biological clock of the mammalian brain, is still very immature at the moment of birth. The above-mentioned considerations lead to the conclusion that fetal circadian rhythms can not be used at present as a measure for the maturity of the fetal brain, since they seem to be determined mainly by the mother.

Other possible relationships between developing fetal brain structures and functions may be sought by the same strategy in order to reveal parameters that can be used to estimate fetal brain maturity, such as the development of fetal handedness (Hepper *et al.* 1990) in relation to the development of the corpus callosum.

Acknowledgements

We want to thank Ms W. Verweij for her secretarial help, and STIPT project 'Ritme meter; MTR 89026' and the Ter Meulen Fund for financial support.

References

Abe, K. and Fukui, S. (1979). The individual development of circadian temperature rhythm in infants. *Journal of Interdisciplinary Cycle Research* **10**, 227–32.

Abe, K., Sasaki, H., and Takebayashi, K. (1978). The development of circadian rhythm of human body temperature. *Journal of Interdisciplinary Cycle Research* **9**, 211–16.

Attanasio, A., Rager, K., and Gupta, D. (1986). Ontogeny of circadian rhythmicity for melatonin, serotonin, and N-acetylserotonin in humans. *Journal of Pineal Research* **3**, 251–6.

Becker, P. T. and Thoman, E. B. (1983). Organization of sleeping and waking states in infants: consistency across contexts. *Physiological Behavior* **31**, 405–10.

Charles, E. (1953). The hour of birth. A study of the distribution of times of onset of labor and of delivery throughout the 24-hour period. *British Journal of Preventive Social Medicine* **7**, 43–59.

Dark, J. G. and Asdourian, D. (1975). Entrainment of the rat's activity rhythm by cyclic light after lateral geniculate lesions. *Physiological Behavior* **16**, 225–301.

Davenne, D. and Adrien, J. (1984). Suppression of PGO waves in the kitten: anatomical effects of the lateral geniculate nucleus. *Neuroscience Letters* **45**, 33–8.

Dawes, G. S., Visser, G. H. A. Goodman, J. D. S., and Levine, D. H. (1981). Numerical analysis of the human fetal heart rate: modulation by breathing and movement. *American Journal of Obstetrics and Gynecology* **140**, 535–44.

Denenberg, V. H. and Thoman, E. B. (1981). Evidence for a functional role for active (REM) sleep in infancy. *Sleep* **4**, 185–91.

Dreyfus-Brisac, C. and Monod, N. (1965) Sleep of premature and full term neonates: A polygraphic study. *Proceedings of the Royal Society of Medicine* **58**, 6–15.

Ducsay, C. A., Cook, M. J., Walsh, S. W., and Novy, M. J. (1983). Circadian patterns and dexamethasone-induced changes in uterine activity in pregnant rhesus monkeys. *American Journal of Obstetrics and Gynecology* **145**, 389–96.

Duncan, M. J., Banister, M. J., and Reppert, S. M. (1986). Developmental appearance of light–dark entrainment in the rat. *Brain Research* **369**, 326–30.

Ellison, N., Weller, J. L., and Klein, D. C. (1972). Development of a circadian rhythm in the activity of pineal serotonin N-acetyltransferase. *Journal of Neurochemistry* **19**, 1335–41.

Fagioli, I. and Salzarulo, P. (1982). Sleep states development in the first year of life assessed through 24h recordings. *Early Human Development* **6**, 215–28.

Fagioli, I., Ricour, C., Salomon, F., and Salzarulo, P. (1981). Weight changes and sleep organization in infants. *Early Human Development* **5**, 395–9.

Figueroa, J. P., Honnebier, M. B. O. M., Jenkins, S., and Nathanielsz, P. W. (1990). Alteration of 24h rhythms in myometrial activity in the chronically catheterized pregnant rhesus monkey following a 6 hour shift in the light-dark cycle. *American Journal of Obstetrics and Gynecology* **163**, 648–54.

Germain, A. M., Ivankovic, M., Orchard, M. F., Brañez, J., Meissner, A., Vergara, M., and Serón-Ferré, M. (1990). A circadian rhythm of uterine activity precedes by several days the onset of labor in humans. *Symposium on uterine contractility: mechanisms of control*, (Abstract 13). St Louis.

Guthmann, H. and Bienhüls, M. (1936). Wehenbeginn, Geburtsstunde und Tageszeit. *Monatschrift für Geburtshülfe und Gynäkologie* **103**, 337–48.

Harbert, G. M. Jr. (1977). Biorhythms of the pregnant uterus (*Macaca mulatta*). *American Journal of Obstetrics and Gynecology* **129**, 40–8.

Harbert, G. M. Jr. and Spisso, K. R. (1980). Biorhythms of the primate uterus (*Macaca mulatta*) during labor and delivery. *American Journal of Obstetrics and Gynecology* **138**, 686–96.

Harbert, G. M. Jr., Croft, B. Y., and Spisso, K. R. (1979). Effects of biorhythms on blood flow distribution in the pregnant uterus (*Macaca mulatta*). *American Journal of Obstetrics and Gynecology* **135**, 828–42.

Hellbrügge, T. (1974). The development of circadian and ultradian rhythms of premature and full term infants. In: *Chronobiology* (ed. L. S. Schevring, F. Halberg, and J. E. Pauly), pp. 339–41. Igaku Shoin, Tokyo.

Hepper, P. G., Shahidullah, S., and White, R. (1990). Origins of fetal handedness. *Nature* **347**, 431.

Hilakivi, L. A., Sinclair, J. D., and Hilakivi, I. T. (1984). Effects of neonatal treatment with clomipramine on adult ethanol related behavior in the rat. *Developmental Brain Research* **15**, 129–32.

Honnebier, M. B. O. M., Swaab, D. F., and Mirmiran, M. (1989a). Diurnal rhythmicity during early human development. In S. M. Reppert (ed.) *Development of circadian rhythmicity and photoperiodism in mammals IX*, pp. 221–44. Perinatology Press, New York.

Honnebier, M. B. O. M., Figueroa, J. P., and Nathanielsz, P. W. (1989b). Variation in myometrial response to pulsatile intravenous oxytocin administration—a pulsatile oxytocin challenge test at different times of the day in the pregnant rhesus monkey at 121 to 138 days' gestational age. *Endocrinology* **125**, 1498–503.

Honnebier, M. B. O. M., Figueroa, J. P., Rivier, J., Vale, W., and Nathanielsz, P. W. (1989c). Studies on the role of oxytocin in late pregnancy in the pregnant rhesus monkey (I): Plasma concentrations of oxytocin in the maternal circulation throughout the 24h day and the effect of the synthetic oxytocin antagonist [1-β-Mpa (β-(CH2)5)1,),)Me)Tyr2, Orn8] OT on spontaneous nocturnal myometrial contractions. *Journal of Developmental Physiology* **12**, 225–33.

Hosemann, H. (1946). Über die Dauer der Geburt. *Deutsche Medizinische Wochenschrifte* **71**, 181–4.

Huisjes, H. J. (1988). Problems in studying functional teratogenicity in man. In: Biochemical basis of functional neuroteratology: permanent effects of chemicals on the developing brain (ed. G. J. Boer, M. G. P. Feenstra, M. Mirmiran, D. F. Swaab, and F. Van Haaren). *Progress in Brain Research* **73**, 51–9.

Huisjes, H. J., Hadders-Algra, M., and Touwen, B. L., (1986). Is clonidine a behavioral teratogen in the human? *Early Human Development* **14**, 43–8.

Inenaga, K. and Yamashita, H. (1986). Excitation of neurones in the rat paraventricular nucleus *in vitro* by vasopressin and oxytocin. *Journal of Physiology* **370**, 165–80.

Jansen, C. A. M., Krane, E. J., Thomas, A. L., Beck, N. F. G., Lowe, K. C., Joyce, P., Parr, M., and Nathanielsz, P. W. (1979). Continuous variability of fetal PO_2 in the chronically catheterized fetal sheep. *American Journal of Obstetrics and Gynecology* **134**, 776–83.

Jenny, E. (1933). Tagesperiodische Einflüsse auf Geburt und Tod. *Schweizerische Medizinische Wochenschrift* **63**, 15–17.

Junge, H. D. (1979). Behavioral states and state related heart rate and motor activity patterns in the newborn infant and the fetus antepartum—a comparative study. I. Technique, illustration of recordings and general results. *Journal of Perinatal Medicine* **7**, (2), 85–107.

Juvancz, P (1981). The sleep of artificially reared newborn rats, effect of alpha-methyldopa treatment on paradoxical sleep and on adult behavior. *Acta Physiologica Academiae Scientiarum Hungarica* **57**, 87–98.

Kaiser, I. H. and Halberg, F. (1962). Circadian periodic aspects of birth. *Annals of the New York Academy of Sciences* **98**, 1056–68.

Kalsbeek, A., Buijs, R. M., Van Heerikhuize, J. J., Arts, M., and van der Woude, T. P. (1992). Vasopressin containing neurons of the suprachiasmatic nuclei control the circadian corticosterone rhythm. Submitted, for publication.

King, P. D. (1956). Increased frequency of births in the morning hours. *Science* **123**, 985–6.

Kirchhoff, H. (1935). Unterliegt der Wehenbeginn kosmischen Einflüssen? *Zentralblatt für Gynäkologie* **59**, 134–44.

Kleitman, N. (1963) *Sleep and wakefulness*, University of Chicago Press, Chicago, Illinois.

Lenn, N. J., Beebe, B., and Moore, R. Y. (1977). Postnatal development of the suprachiasmatic hypothalamic nucleus of the rat. *Cell and Tissue Research* **178**, 463–75.

Main, D. M., Honnebier, M. B. O. M., Grandberry, P., Reganstein, A., and Nathanielsz, P. W. (1989). The use of a pulsatile oxytocin (OT) challenge test to determine variation in myometrial response to OT at different times of day in the human at 30 to 40 weeks gestation. *Society for gynecologic investigation*, Abstract 395. St Louis.

Malek, J. (1952). The manifestation of biological rhythms in delivery. *Gynaecologia* **133**, 365–72.

Mann, N. P., Haddow, R., Stokes, L., Goodley, S., and Rutter, N. (1986). Effect of night and day on preterm infants in a newborn nursery: randomized trial. *British Medical Journal* **293**, 1265–7.

Martin-du-Pan, R. (1970). Le rôle du rythme circadian dans l'alimentation sur nourission. *La Femme l'Enfant* **4**, 23–30.

Minors, D. S. and Waterhouse, J. M. (1979). The effect of maternal posture, meals and time of day on fetal movements. *British Journal of Obstetrics and Gynecology* **86,** 717–23.

Mirmiran, M. (1986). The importance of fetal/neonatal REM sleep. *European Journal of Obstetrics and Gynecology and Reproductive Biology* **21,** 283–91.

Mirmiran, M., Poll, N. E. van de, Corner, M. A., Van Oyen, H. G., and Bour, H. L. (1981). Suppression of active sleep by chronic treatment with chloromipramine during early postnatal development: effects upon sleep and behavior in the rat. *Brain Research* **204,** 129–46.

Mirmiran, M., Kok, J. H., Kleine, M. J. K. de, Koppe, J. G., Overdijk, H., and Witting, W. (1990). Circadian rhythms in preterm infants: a preliminary study. *Early Human Development* **23,** 139–46.

Moar, V. A., Jefferies, M. A., Mutch, L. M. M., and Redman, C. W. G. (1978). Neonatal head circumference and the treatment of maternal hypertension. *British Journal of Obstetrics and Gynaecology* **85,** 933–7.

Moore, R. Y. (1983). Organization and function of a central nervous system circadian oscillator: the suprachiasmatic nucleus. *Federation Proceedings* **42,** 278–80.

Moore, R. Y. and Lenn, N. J. (1972). A retinohypothalamic projection in the rat. *Journal of Comparative Neurology* **146,** 1–14.

Moore, R. Y., Shibata, S., and Bernstein, M. E. (1989). Developmental anatomy of the circadian system. In: *Development of circadian rhythmicity and photoperiodism in mammals* (ed. S. M. Reppert), pp. 1–24. Perinatology Press, New York.

Nathanielsz, P. W., Bailey, A., Poore, E. R., Thorburn, G. D., and Harding, R. (1980). The relationship between myometrial activity and sleep state and breathing in fetal sleep throughout the last third of gestation. *American Journal of Obstetrics and Gynecology* **138,** 653–9.

Nathanielsz, P. W., Jansen, C. A. M., Yu, H. K., and Cabalum, T. (1984). Regulation of myometrial function throughout gestation and labor: Effect on fetal development. In: *Fetal physiology and medicine: the basis of perinatology* (ed. R. W. Beard and P. W. Nathanielsz), pp. 629–53. Perinatology Press, New York.

Ounsted, M. K., Moar, V. A., Good, F. J., and Redman, C. W. G. (1980). Hypertension during pregnancy with and without specific treatment: the development of the children at the age of four years. *British Journal of Obstetrics and Gynaecology* **87,** 19–24.

Parmelee, A. H. Jr., Akiyama, Y., Scultz, M. A., Werner, W. H., Schulte, F. J., and Stern, E. (1968). The electroencephalogram in active and quiet sleep in infants. In: *Clinical electroencephalography of children* (ed. P. Kellaway and I. Petersen). Almqvist and Wiksell, Stockholm.

Patrick, J., Challis, J., Natale, R., and Richardson, B., (1979). Circadian rhythms in maternal plasma cortisol, strone, estradiol, and estriol at 34 to 35 weeks' gestation. *American Journal of Obstetrics and Gynecology* **135,** 791–8.

Patrick, J., Campbell, K., Carmichael, L., Natale, R., and Richardson, B. (1982). Patterns of gross fetal body movements over 24 hour observation during the last 10 weeks of pregnancy. *American Journal of Obstetrics and Gynecology* **142,** 363–71.

Patrick, J., Carmichael, L., Ches, L., and Staples, C. (1984). Accelerations of the human fetal heart rate at 38 to 40 weeks' gestational age. *American Journal of Obstetrics and Gynecology* **148,** 35–40.

Porte, J. V. de (1932). The prevalent hour of stillbirth. *American Journal of Obstetrics and Gynecology* **23**, 31–7.

Prechtl, H. F. R. (1974). The behavioral states of the newborn infant. *Brain Research* **76**, 185–212.

Price, D. A., Close, G. C., and Fielding, B. A. (1983). Age of appearance of circadian rhythm in salivary cortisol values. *Archives of Diseases in Childhood* **58**, 454–6.

Reppert, S. M. (ed.) (1989). *Development of circadian rhythmicity and photoperiodism in mammals*, p.262. Perinatology Press, New York.

Reppert, S. M. and Schwartz, W. J. (1983). Maternal coordination of the fetal biological clock *in utero*. *Science* **220**, 969–71.

Reppert, S. M. and Schwartz, W. J. (1984a). The suprachiasmatic nuclei of the fetal rat: characterization of a functional circadian clock using 14C-labeled deoxyglucose. *Journal of Neuroscience* **4**, 1677–82.

Reppert, S. M. and Schwartz, W. J. (1984b). Functional activity of the suprachiasmatic nuclei in the fetal primate. *Neuroscience Letters* **46**, 145–9.

Reppert, S. M. and Uhl, G. R. (1987). Vasopressin messenger ribonucleic acid in supraoptic and suprachiasmatic nuclei: appearance and circadian regulation during development. *Endocrinology* **120**, 2483–7.

Roberts, A. B., Little, D., Cooper, D., and Campbell, S. (1979). Normal patterns of fetal activity in the third trimester. *British Journal of Obstetrics and Gynaecology* **86**, 4–9.

Roffwarg, H. F., Muzio, J., and Dement, W. C. (1966). Ontogenetic development of the human sleep-wakefulness cycle. *Science* **152**, 604–19.

Rusak, B. and Zucker, I. (1979). Neural regulation of circadian rhythms. *Physiological Reviews* **59**, 449–526.

Sadun, A. A., Schaechter, J. D., and Smith, L. E. H. (1984). A retinohypothalamic pathway in man: light mediation of circadian rhythms. *Brain Research* **302**, 371–7.

Sander, L. W. and Julia, H. L. (1966). Continuous interactional monitoring in the neonate. *Psychosomatic Medicine* **28**, 822–35.

Sander, L. W., Julia, H. L., Stechler, G., and Burns, P. (1972). Continuous 24-hour interactional monitoring in infants reared in two caretaking environments. *Psychosomatic Medicine* **34**, 270–82.

Saucier, D. and Astic, L. (1975). Effects de l'alpha-methyldopa sur le someil du chat nouveau-né. *Psychopharmacology* **42**, 299–303.

Schwartz, W. J., Busu, N. A., and Tessa Hedley-Whyte, E. (1986). A discrete lesion of ventral hypothalamus and optic chiasm that disturbed the daily temperature rhythm. *Journal of Neurology* **233**, 1–4.

Shettles, L. B. (1960). Hourly variation in onset of labor and rupture of membranes. *American Journal of Obstetrics and Gynecology* **79**, 177–9.

Shibata, S. and Moore, R. Y. (1987). Development of neuronal activity in the rat suprachiasmatic nucleus. *Developmental Brain Research* **34**, 311–5.

Shimohira, M., Kohyama, J., Kawano, M., Suzuki, H., Ogiso, M., and Iwakawa, Y. (1986). Effect of alpha-methyldopa administration during pregnancy on the development of a child's sleep. *Brain and Development* **8**, 416–23.

Stanfield, B. and Cowan, W. M. (1976). Evidence for a change in the retinohypothalamic projection in the rat following early removal of one eye. *Brain Research* **104**, 129–36.

Swaab, D. F. and Mirmiran, M. (1984). Possible mechanisms underlying the teratogenic effects of medicines on the developing brain. In: *Neurobehavioral Teratology* (ed. J. Yanai), pp. 55–71. Elsevier, Amsterdam.

Swaab, D. F. and Fliers, E. (1986). Clinical strategies in the treatment of Alzheimer's disease. In: Aging of the Brain and Alzheimer's disease (ed. D. F. Swaab *et al.*). *Progress in Brain Research* **70**, 413–27.

Swaab, D. F., Fliers, E., and Partiman, T. S. (1985). The suprachiasmatic nucleus of the human brain in relation to sex, age and dementia. *Brain Research* **342**, 37–44.

Swaab, D. F., Hofman, M. A., and Honnebier, M. B. O. M. (1990). Development of vasopressin neurons in the human suprachiasmatic nucleus in relation to birth. *Developmental Brain Research* **52**, 289–93.

Taylor, N. F., Martin, M. C., Nathanielsz, P. W., and Serón-Ferré, M. (1983). The fetus determines circadian oscillation of myometrial electromyographic activity in the pregnant rhesus monkey. *American Journal of Obstetrics and Gynecology* **146**, 557–67.

Timor-Tritsch, I., Zador, I., Hertz, R. H., and Rosen, M. G. (1977). Human fetal respiratory arrhythmia. *American Journal of Obstetrics and Gynecology* **127**, 662–6.

Visser, G. H. A., Goodman, J. D. S., Levine, D. H., and Dawes, G. S. (1982). Diurnal and other cyclic variations in human fetal heart rate near term. *American Journal of Obstetrics and Gynecology* **142**, 533–44.

Vogel, G., Neill, D., Hagler, M., and Kors, D. (1990). A new animal model of endogenous depression: a summary of present findings. *Neuroscience and Biobehavioral Reviews* **14**, 85–91.

Vries, G. J. de, Buijs, R. M., and Swaab, D. F. (1981). Ontogeny of the vasopressinergic neurons of the suprachiasmatic nucleus and their extrahypothalamic projections in the rat brain—presence of a sex difference in the lateral septum. *Brain Research* **218**, 67–78.

Vries, J. I. P. de, Visser, G. H. A., and Prechtl, H. F. R. (1985). The emergence of fetal behavior. II. Quantitative aspects. *Early Human Development* **12**, 99–120.

Walsh, S. W., Stanczyk, F. Z., and Novy, M. J. (1984). Daily hormonal changes in the maternal, fetal, and amniotic fluid compartments before parturition in a primate species. *Journal of Clinical Endocrinology and Metabolism* **58**, 629–39.

Yerushalmy, J. (1938). Hour of birth and stillbirth and neonatal mortality rates. *Child Development* **9**, 373–8.

8

Central nervous control

G. S. DAWES

During the past 20 years it has become evident from observations, initially on animals and more recently on man, that the variable phenomena that can be observed as signs of health *in utero* are extensively modulated by the emergence of fetal behavioural states. From 20 weeks of gestation, when maternal perception of fetal movements (quickening) first becomes evident, until about 28 weeks fetal movements occur randomly, the pattern of fetal heart-rate (FHR) with time is heterogeneous, and there is no evidence of clustering of fetal movements, breathing or other muscular activity over short periods. From 28 to 36 weeks of gestation, in man, a gradually developing inhibitory influence is superimposed, concurrent with the descending inhibition of spinal cord activity recorded late in gestation or after birth (variable in time with species). The development of fetal states has become well co-ordinated in man by 36 weeks' gestation (Nijhuis *et al.* 1984), and evidence of fetal behavioural states persists in labour and postnatally. The emergence of behavioural states before birth seems to be associated with lengthy gestation rather than precocity, since the sheep is precocial, but man is altricial, yet it is present in both. We should also note that in both sheep and man, active (REM) sleep states persist for a high proportion of the time, approximately 40 per cent towards term. Two points arise: firstly the question of why so much time is taken up by REM sleep early in life, to which there is as yet no answer; and secondly, the presence of these behavioural states *in utero* in the absence of gross environmental stimuli provides favourable conditions for studying their control mechanisms.

Normal phenomena associated with changes in fetal behaviour

The criteria used in determining human fetal behaviour from 36 weeks' gestation onwards are derived from studies of FHR, and of fetal eye, breathing, and body or limb movements, recorded by ultrasound imaging. In fetal lambs these phenomena can also be related to episodic changes in fetal electrocortical activity *in utero*. In association with changing electrocortical activity near term, the modulation of breathing movements, of the activity of the limb and genioglossus muscles, and of spinal or cranial reflexes, are different. Thus fetal breathing, the activity of the genioglossus muscle, and the digastric reflex, are inhibited in high-voltage electrocortical activity (that is in quiet sleep), while the lumbar (L4 to L5) spinal flexor and thyro-arytenoid reflexes are inhibited in low-voltage electrocortical activity characteristic of REM sleep (Dawes 1986). No comparable studies are yet available in man.

Secondly, during low-voltage electrocortical activity in sheep, blood-flow (measured by using isotope-labelled microspheres) is increased by about 25 per cent to the pons, medulla, and areas in the brain stem associated with the reticular formation (Richardson et al. 1985; Jensen et al. 1986). This suggests an increase in metabolic activity in these areas during REM sleep. With present methods it seems unlikely that this phenomenon can be studied in man.

Thirdly, there is a suggestion (Slotten et al. 1989) that in sheep umbilical flow may be a little greater during low-voltage electrocortical activity, associated with increased muscular activity in the diaphragm and elsewhere. However the difference, if present in man, may be too small to be detected by flow velocity waveform analysis.

Effect of transection of the brain stem

In his classic book Sir Joseph Barcroft (1946) describes early experiments in which the brain stem of fetal lambs was transected by Barron at different levels, as a means of discriminating higher and lower brain stem mechanisms of neural control. Unfortunately their experiments were terminated by the onset of war in 1939 and hence diversion to other activities. In the early 1980s we came to employ the same method of investigation through the following argument. It was by then known that whereas fetal breathing movements were episodic in character near term, and associated with the changing level of electrocortical activity, earlier in gestation (before 110 days) breathing movements were almost continuous. This suggested that with the development of fetal behavioural states there might be episodic descending inhibition of fetal breathing. If this hypothesis is correct then transection of the fetal brain stem above the pons should dissociate electrocortical activity and fetal breathing movements; the latter might then become almost continuous again, as they were before 110 days. This proved to be so. After transection at the upper pons, or at the level of the lower colliculi, fetal electrocortical activity became dissociated from fetal breathing activity and, after several days of recovery, there was a progressive increase in fetal breathing activity, which tended to become continuous (Dawes et al. 1983). When the sections were made more rostrally, both electrocortical activity and fetal breathing activity remained synchronous near term. This suggested that the origin of episodic electrocortical activity depended on the integrity of central nervous structures only a little rostral of the inferior colliculi. However we readily concede that these were gross surgical interventions, which can only delimit the structures involved in a most general way. The simplest explanation of the dissociation between episodic sleep states and fetal breathing movements by transection in the upper pons, is that the transection has interrupted a descending inhibitory pathway or pathways. There are more complex explanations, such as interference with an ascending–descending neural loop, or the wider effects of vascular section and spreading degeneration, with consequences not topographically limited to the area of section. None the less the experiments do show that there is something interesting to be discovered, and they have been the starting point for more detailed studies.

A considerable effort has been made in the last eight years to identify the different pathways involved in the descending inhibition of fetal breathing. This has two components. First, there is the descending inhibition of fetal breathing movements associated with low-voltage electrocortical activity. Secondly, there is the inhibition of both fetal breathing and limb movements associated with acute mild isocapnic hypoxia (e.g. a reduction of fetal P_aO_2 from 23 to 12 mm Hg in lambs *in utero* near term over one hour). This degree of hypoxaemia, caused by giving the ewe a gas mixture low in oxygen to breathe, or by reduction of uterine blood flow, is not inevitably accompanied by metabolic acidaemia. If the hypoxaemia is continued for a day, there is fetal adaptation; breathing, body, and limb movements are restored in spite of persistent chronic hypoxaemia (reduced P_aO_2), even though there is as yet no rise in haemoglobin concentration.

As to the first type of inhibition of fetal breathing (in association with high-voltage electrocortical activity characteristic of quiet sleep), few further experiments have been reported. Parkes *et al.* (1984) found that bilateral *centrally located* lesions of relatively large size (several mm, using cautery) in the upper pons restored fetal breathing during low-voltage electrocortical activity, although hypoxia still caused arrest of breathing. This suggested that there might be two descending inhibitory pathways serving different functions. It is desirable that these experiments should be either confirmed or disproved using smaller lesions to delineate more precisely the presumptive descending tracts.

More work has been carried out in an attempt to define the site of action of hypoxaemia in causing respiratory arrest either before or after birth. Cross and his colleagues (Cross and Warner 1951; Cross and Oppé 1952) showed that mild hypoxia (exposure of a human neonate to 15 per cent oxygen) caused a biphasic response; brief hyperventilation for a few minutes was followed by a reduction in minute volume down to, or sometimes below, the initial value. The secondary response is now attributable to the same mechanism as in fetal hypoxia, since it is also abolished by decerebration, and is unaffected by denervation of the carotid chemoreceptors (Martin-Body 1988; Martin-Body and Johnston 1988). This has widened the field of inquiry to use neonatal or adult animals as well as fetuses, even though after birth the breathing response is normally confounded by the activity of the systemic arterial chemoreceptors.

Interest in locating this 'new'central chemoreceptor has received a further impetus from two sets of observations. First, Hanson and his colleagues have shown that almitrine (a drug known to excite the carotid chemoreceptors of adult cats) administered to fetal lambs near term causes arrest of fetal breathing (Moore *et al.* 1989), unaffected by carotid denervation or vagotomy, but abolished by upper pontine lesions, which prevent the arrest of breathing by hypoxia. This may provide a tool for localization in the central nervous system in or above the pons. It seems unlikely that almitrine has a systemic action (for example, by releasing a substance in the systemic circulation which is then carried to the brain). Secondly there is the observation by Koos (1985) that administration of adenosine, peripherally, or in small doses into the lateral ventricles, also arrests fetal breathing in sheep; and likewise, this inhibition is abolished by section of the upper pons. Adenosine is believed to be released locally as a consequence of hypoxaemia. We need to know its central site(s) of action in these respects.

Such experiments reported so far do not point clearly to a single descending pathway or nucleus responsible for the effects of acute isocapnic hypoxia in arresting fetal breathing movements. Gluckmann and Johnston's work (1987) suggests a lateral location in the rostral pons close to the parabrachial nucleus, as identified by small bilateral lesions placed by stereotaxic instrumentation. Infusion of lactic acid intravenously causes continuous fetal breathing after such lesions (Johnston and Gluckmann 1989), but not otherwise. However their maps were not constructed at right angles to the brain stem, which makes location, and comparison with the work of others, difficult. In newborn lambs Noble and Williams (1989) found electrical activity in neurones located more centrally in the rostral pons; this was increased by hypoxia, but not by intense transient excitation of the carotid chemoreceptors (Noble *et al.* 1990). Electrical stimulation of this area caused arrest of breathing (Coles *et al.* 1989), and local cooling (by a single thermode) abolished the arrest of breathing by hypoxia (Parkes *et al.* 1990). So there are two competing sites for consideration; laterally or more centrally in the rostral pons; and it might be profitable for the two groups to sort out the technical differences by collaboration. We need to improve on the gross lesions associated with brain stem section.

Sites of drug actions

With all the reservations expressed above, we are nevertheless in a position to draw some crude conclusions as to the site of actions of some drugs on the fetal nervous system. We are still uncertain of the location of the nuclei, or group of nuclei, responsible for generating electrocortical activity in the fetus. This activity can be recorded from the surface of the cortex, but we should not assume its topographical origin is close to the cortex. Thus van der Wildt (1982), in an article that deserves wider publication, showed that administration of atropine sulphate to the fetal lamb induces prolonged high-voltage electrocortical activity, while episodic fetal breathing movements persist. We confirmed this (Bamford *et al.* 1985) and also showed the same effect with hyoscine, but not with atropine-methonitrate, which blocks systemic muscarinic pathways, but does not cross the blood–brain barrier. This suggests that there is a (hypothetical) state generator in the fetal lamb, communicating with the source of electrocortical activity (perhaps beneath the parietal cortex) by a muscarinic central nervous pathway to cause desynchronization of activity. It also follows that its connection caudally, with the pons and medulla to inhibit fetal breathing episodically, is non-muscarinic. It would be interesting to know the nature of the putative neurotransmitter to the pons. An antagonist might have clinical application in blocking the potentially lethal effect of respiratory depression by hypoxia postnatally.

We should also consider the prostaglandin synthetase inhibitors (indomethacin, meclofenamate, and acetyl salicylate), which cause prolonged continuous deep fetal breathing, even during high-voltage electrocortical activity. The action can be reproduced by administration of small doses into the cerebrospinal fluid via a lateral ventricle, so must be due to direct central nervous system (CNS) action. Yet since this persists after dividing the afferent nerves from the systemic arterial chemoreceptors, or the brain stem (in the upper or lower pons; Koos 1985), it is likely to be attributable to a direct effect on the medulla or/and the spinal cord.

There is a third type of action, illustrated by the effect of small doses of pentobarbitone (5 mg/kg) given intravenously to a pregnant ewe. These cause a long episode of high-voltage electrocortical activity and arrest of fetal breathing movements (with no evident effect on the mother or changes in fetal blood gases). The arrest of fetal breathing was abolished by transection of the pons and is thus indirect (that is, by a suprapontine effect, perhaps on the state-generator).

In contrast morphine, infused intravenously to the fetus, has two effects, producing a shorter period of vigorous continuous breathing movements superimposed on a much longer period of respiratory depression or inhibition (Olsen and Dawes 1985). Bennet *et al.* (1986) have shown that on administration into a lateral cerebral ventricle these effects are dose related. These central actions have been separated by Hasan *et al.* (1989) who have shown that after transection of the brain stem in the upper pons the stimulation by morphine is abolished, but the long period of depression persists. Hence there are at least two sites of action, above and below the level of the transection.

Indeed, the same may be true of hypoxaemia in relation to electrocortical activity. In our first efforts at understanding the effect of isocapnic hypoxaemia on electrocortical activity we found that it caused a switch to high-voltage (Boddy *et al.* 1974; Clewlow *et al.* 1983), which thus might have contributed to the reduction in or arrest of breathing. Subsequent workers have not always confirmed these results. Comparison of the methods used did not explain the differences, and we began to wonder whether there were mixed effects which could lead to different conclusions by chance. In a more recent study there was a clear effect of hypoxia in enhancing high-voltage electrocortical activity in fetal lambs after section of the brain stem in the upper pons (Bamford and Dawes 1990). So there may be two sites of action, above the pons and elsewhere

There is an additional complication in designating the site of action of ethyl alcohol, which in small doses arrests fetal breathing movements, an effect which persists after transection of the brain stem, and is therefore elicited at or below the pons. Sometimes after these operations the whole brain stem down to the upper spinal cord (C1) was destroyed by haemorrhage; the intermittent diaphragmatic electromyographic (emg) activity which persisted was also arrested by ethyl alcohol (Bamford *et al.* 1984).

Hence in considering just this one variable, fetal breathing, multiple sites of CNS action must be considered in drug action alone; in, above, or below the brain stem; without or with the involvement of the (hypothetical) state-generator.

Other aspects of central control: the fetal heart-rate

To the clinician a principal method of determining fetal health has been visual analysis of the FHR. And although behavioural modulation of the FHR has been recognized for the past 10 years, it is surprising that not all the implications of this confounding factor have been considered (e.g. in the persistence of behavioural states in labour).

We still have comparatively few basic facts. Of course the FHR is modulated through the autonomic nervous system, though when that is blocked on both sides by propranolol and atropine, FHR variation is reduced by only about 60 per cent in sheep (Dalton *et al.* 1983). Some of the remaining variation is instrumental in origin, or due to fetal movements (especially when recording externally by ultrasound) and other factors, including changes in temperature, blood volume, and atrial pressure. The centrally determined accelerations, in association with fetal movements, are of indirect origin, since muscular paralysis does not abolish accelerations in sheep (Clewlow and Dawes 1985; Bocking *et al.* 1985). And we notice, with perhaps some surprise, that administration of an alpha-2 blocker acting centrally, such as clonidine, causes a gross decrease in FHR variation (Bamford *et al.* 1986). So we must reserve the possibility that changes, upwards or downwards, in FHR variables due to central factors, may be the consequences of pathophysiological processes that are not yet fully understood. How else can we explain the progressive decrease in short-term human FHR variation measured by computer to give warning of impending intrauterine death (Street *et al.* 1991) in chronic hypoxaemia or developing acidaemia, in growth retardation, and in maternal hypertension or pre-eclampsia? For in animal experiments (Dalton *et al.* 1977) hypoxaemia caused an increase in FHR variation, as we have also recorded during human labour (Pello *et al.* 1991). This increase is attributed to catecholamine release. We evidently need more information to understand even the simple FHR variables, which have been so important to clinical practice.

References

Bamford, O. S. and Dawes, G. S. (1990). The effects of hypoxia on electrocortical activity in the fetal lamb. *Journal of Developmental Physiology* **13**, 271–6.

Bamford, O. S., Dawes, G. S., Hofmeyr, G. J., Parkes, M. J., and Quail, A. W. (1984). Effects of maternally administered ethanol on fetal sheep. *Proceedings of the Society for the Study of Fetal Physiology*, p. 13.

Bamford, O. S., Dawes, G. S., and Ward, R. A. (1985). A possible dopaminergic pathway stimulating breathing in fetal lambs. *Journal of Physiology* **365**, 271–6.

Bamford, O. S., Dawes, G. S., Danny, R., and Ward, R. A. (1986). Effects of the alpha$_2$-adrenergic agonist clonidine and its antagonist idazoxa on the fetal lamb. *Journal of Physiology* **381**, 29–37.

Barcroft, Sir J. (1946). *Researches on pre-natal life* Blackwell Scientific Publications, Oxford.

Bennet, L. Johnston, B. M., and Gluckmann, P. D. (1986). The central effects of morphine on fetal breathing movements in the fetal sheep. *Journal of Developmental Physiology* **8**, 297–305.

Bocking, A. D., Harding, R., and Wickham, P. J. D. (1985). Relationships between accelerations and decelerations in heart rate and skeletal muscle activity in fetal sheep. *Journal of Developmental Physiology* **7**, 47–54.

Boddy, K., Dawes, G. S., Fisher, R., Pinter, S., and Robinson, J. S. (1974). Foetal respiratory movements, electrocortical and cardiovascular responses to hypox-aemia in sheep. *Journal of Physiology* **243**, 599–618.

Clewlow, F. and Dawes, G. S. (1985). The association between cardiac accelerations and movements in fetal sheep. *Journal of Developmental Physiology* **7**, 281–7.

Clewlow, F., Dawes, G. S., Johnston, B. M., and Walker, D. W. (1983). Changes in breathing, electrocortical and muscle activity in unanaesthetized fetal lambs with age. *Journal of Physiology* **341**, 463–76.

Coles, S. K., Kumar, P., and Noble, R, (1989). Pontine sites inhibiting breathing in anaesthetized neonatal lambs. *Journal of Physiology* **409**, 66p.

Cross, K. W. and Warmer, P. (1951). The effect of inhalation of high and low oxygen concentrations on the respiration of the newborn infant. *Journal of Physiology* **114**, 238–95.

Cross, K. W. and Oppé, T. E. (1952). The effect of inhalation of high and low concentrations of oxygen on the respiration of the premature infant. *Journal of Physiology* **117**, 38–55.

Dalton, K. J., Dawes, G. S., and Patrick, J. E. (1977). Diurnal, respiratory and other rhythms of fetal heart rate in lambs. *American Journal of Obstetrics and Gynecology* **127**, 414–24.

Dalton, K. J., Dawes, G. S., and Patrick, J. E. (1983). The autonomic nervous system and fetal heart rate variability. *American Journal of Obstetrics and Gyne-cology* **146**, 456–62.

Dawes, G. S. (1986). The central nervous control of fetal behaviour. *European Journal of Obstetrics and Gynecology and Reproductive Biology* **21**, 341–6.

Dawes, G. S., Gardner, W. N., Johnston, B. M., and Walker, D. W. (1983). Breathing in fetal lambs: the effect of brain stem transection. *Journal of Physiology* **335**, 535–53.

Gluckmann, P. D. and Johnston, B. M. (1987). Lesions in the upper lateral pons abolish the hypoxic depression of breathing in unanaesthetized fetal lambs *in utero*. *Journal of Physiology* **283**, 373–83.

Hasan, S. V., Bamford, Q., Hawkins, R., Gibson, D. A., Nowaczyk, B., Cates, D., and Rigatto, H. (1989). The effect of midbrain section on the breathing response to morphine in the fetal sheep. *Proceedings of the Society for the Study of Fetal Physiology* G9.

Jensen, A., Bamford, O. S., Dawes, G. S., Hofmeyr, G. J., and Parkes, M. J. (1986). Changes in organ blood flow between high and low voltage electrocorti-cal activity in fetal lambs. *Journal of Developmental Physiology* **8**, 187–94.

Johnston, B. M. and Gluckmann, P. D. (1989). Lateral pontine lesions affect central chemosensitivity in unanaesthetized fetal lambs. *Journal of Applied Physiology* **67**, 1113–18.

Koos, B. J. (1985). Central stimulation of breathing movements in fetal lambs by prostaglandin synthetase inhibitors. *Journal of Physiology* **362**, 455–66.

Martin-Body, R. L. (1988). Brain transections demonstrate the central origin of hypoxic ventilatory depression in carotid body-denervated rats. *Journal of Physiology* **407**, 41–52.

Martin-Body, R. L. and Johnston, B. M. (1988). Central origin of the hypoxic depression of breathing in the newborn. *Respiratory Physiology* **71**, 25–32.

Moore, P. J., Hanson, M. A., and Parkes, M. J. (1989). Almitrine inhibits breath-ing movements in fetal sheep *in utero*. *Journal of Developmental Physiology* **11**, 277–81.

Nijhuis, J. G., Martin, C. B., and Prechtl, H. F. R. (1984). Behavioural states of the human fetus. In: Continuity of neural functions from prenatal to postnatal life. *Clinics in Developmental Medicine* (ed. H. F. R. Prechtl) **94**, 65–78.

Noble, R. and Williams, B. A. (1989). Excitation of neurones in the rostral pons during hypoxia in anaesthetized neonatal lambs. *Journal of Physiology* **417**, 146P.

Noble, R. Williams, B. A., Hanson, A., and Smith, J. A. (1990). Transient intense carotid chemoreceptors stimulation does not affect discharge of rostral pontine neurones found to be excited in anaesthetized newborn lambs. *Journal of Physiology*, **429**, 81P.

Olsen, G. D. and Dawes, G. S. (1985). Morphine-induced depression and stimulation of breathing movements in the fetal lamb. In: *The Physiological development of the fetus and newborn* (ed. C. T. Jones and P. W. Nathanielsz), pp. 633–8. Academic Press, London.

Parkes, M. J., Bamford, O. S., Dawes, G. S., Hofmeyer, G. J., Gianopoulos, J. C., and Quail, A. W. (1984). The effects of removal of the cerebellum and brainstem lesions in fetal lambs. *Proceedings of the Society for the Study of Fetal Physiology*. p.8.

Parkes, M. J., Moore, P. J., Noble, R., and Hanson, M. A. (1990). Reversible blockade of the secondary fall of ventilation during hypoxia in newborn sheep. *Proceedings of the Society for the Study of Fetal Physiology* **11**, 4.

Pello, L. C., Rosevear, S. K., Dawes, G. S., Moulden, M., and Predman, G. W. G. (1991). Computerized fetal heart rate analysis in labor. *Obstetrics and Gynecology* **78**, 602–10.

Richardson, B. S., Patrick, J. E., and Abdulljabbar, H. (1985). Cerebral oxidative metabolism in the fetal lamb: relationship to electrocortical state. *American Journal of Obstetrics and Gynecology* **153**, 426–31.

Slotten, P., Phermetton, T. M., and Rankin, J. H. G. (1989). Relationship between fetal electrocorticographic changes and umbilical blood flow in the near-term sheep fetus. *Journal of Developmental Physiology* **11**, 19–23.

Street, P., Dawes, G. S., Moulden, M. and Redman, C. W. G. (1991). Short term variation in abnormal antenatal fetal heart rate records. *American Journal of Obstetrics and Gynecology*, **165**, 515–23.

Van der Wildt, B. (1982). Heart rate, breathing movements and brain activity in fetal lambs. Doctoral Thesis, University of Nijmegen.

9
Animal investigations
P. J. MOORE and M. A. HANSON

Introduction

Any investigation of fetal behaviour tends to be based on a desire to determine whether a particular individual is healthy, acutely distressed, or bearing some chronic abnormality or dysfunction. Clinically, attempts have been made to use the gross behaviour of a fetus to assess its condition during the last few weeks of pregnancy. In particular it is hoped that this approach will indicate the condition of the processes underlying that behaviour, namely those of the central nervous system (CNS). Patterns of physical activity would thus be of particular value if they could reflect the development and health of the CNS. However, to ascertain a link between CNS activity and gross behaviour is difficult.

Observations conducted on the human fetus are restricted to those variables that are available for non-invasive measurement. These variables are recorded by an observer and placed into categories, according to recurrent coincidence of behaviour patterns. These categories are called 'behavioural states' and are deemed to be similar in concept to 'states of consciousness' in adults. However to make sense of these groupings much data is required. Measurements must be made in both undisturbed and disturbed situations to determine not only the coincidence of behaviour and CNS activity, but also to see how this relationship is affected by distress or disability.

Such investigation has been hindered by the physical inaccessibility of the fetus. To make progress we need to be able to make continuous recordings of fetal activity for many days, and to include within our protocol the direct recording of the activity of specific parts of the fetal brain. As it is not possible to make prolonged recordings in the human, much less make direct recordings of neuronal activity, and it is not permissible to disturb the fetus deliberately in such a way as to cause disability or distress, we must necessarily approach this investigation using an animal model.

In moving to an animal model, we have a number of distinct advantages combined with a few very important disadvantages. Chronically implanting recording devices on to fetuses allows prolonged recordings that are not influenced by the presence of anaesthetic or other drugs which may modify behaviour. The electrical activity of muscles, and the massed activity of individual nerves or the electrocorticogram (ECoG), can be recorded along with variables such as blood flow through a particular artery or organ, gross movement of one part of the body relative to another, and the vast array of biochemical variables that can be monitored in blood samples. Such recordings benefit from being relatively free of the problems of subjectivity introduced by the more remote forms of observation employed in clinical measurements. Because they are recorded continuously and simultaneously for many days at a time, the patterns of coincidence can be determined and established, and correlated with various measures of fetal health.

Against these advantages it must not be forgotten that there are great differences in the development of behaviour between species, for example, the different effects of sounds on the FHR between human and sheep fetuses (Parkes *et al.* 1991). However, to understand the ontology of behaviour in any one species would be an important scientific advance in itself. Only then can considerations of comparability be made.

Much time and effort has been devoted to establishing the existence of different behavioural states in fetuses. Before looking at the importance of this approach let us look at the underlying philosophy. It is not sufficient to look for states that merely appear to show similarities with postnatal behaviour, as behaviour is essentially governed by functional requirements. A fetus exists in an environment that is crucially different from that to which it will be exposed postnatally. It has no need to search for food or escape predation, and gaseous exchange is dependent upon its mother's respiratory and circulatory systems. *A priori*, there is no reason to assume that the fetus requires behavioural states at all. Furthermore, to use terms like fetal 'sleep states' to describe fetal behaviour patterns, sadly precludes any discussion about whether or not a fetus is ever awake or asleep—a problem that is far from being resolved (Parkes 1991). Also, it must not be assumed that a change in physical activity denotes a change in state; an adult may, at will, sit without moving for many hours and then decide to stand up, all of which has been performed whilst being 'awake'. Moreover, different states may easily share behavioural attributes (e.g. postnatally limb movement can occur in both sleep and wakefulness). Thus to define transitions between states simply by reference to the commencement or cessation of a particular pattern of physical activity is very limited.

So what do we need to know to be convinced of the presence of a state? Ideally one needs to determine the response of a fetus to external stimuli. This requires a stimulus–response relationship that is strongly 'state-related'. If we can only observe the fetus, then great care must be taken in choosing the number and type of variables observed. If one can observe only one variable and must decide whether it is present or absent, then fetal behaviour can be divided into only 2^1, (i.e. two) categories; if two such variables are observed simultaneously, and each is totally independent of the other, then there are 2^2 (i.e. four) possible combinations to choose from; three independent variables gives eight possible combinations, and so on. Thus to allocate a fetus into one of four possible 'states' with any hope of accuracy requires observation of at least three independent variables at any one time. Fewer than this would provoke criticism that the fetus has to be in one of the four categories. The groupings could then be entered arbitrarily, without implying any organization underlying the concurrence.

The requirement for variables to be independent must be stressed if they are to be used as separate determinants of behaviour and not merely as behavioural concomitants. One can not, for example, employ tracheal pressure changes and diaphragm activity as separate variables. Similarly, caution is needed before using certain movements with variables of fetal heart-rate (FHR), as the former may influence the latter (Dawes *et al.* 1981; Patrick *et al.* 1984). Indeed, it is difficult to find many variables that can be claimed confidently as independent. Figure 9.1 lists the variables commonly monitored, indicating those that are likely to influence each other. If two variables that can be measured clinically are required, then any pair not shown to influence each other would be suitable, for example,

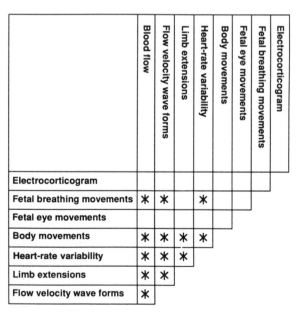

	Blood flow	Flow velocity wave forms	Limb extensions	Heart-rate variability	Body movements	Fetal eye movements	Fetal breathing movements	Electrocorticogram
Electrocorticogram								
Fetal breathing movements	✶	✶		✶				
Fetal eye movements								
Body movements	✶	✶	✶	✶				
Heart-rate variability	✶	✶	✶					
Limb extensions	✶	✶						
Flow velocity wave forms	✶							

Fig. 9.1. Listing of variables commonly used for the description of fetal behaviour, indicating those that are likely to influence each other.

FHR and fetal eye movements (FEM). To find three such variables is more difficult, but at first sight FEM, fetal breathing movements (FBM), and body movements, would be a permissible choice. It is interesting to note that presence or absence of FBM occur in all of the current definitions of human fetal states. FBM has therefore been assigned the status of a state concomitant, and is not a state variable. In animal experiments the choice is increased by the inclusion of the ECoG.

To supplement the paucity of truly independent variables, weight is sometimes placed upon the coincidence of change in activity. But how tight do these boundaries between states need to be, as it is unusual to see a number of activities change at exactly the same time? Such an appraisal of activity does not allow for two consecutive states sharing a common feature. Furthermore, if disturbed, a fetus may only gradually return to a normal pattern of behaviour with variables regrouping over an extended period. In that case it would be difficult to assign the fetus to a state, as no 'switch' has occurred. As behavioural observations are often made to establish the time taken for a fetus to recover from a given procedure, this is more than an academic problem.

Another necessary consideration is the required duration of coincidence of specific activity of independent variables for differentiation between a stable state and a merely arbitrary and transient incident.

With these considerations in mind it is not surprising that the only animals in which reasonably extensive studies of behavioural states have been performed are the rhesus monkey (Martin *et al.* 1974), baboon (Myers *et al.* 1990), and sheep. Whilst the fetuses of other species have been successfully studied for other purposes, their size or susceptibility to chronic instrumentation has made them unsuitable for recording multiple variables for a prolonged time without the use of anaesthetics. In the case of the rhesus monkey, Martin *et al.* (1974) have proposed the existence of two states, based on observations of FHR, FBM, and FEM. There is little other data available for the rhesus monkey, and the variables of FHR and FBM may not be completely independent. In the sheep, much data exists for multiple, concurrently recorded variables which have been taken at least four days after any operative procedure. It is therefore worth considering whether or not states exist in the sheep.

Knowledge of fetal behaviour in late gestation in the sheep—is it appropriate to group this behaviour into states?

Through the placement of catheters, electrodes, and other specialized transducers onto the sheep fetus, an extensive picture of fetal behaviour has been established.

ECoG

The ECoG is measured by placing electrodes bilaterally on the parietal
dura and recording differential activity in relation to an indifferent electrode
placed elsewhere on the fetal body. The recordings have classically been
divided into two categories, one characterized by low-voltage, high-
frequency waveforms (usually termed LV), and the other by high-voltage,
low-frequency waveforms (termed HV) (Dawes *et al.* 1972). Ruckebusch *et
al.* (1977) describe a third pattern, similar to LV, but with an increased
amplitude. Because of other concurrent activity of the fetus they were bold
enough to suggest that during these times the fetus was awake. However
other studies have failed to find evidence for wakefulness (Parkes 1991).
McNerney and Szeto (1990) have suggested an approach for dividing
ECoG activity into four separate conditions, the two categories additional
to LV and HV being intermediate in character between them and being
inherently unstable in nature (i.e. short-lived). The short time span of their
duration must bring into question whether these can indeed be termed
states, or are just transient incidents in activity, as discussed above. Even
in the sheep, differentiation of ECoG patterns occurs only relatively late
(after about 119 days) in gestation. After this time HV or LV activity are
strongly associated with different fetal behaviour. Does this mean that
states do not exist before this time, or does it merely highlight our lack of
methods for measuring them?

Of all the currently recorded variables ECoG is possibly the most con-
fused and confusing. Little is known of its origin and even less of its
function, if any. However, owing to the association of several features of
fetal behaviour with either HV or LV activity it is easy to slip into the
assumption that ECoG activity actually determines fetal behaviour and
thus state, as opposed to being merely one aspect of behaviour. In fact the
association between ECoG and other aspects of behaviour is not rigid and
it can be disturbed with relative ease, for example by giving atropine or
hyoscine, which dissociates ECoG activity from fetal behaviour (Dawes
1986). Thus, it would appear that the ECoG and other behaviour are
independently influenced by a separate 'state-generator'. It is for this reason
that no coincidence markers have been placed against ECoG in Fig. 9.1.

Fetal breathing movements

In the fetal sheep, FBM are measured by placing a bipolar electrode on
the diaphragm and by monitoring pressure changes in the trachea via an
implanted catheter.

They first occur at about 40 days of gestation, becoming virtually continuous at 95 to 115 days. After this they assume an episodic pattern with

the periods of rapid movements being associated with LV ECoG (Dawes 1984). FBM may be influenced pharmacologically or by acutely altering the fetal PaO_2.

As FBM are episodic in late gestation, their presence or absence could be useful as a monitor of fetal behaviour, or possibly even of well-being. However the use of FBM in this way is associated with problems. FBM adjust to changes in fetal condition or environment very rapidly. For instance, in prolonged hypoxia FBM return to a 'normal' pattern after 4 or 5 hours (Koos *et al.* 1988), and after almitrine, a drug which stimulates respiration for 24 hours or more in adults, and like hypoxia inhibits FBM, FBM return to a 'normal' pattern after only 4 or 5 hours (Moore *et al.* 1989). Whether this means that the fetus has successfully adapted to its new *milieu interieur* adequately and hence normal behaviour patterns have returned, or whether it means that fetal behaviour occurs irrespective of fetal condition, is yet to be resolved. Clearly some care is required in interpreting such data.

Eye movements

In fetal sheep FEM are monitored by placing one electrode on the upper eyelid and one beneath the lower eyelid. Differential recordings are made from the electrodes with reference to an indifferent electrode placed elsewhere on the fetus.

Rapid movements of the eyeball occur in an episodic pattern, concomitantly with both LV ECoG and with FBM (Dawes *et al.* 1972). As these movements occur in grouped episodes, they may thus be indicators of a particular pattern of behaviour. These eye movements have many of the characteristics of the movements that occur in rapid eye movement (REM) sleep, and they occur concomitantly with a LV pattern of ECoG, which is also characteristic of REM sleep in the adult; there has, therefore, been a tendency to refer to this activity as fetal REM sleep. Whilst this is a convenient term, its extensive use is unfortunate as it pre-empts any discussion about the existence of sleep in the fetus.

Body and limb movements

Prior to 115 days of gestation, forelimb movements and nuchal muscle contraction occur randomly. As gestation progresses these movements become grouped into episodes, which are correlated with LV ECoG activity. Again their episodic nature suggests that their presence or absence may be used within a description of fetal activity.

It is easy to view these movements as prenatal equivalents of movements that occur postnatally, yet this approach has pitfalls. Postnatally, phasic movements are often superimposed on posture, and even human neonates show placing and stepping reflexes that have an important postural element. However, the available evidence suggests that the CNS elements of postural control may operate rather differently in the fetus than in the neonate. Obviously, in late gestation the range of postures available to the fetus is limited, even though activity of neck or limb extensor muscles, and movements of the trunk, are associated with posture. But the most striking example of the difference comes from the effects of decerebration pre- or postnatally; in the neonate this produces greatly enhanced tone in postural extensor muscles (decerebrate rigidity), whereas in the fetus no such increased tone occurs (Dawes *et al.* 1983). Clearly much more needs to be known about the development of reflex control at spinal and supraspinal levels. A start was made by Rigatto *et al.* (1983) who showed that the magnitude of lumbar polysynaptic flexor reflexes is enhanced during times when the fetus is also in HV ECoG. The gain of the reflex is also much reduced in intensity by hypoxia as are all body movements (Dawes 1984).

Fetal heart-rate variability

Heart-rate variability is episodic in nature and many workers now envisage that different patterns of FHR variability are synonymous with different fetal states. Sadly there is little known about FHR variations in animals. Dalton *et al.* (1977) monitored FHR variations in 28 fetal sheep and showed that variation in it occurred. Periods of high variability were associated with either body movements or FBM. Of importance to the present discussion is that they reported no difference in FHR variations between times in which the fetus was in HV or in LV ECoG when FBM were absent. The only differences found were attributed not to the ECoG state itself, but to the FBM that were occurring during LV.

Prolonged loss of variability in FHR traces is now recognized as a sign of serious fetal distress. This is often said to be due to fetal hypoxia. However Dalton *et al.* (1977) and Bocking *et al.* (1986) investigated this and found that FHR variability in sheep increased, rather than decreased, during acute hypoxia. A subsequent paper showed that FHR patterns return to normal after 24 hours in chronic hypoxia (Bocking *et al.* 1989). Therefore in the sheep it would appear that FHR is not a good indicator of hypoxaemia, and its role in determining fetal state is yet to be confirmed.

Blood flow

Blood flow to the brain can be measured most accurately using radio-labelled microspheres. This technique has shown that regional cerebral blood flow is not constant. The episodes of highest flow are concurrent with increased cerebral oxidative metabolism and also with LV ECoG. The link between blood flow, oxygen delivery, and the metabolic demands of brain tissue, is consistent with the idea that LV ECoG occurs during greater neuronal activity (Richardson *et al*. 1989).

Blood flow to other organs of the body seems to be more constant, and there is no consistent pattern of flow changes concomitant with other potential indicators of fetal state, for example there are no differences in organ blood flows between times occupied by HV and LV ECoG activity (Jansen *et al*. 1989).

Circadian rhythm

It must not be forgotten that any of the above variables may be influenced by a diurnal rhythm. This could variously be described as something imposed on an underlying pattern of fetal behaviour, or as a facet of fetal behaviour *per se*.

There has been a considerable amount of work done to try to establish the nature of the cue that transmits the circadian clock to the fetus. Much of the work has centred around FBM, which are reported to have a diurnal variation, to see if a hormonal influence from the mother can be established. The prostaglandins have a diurnal fluctuation in concentration, and if their synthesis is inhibited, prolonged FBM occur. These movements persist through times in which HV ECoG is occurring (Koos 1985). Prostaglandins would appear to be likely candidates for the transmission of a signal to the fetus, but Callea *et al*. (1990) showed that if the feeding regimen was disturbed so as to alter the diurnal fluctuation in prostaglandin concentration, FBM were not affected. By the same experiments these workers also showed that fluctuations in the concentrations of glucose caused by maternal feeding did affect FBM.

Another hormone with a diurnal variation in its concentration is prolactin. N. S. Bassett *et al*. (1989) showed that changes in maternal nutrition could effect fetal prolactin levels, and fetal and maternal prolactin levels are also affected by the time of year (Serón-Ferré *et al*. 1989). So if prolactin is important in determining fetal behaviour patterns, the feeding regimen of the mother would need to be considered. That the diurnal rhythm is derived from the mother was shown by McMillen *et al*. (1990) who demonstrated that pinealectomy abolished fetal circadian rhythm in plasma prolactin concentration.

Melatonin has a circadian and a seasonal rhythm, and it is implicated in the reproductive development, and circadian and seasonal activity in many animals, including the sheep. Its release increases during periods of darkness, and is diminished when the mother is exposed to light. This rhythm is present in both mother and fetus, and can be abolished by maternal pinealectomy (Yellon and Longo 1988). Furthermore fetal plasma prolactin is reduced on maternal administration of melatonin, giving evidence that melatonin acts as a transmitter of photoperiodic information to the fetus (J. Bassett *et al.* 1989).

Emphasizing the need for caution in determining causal links, Dalton *et al.* (1977) report diurnal rhythm in FHR. However this seems to be due to the influence of FBM and body movement on FHR, and is not a unique circadian rhythm.

Thus activity cycles with a 24-hour time-period are present in many variables. The underlying mechanisms of transmission of this 'clock' to the fetus are not totally understood. Until the mechanism is established, any analysis of fetal behaviour in sheep that does not take account of the time of day, or even of year, should be interpreted with care.

Effects of disturbance of 'state'

Thus all the above variables follow an episodic pattern of behaviour (i.e. they are present only some of the time). However, this does not allow us to distinguish whether these are states of consciousness or just activity cycles, much in the same way as adult activity cycles through the day do not necessarily indicate a change in state of consciousness. In order to address this, experiments that involve applying a stimulus to the fetus have been employed to see if the response is different if the stimulus is applied during different 'states'.

Parkes *et al.* (1990) applied sound to the maternal flank in sheep and caused the fetal ECoG state to change from HV to LV. This response was abolished by ablation of the cochlea, showing it to be a vibro-acoustic rather than a vibro-tactile stimulus. This stimulus also tended to cause increased FBM and FEM activity, supporting the concept that a change in activity, and possibly in state, had been caused. As the change was from HV to LV, but never from LV to HV, and as LV is associated with greater fetal activity, the response is consistent with the notion that vibro-acoustic stimulation arouses the fetus. However, as this stimulus caused a change in apparent state (HV to LV) it is not possible to compare and contrast the effect of the stimulus on fetuses in LV and in HV, as applying the stimulus in LV clearly did not produce an effect. We are therefore left in the dark as to whether or not the fetal sheep can detect a vibro-acoustic stimulus in LV. It is interesting to note that in these experiments there was no change in FHR on application of the stimulus. This is in marked contrast with the effect reported in the human fetus (Jensen 1984; Johansson *et al.* 1979).

Thus to show that a stimulus has a different effect in different states requires that the stimulus does not itself cause a change in state. This has possibly been best shown by Rigatto *et al.* (1983) who, as already mentioned, applied electrical stimulation to the hind limb of fetal sheep. They found that the reflex response to the stimulus was enhanced during HV ECoG.

Attempts to disturb the system pharmacologically have had little more success in clarifying the situation. The main conclusion that can be drawn from such studies is that the variables are controlled separately and that their activity can be isolated from each other with relative ease. For example, almitrine causes a decrease in FBM for 4 to 12 hours but affects ECoG for only 1 to 2 hours. Atropine causes a prolonged episode of HV ECoG, but FBM are unaffected and continue to be episodic (Moore *et al.* 1989). L-5-hydroxytryptophan causes the fetus to assume HV ECoG and prolonged FBM (Fletcher *et al.* 1988). Ethanol induces HV ECoG, and abolishes FBM and FEM. However, the reduction in FBM lasts for 8 hours, but ECoG and FEM are affected for only 3 hours (Smith *et al.* 1989*a*). Furthermore, if indomethacin is given after ethanol, the suppression of FBM is removed and, indeed, replaced with stimulation for 18 hours, but the ethanol-induced inhibition of LV and FEM activity is not affected (Smith *et al.* 1989*b*).

The list could be continued, but to date there is no drug that can be used to clearly indicate either the presence or absence of behavioural states. None of the drugs have a coherent action on a group of variables that would enable one to say with any confidence that the fetus had either changed state or modulated its response to the drug according to the state in which the drug was given.

Conclusion

In 1974 when the concept of behavioural states was established, Prechtl (1974) defined states as 'any well-defined conditions or properties that can be recognised if they occur again'. Within the fetal sheep it is clear that there are conditions that can be defined as occurring repeatedly (e.g. FBM with LV ECoG and FEM). What has not, however, been determined is whether these are indeed 'states' with any functional significance, or are simply cycles of activity, which may be controlled by the CNS (may even be 'programmed'), but which do not correspond to the behavioural states that occur postnatally. Caution is needed in thinking of fetal behavioural states occurring in any species in view of the lack of a clear demonstration to date of their existence in the sheep fetus. But this merely stresses the need for further work. After all, absence of evidence is not in itself evidence of absence.

References

Bassett, J. M., Curtis, N., Hanson, C., and Weeding, C. M. (1989). Effects of altered photoperiod or maternal melatonin administration on plasma prolactin concentration in fetal lambs. *Journal of Endocrinology* **122**, 633–43.

Bassett, N. S., Bennet, L., Ball, K. T., and Gluckmann, P. D. (1989). Presence of a diurnal rhythm in fetal prolactin secretion and influence of maternal nutrition. *Biology of the Neonate* **55**, 164–70

Bocking, A. D., Harding, R., and Wickham, J. D. (1986). Effects of reduced uterine blood flow on accelerations and decelerations in heart rate of fetal sheep. *American Journal of Obstetrics and Gynecology* **154**, 329–35.

Bocking, A. D., White, S., Gagnon, R., and Hansford, H. (1989). Effects of prolonged hypoxia on fetal heart rate accelerations and decelerations in sheep. *American Journal of Obstetrics and Gynecology* **161**, 722–7.

Callea, J., McMillen, I. C., and Walker, D. W. (1990). Effect of feeding regime on diurnal variation of breathing movements in late-gestation fetal sheep. *Journal of Applied Physiology* **68**, 1786–92.

Dalton, K. J., Dawes, G. S., and Patrick, J. E. (1977). Diurnal respiratory and other rhythms of fetal lambs. *American Journal of Obstetrics and Gynecology* **127**, 414–24.

Dawes, G. S. (1984). The central control of fetal breathing movements and skeletal muscle movements. *Journal of Physiology* **346**, 1–18.

Dawes, G. S. (1986) The central nervous control of fetal behaviour. *European Journal of Obstetrics and Gynecology and Reproductive Biology* **21**, 341–6.

Dawes, G. S., Fox, H. E., Leduc, B. M., Liggins, G. C., and Richards, R. T. (1972). Respiratory movements and REM sleep in the fetal lamb. *Journal of Physiology* **220**, 119–43.

Dawes, G. S., Visser, G. H. A., Goodman J. D. S., and Levine, D. H. (1981). Numerical analysis of the human fetal heart rate: modulation by breathing and movement. *American Journal of Obstetrics and Gynecology* **140**, 525–44.

Dawes, G. S., Gardner, W. G., Johnston, B. M., and Walker, D. W. (1983). Breathing in fetal lambs: effects of brain stem section. *Journal of Physiology* **335**, 535–53.

Fletcher, D. J., Hanson, M. A., Moore, P. J., Nijhuis, J. G., and Parkes, M. J. (1988). Stimulation of breathing movements by L-5-hydroxytryptophan in fetal sheep during normoxia and hypoxia. *Journal of Physiology* **404**, 575–89.

Jansen, A. H., Belik, J., Ioffe, S., and Chernick, V. (1989). Control of organ blood flow in fetal sheep during normoxia and hypoxia. *American Journal of Physiology* **257**, 1132–9.

Jensen, O. H. (1984). Fetal heart rate response to controlled sound stimuli during the third trimester of normal pregnancy. *Acta Obstetrica Gynaecologica Scandinavcia* **63**, 193.

Johansson, B., Wedenberg, E., and Westin, B. (1979). Measurements of tone response by the human fetus. A preliminary report. *Acta Otolaryngologica* **57**, 188.

Koos, B. J. (1985). Central stimulation of breathing movements in fetal lambs by prostaglandin synthetase inhibitors. *Journal of Physiology* **362**, 455–66.

Koos, B. J., Kitanaka, T., Gilbert, R. D., and Longo, L. D. (1988). Fetal breathing adaptation to prolonged hypoxaemia in sheep. *Journal of Developmental Physiology* **10**, 161–6.

Martin, C. B., Murata, Y., Petrie, R. H., and Parer, J. T. (1974). Respiratory movements in fetal rhesus monkeys. *American Journal of Obstetrics and Gynecology* **119**, 939–48.

McMillen, I. C., Nowak, R., Walker, D. W., and Young, I. R. (1990). Maternal pinealectomy alters the daily pattern of fetal breathing in sheep. *American Journal of Physiology* **258**, R284–7.

McNerney M. E. and Szeto H. H. (1990). Automated identification and quantification of four patterns of electrocortical activity in the near-term fetal lamb. *Pediatric Research* **28**, 106–10.

Moore, P. J., Hanson, M. A., and Parkes, M. J. (1989). Almitrine inhibits breathing movements in fetal sheep *in utero*. *Journal of Developmental Physiology* **11**, 277–81.

Myers, M. M., Fifer, W., Haiken, J., and Stark, R. I. (1990). Relationships between breathing activity and heart rate in fetal baboons. *American Journal of Physiology* **258**, R1479–85.

Parkes, M. J. (1991). Sleep and wakefulness—do they occur *in utero*? In: *Fetal and neonatal brain stem* (ed. M. A. Hanson), pp. 230–57. **164**, 1336–43. Cambridge University Press, Cambridge.

Parkes, M. J., Moore, P. J., Moore, D. R., Fisk, N. M., and Hanson, M. A. (1991). Behavioural changes in fetal sheep caused by vibro-acoustic stimulation; the effects of cochlear ablation. *American Journal of Obstetrics and Gynecology* **164**, 1336–43.

Patrick, J., Carmichael, L., Chess, L., and Staples, C. (1984). Accelerations of the human fetal heart rate at 38–40 weeks gestational age. *American Journal of Obstetrics and Gynecology* **148**, 35–41.

Prechtl, H. F. R. (1974). The behavioural states of the newborn infant. *Brain Research* **5**, 477–93.

Richardson B. S., Carmichael, L., Homan, J., and Gagnon, R. (1989). Cerebral oxidative metabolism in lambs during the perinatal period: relationship to electrocortical state. *American Journal of Physiology* **257**, R1251–7.

Rigatto, H., Blanco, C. E., and Walker, A. M. (1983). The response to stimulation of hind-limb nerves in fetal lambs, *in utero*, during the different phases of electrocortical activity. *Journal of Developmental Physiology* **3**, 175–85.

Ruckebusch, Y., Ganjox, M., and Eghbali, B. (1977). Sleep cycles and kinesis in the foetal lamb. *Electroencephalographic Clinical Neurophysiology* **42**, 226–37.

Serón-Ferré, M., Vergara, M., Parraguez, V. H., Riquelme, R., and Llanos, A. J. (1989). The circadian variation of prolactin in fetal sheep is affected by the seasons. *Endocrinology* **125**, 1613–16.

Smith, G. N., Brien, J. F., Carmichael, L., Homan, J., Clarke D. W., and Patrick, J. (1989*a*). Development of tolerance to ethanol-induced suppression of breathing movements and brain activity in the near-term fetal sheep. *Journal of Developmental Physiology* **11**, 189–97.

Smith, G. N., Brien, J. F., Homan, J., Carmichael, L., and Patrick. J. (1989). Indomethacin antagonizes the ethanol-induced suppression of breathing activity but not the suppression of brain activity in the near-term fetal sheep. *Journal of Developmental Physiology* **12**, 69–75.

Yellon, S. M. and Longo, L. D. (1988). Effect of maternal pinealectomy and reverse photoperiod on the circadian melatonin rhythm in the sheep and fetus during the last trimester of pregnancy. *Biology of Reproduction* **39**, 1093–9.

10
Effects of perinatal medication on the developing brain

M. MIRMIRAN and D. F. SWAAB

During the third trimester of pregnancy the brain of the fetus is able to display complex neurobehavioural functions. At the same time this rapidly developing brain is very susceptible to chemicals used by the mother. In addition to self-medication, there is widespread (80 per cent) drug administration to pregnant and lactating women for the treatment of, for example, hypertension, epilepsy, depression, and premature labour (Eskes *et al*. 1983). Disturbances caused by such chemicals used during the third trimester are not usually of a grossly physical nature, but are based upon permanent microscopic and biochemical alterations in the formation of neurones, their migration, formation of neurites, synapses, transmitters, receptors, and behavioural states. The effect of functional deficits induced in the child in this way is called behavioural teratogenicity, or rather functional neuroteratology, since neuroendocrine systems or temperature regulation, for example, may be affected. This topic has recently received much attention and its potentiality has been reviewed in a volume of the series of *Progress in Brain Research* (Boer *et al*. 1988). The intention of this chapter is to update our knowledge of the subtle changes induced in the developing brain of the unborn child by drugs used during the last trimester of gestation. We limit ourselves to the sequelae of a number of drugs, and for further reading on this topic we refer to earlier reviews (Benesova 1989; Eskes and Finster 1983; Hutchings 1978; Mirmiran and De Boer 1988; Mirmiran and Swaab 1987; Riley and Vorhees 1986; Swaab and Mirmiran 1984, 1988; Swaab *et al*. 1988; Yanai 1984). We want especially to point out the sensitivity of man to the hazards of medicines and to put forward the hypothesis that neurotransmitter, neuroendocrine, and behavioural state changes in response to drugs may indeed mediate the occurrence of a macroscopically normal but functionally handicapped brain.

Effects of drugs on brain neurotransmitters

Monoamines (i.e. noradrenaline (NA), serotonin (5HT), and dopamine

(DA)) are among the best-studied brain neurotransmitters. Rats, the experimental animal model generally used for behavioural teratology experiments, are very immature when born. For example, the cerebral cortex of a newborn rat is comparable to that of a 7-month-old human fetal brain (Dobbing and Sands 1979), although this might not always be a good comparison (see later). In the rat, which has a gestational period of about 21 days, NA, DA, and 5HT neurones are already born and functionally responsive to pharmacological manipulations by day 15 of gestation (Lauder and Bloom 1974; Mirmiran 1986; Mirmiran *et al*. 1988). An early appearance of monoamines has been shown by mid-term in the human fetus (Hyppä 1972; Masudi and Gilmore 1983; Nobin and Björklund 1973; Olson *et al*. 1973; Pearson 1983; Pearson *et al*. 1980). A similar early development of neurotransmitters in fetal human brain has been shown for other neurotransmitters: e.g. acetylcholine, by as early as 18 weeks of gestation (Brooksbank *et al*. 1978; Schlumpf and Lichtensteiger 1987); amino acids as early as mid-gestation (Brooksbank *et al*. 1981; Repressa *et al*. 1989); and a variety of peptides before mid-gestation (Aubert 1979; Bloch *et al*. 1978; Bugnon *et al*. 1977; Paulin *et al*. 1986; Siler-Khodr and Khodr 1978; Winters *et al*. 1974). However, there are two factors to bear in mind. First there are considerable regional differences in the developmental time of each given neurotransmitter in the brain. Secondly, although in a particular period of development an excess of a neurotransmitter may be trophic for the maturation of a certain brain area, in an earlier period it may be insensitive, or in a later period toxic, to the maturation or survival of the neurones (Balázs *et al*. 1989).

In order to demonstrate the functional capacity and sensitivity of the monoaminergic neurons to drugs in the developing brain, several biochemical and electrophysiological studies have been carried out in rats. Drugs such as reserpine, alpha-methyldopa, and clonidine, which are used for the treatment of hypertension, upset the balance of the monoamine levels and/or influence the sensitivity of the receptors as effectively in fetal and newborn rats as in adults (Feenstra *et al*. 1991; Nomura *et al*. 1982; Tennyson *et al*. 1983). Another antihypertensive drug, propranolol, significantly reduced NA content and turnover in the brain of the developing rat when administered from day 1 to 21 postnatally (Erdstieck-Ernste *et al*. 1991). Feenstra *et al*. have shown that clonidine is as effective in reducing the amount of NA activity in many brain areas of the rat throughout development as it is in adulthood (Boer *et al*. 1990). Tricyclic antidepressants, such as imipramine and clomipramine, inhibit the re-uptake of both NA and 5HT in the developing brain to the same extent as in adulthood (Nomura *et al*. 1978).

Animal studies have indeed improved our knowledge of neurotransmitter disturbances as one of the mechanisms of the neuroteratological disturbances induced by chemicals. Such systematic, well-controlled, develomental studies on drug administration can not of course be carried out in humans. However, in the near future some parameters of neurotransmitter activity may be sought in humans, for example the content of neurotransmitters and their breakdown products in the cerebrospinal fluid, receptor binding studies using blood platelet or placental tissue, PT scan and NMR techniques, and—if brain material is available—immuno-cytochemical and biochemical studies. Recent studies by Perry *et al.* (1984), and Perry (1988) using human placental tissues have strengthened the hypothesis that prenatal drug exposure in man may result in neurotransmitter system changes, which in turn, cause behavioural teratology. On the assumption that placental tissue neurotransmitter regulation may mirror fetal brain receptor regulation, placental neurotransmitter receptors from opioid-drug-abusing pregnant women and controls have been examined by these investigators. Increased amounts of opiate receptors and adrenergic receptors were found in the placentas of women who had used opiates and amphetamines during gestation.

Effects of drugs on behavioural states

Behavioural sleep–wake states of the fetus are manifest by the third trimester of pregnancy (see Chapter 3). Fetal behavioural states are: state 1F (quiet sleep); state 2F (rapid eye movement (REM) sleep); state 3F (quiet wakefulness); and state 4F (active wakefulness). Since the behavioural states are generated in the brain and show a very close relationship to the stage of brain development, they may be used as a good indicator of chemical hazards to the brain. Unfortunately, so far the effects of only a few drugs on behavioural states during development have been tested, and mainly following drug withdrawal (Hutchings *et al.* 1979). Our own studies have shown clear disturbances of sleep–wake patterns during chronic administration of antidepressant drugs, such as clomipramine or antihypertensives, such as clonidine or alpha-methyldopa, in the developing rat (Mirmiran 1986; Mirmiran *et al.* 1981, 1983*a*, 1985). Chronic administration of each of these drugs to developing rats dramatically reduced the amount of time spent in state 2, as well as the amount of eye movement during this state. Similar results were found by other investigators (Hilakivi *et al.* 1988; Vogel *et al.* 1990).

Although ultrasound techniques are frequently used in clinics, very few studies have attempted to investigate systematically the influence of drugs used by pregnant women on fetal behaviour during chronic exposure. Such tests would yield very straightforward evidence of the amount of functional damage inflicted on the fetal brain as a result of maternal medication. In a study by Arduini *et al.* (1987) a clear-cut reduction of fetal states 1 and 2 was found on naloxone administration to pregnant women near term. In an ongoing study by the group of van Geijn at the Free University of Amsterdam, changes in fetal behavioural states were found in women treated with anti-epileptics.

Most drugs easily pass the placenta and fetal blood–brain barrier, and their concentration in the fetal brain may be much higher than in the maternal plasma (Mirmiran and Swaab 1987; Mirmiran *et al.* 1985). The majority of these compounds suppress state 2 and disturb the normal sleep–wake cycle rhythms (Swaab and Mirmiran 1984). There are drugs that influence sleep by affecting different brain neurotransmitters, such as NA (e.g. alpha-methyldopa, clonidine, and propranolol), 5HT (e.g. imipramine, clomipramine, and zimelidine), and gamma-aminobutyric acid (e.g. diazepam). Several investigators have examined behavioural states of passively-dependent human infants during opiate withdrawal. A significant decrease in state 1 was found in neonates prenatally exposed to opiates, and this profile is shared by many neonates with a high risk of central nervous system impairment (Dinges *et al.* 1980; Schulman 1969). A decrease in both state 1 and 2 was found in the neonates of addicted women (Sisson *et al.* 1974). Sisson *et al.* concluded that since protein synthesis is stimulated during state 2, withdrawal treatment may be essential not only to relieve the symptoms, but also to promote normal and necessary sleep patterns required for brain development (Mirmiran *et al.* 1983*a*).

Long-term consequences

Animal studies

We have studied the long-lasting effects of several drugs chronically administered to the developing rat, at biochemical and electrophysiological levels in adult animals (Boer *et al.* 1990; Gorter *et al.* 1989; Mirmiran *et al.* 1985, 1988, 1990). Clonidine reduced NA turnover in the adult brain of neonatally-treated rats. In the hippocampus we found a supersensitivity of the pyramidal neurones to the depressive effects of NA, whereas the cortical neurones were more inhibited by GABA, compared to the controls. Long-lasting changes in rats after perinatal exposure to antidepressants were also reported by Del Rio *et al.* (1988). These changes include a decreased number of NA and 5HT receptors following perinatal exposure to chlorimipramine, imprindole, mianserin, and nomifensine during the second half of gestation in rats. Similar brain monoamine disturbances were also reported by Hilakivi *et al.* (1988).

Table 10.1 Sequelae of chronic drug exposure during gestation and lactation in man and other mammals

Drugs	Brain and behavioural alterations in man	Brain and behavioural alterations in other mammals
Alpha-methyldopa	Smaller head circumference, questionable neurological status, increased myoclonic jerks during sleep	Hyperactivity, delayed motor co-ordination, hyperanxiety in novel environment
Propranolol	Smaller head circumference, light for date	Reduced brain weight and brain body–weight ratio
Clonidine	Increased myoclonic jerks during sleep, hypotonia, hyperanxiety, minor neurological dysfunction	Supersensitivity of hippocampal neurons to noradrenaline, reduced level of hippocampal plasticity
Barbiturates	Hyperactivity, restlessness, disturbed sleep, hyperreflexia, reduced responsiveness to sensory stimuli	Hyperactivity, hyperanxiety, reduced masculine sexual behaviour, impairment of learning, reduced responsiveness to sensory stimuli, smaller brain
Reserpine	Anorexia, lethargy	Smaller brain
Diazepam	Low Apgar, reluctance to eat	Hyperactivity, learning impairment, reduced acoustic startle reflex
Imipramine-like compounds	Poor suckling, irritability	Hyperactivity, hyperanxiety, reduced masculine sexual behaviour, increased voluntary alcohol consumption, smaller brain
Chlorpromazine	Extrapyramidal dysfunction, tremor, hypertonus	Hyperactivity, reduced exploratory behaviour, learning impairment, smaller brain
Amphetamine	Withdrawal symptoms	Marked reduction in ability to habituate to new surroundings, reduction of dendritic spines and dendritic arborization of cortical neurons

Not only in development, but also in adulthood behavioural states are affected by drugs administered during rapid brain maturation. Developing rats treated with either clomipramine or clonidine show a high level of myoclonic jerks during state 2, as well as disturbances in sleep–wake cyclicity as adults (de Boer *et al.* 1989; Mirmiran *et al.* 1981, 1983*a*; Vogel *et al.* 1990). Following six days of valium exposure during the last week of gestation, mature prenatally exposed rats displayed significantly less quiet sleep at four months of age than controls (Livezey *et al.* 1985). Furthermore, the amplitude of circadian rhythmicity of sleep and wakefulness was also reduced. It is interesting to note that the amplitude of the circadian rhythm of maternal body temperature, and thereby that of the fetus, is significantly reduced in genetically hypertensive rats treated with clonidine during gestation. Moreover, male sexual behaviour was impaired while emotionality was increased in neonatally chlorimipramine- or clonidine-treated animals (Mirmiran *et al.* 1981, 1983; Vogel 1990). Neonatal treatment with clomipramine or clonidine reduced the size of the brain studied in adulthood (Mirmiran *et al.* 1983*a*). On the other hand, brain plasticity, measured either by environmental stimulation, or by electrical stimulation of the hippocampus, was reduced in clonidine-treated rats (Gorter *et al.* 1990; Mirmiran *et al.* 1983*b*; Nelson *et al.* 1985). Similar impairment of brain plasticity in response to environmental novelty was reported earlier by Coyle and Singer (1975) in rats prenatally exposed to imipramine.

Human studies

Human studies on the long-term consequences of drug use during pregnancy on the development of the child are rare. Nevertheless there are certain data suggesting similar deleterious drug effects as found in animal studies (Table 10.1; Mirmiran *et al.* 1985; Swaab and Mirmiran 1984; Swaab *et al.* 1988). Prenatal exposure of hypertensive pregnant women to alpha-methyldopa causes smaller head circumference, minor neurological dysfunctions, and increased myoclonic jerks during sleep in the child (Shimohira *et al.* 1986). Propranolol also causes a smaller head circumference and a higher incidence of babies who are smaller than average for their gestational age (i.e. small gestational age, SGA). Prenatal exposure to clonidine does not cause smaller head circumference, but it does lead to sustained hypertension in the neonate during the first three days of life (Boutroy *et al.* 1988), increased myoclonic jerks during sleep, and enhanced sleep terrors in children of 3 to 9 years of age (Huisjes 1988; Huisjes *et al.* 1986). Hadders-Algra *et al.* (1986) of the Groningen prenatal group have carefully studied the physical, neurological, and behavioural development of a large group (n=78) of 6-year-old children who were prenatally exposed to ritodrine. No neurological differences were found between the ritodrine and the control group.

However, all of the drug-exposed children showed inferior school performance in motor and social skills, emotional development, and cognitive
development. Drugs such as barbiturates induce withdrawal symptoms in
neonates, for example hyperactivity, restlessness, disturbed sleep, hyper-
reflexia, and reduced responsiveness to sensory stimuli. A recent study by
Dessens *et al.* (unpublished observation) at the Academic Medical Centre
of the University of Amsterdam demonstrated that the children of epileptic
women had a smaller head circumference due to barbiturate exposure
during pregnancy. Diazepam exposure results in neonates with a low Apgar
score, hypotonia, and poor suckling. No follow-up studies were carried out
in children prenatally exposed to tricyclic antidepressants, although poor
suckling and irritability are reported in these children at birth.

Concluding remarks

Some data on functional teratology of drugs used during human gestation certainly point to deleterious effects such drugs might have at the
neurobehavioural level, in a manner similar to that observed in animal
experiments. However, the available data on humans are scarce. There are
also certain problems with respect to applying animal (particularly rat)
data to humans (Swaab *et al.* 1988). In the first place there is no good
animal model for humans taking into account the degree of human vulner-
ability, a comparable stage of brain development at the moment of birth,
etc. Although, in contrast to what is generally believed, humans are often
more sensitive than animals to the teratogenicity of drugs (Council on
Environmental Quality 1981), there are certain unexpected observations.
For example a single injection of glucocorticoids to neonatal rats induces
adulthood behavioural abnormalities such as hyperactivity, stereotypy,
emotional hyperactivity, decreased adaptability, motor incoordination,
and impaired reproductive functions (Benesova 1989; Benesova and Pavlik
1989). Moreover, this single injection of glucocorticoid resulted in morphological and biochemical alterations of the brain, reduced cerebellar and
hippocampal size, and decreased NA in the hypothalamus. On the other
hand, in follow-up studies on premature babies treated with glucocorticoids for the prevention of lung disorders, no significant differences in the
medical history or psychological/neurological development of these infants
were found compared to non-treated controls (Schmand *et al.* 1990;
Smolders-de Haas *et al.* 1990); it should be noted that prenatal infusion of
dexamethasone in monkeys disturbs the circadian rhythms of maternal
uterine activity as well as the fetal hormonal rhythms (Ducsay *et al.* 1983).
However, prenatal exposure to antihypertensive drugs such as clonidine
might make the child susceptible to developing hypertension or sleep

disturbances (Boutroy *et al.* 1988; Huisjes *et al.* 1986), while similar pre-natal treatment in rats induces little effect (Ali *et al.* 1988).

Secondly, the drugs are administered to healthy animals, while in the human situation, except in the case of addicted women, they are prescribed to pregnant women with disorders such as epilepsy, hypertension, and depression. Although there are exceptions, a study of continuous clonidine infusion to pregnant hypertensive rats has shown a clear reduction of the amplitude of circadian rhythms of body temperature in the mother. As it is known that the maternal circadian rhythm is one of the main factors in the generation of fetal circadian rhythms (see Part 2), one might expect to see a deleterious effect of drug therapy on the fetus under pathological condi-tions comparable to those of the human. In general, we do not know exactly to what extent disorder, treatment, and a combination of the two, affect the developing brain of the unborn child.

Huisjes reviewed the problems of studying functional teratogenicity in man (Huisjes 1988). He pointed out a number of important issues to be considered. On the one hand, although structural defects in man can be recognized within one year after birth, recognition of neurobehavioural abnormalities may require a follow-up study of more than 10 years. One of the main problems of recognizing symptoms of funtional teratology is the long time interval between the moment when chemicals act upon the developing brain and the occurrence of symptoms. Furthermore, although morphological defects can be identified on the basis of known normal morphology, a description of what constitutes normal neurobehavioural function in an individual cannot always be given. Another important issue is the phase of gestation in which drugs may induce neurobehavioural teratogenicity. While the first trimester of gestation is considered to be more associated with gross morphological abnormalities, the third tri-mester may be closely associated with functional teratogenicity, since this is the period of rapid growth of the brain. However, it is sometimes hard to find cases in which the drug is administered during only one phase of gestation and not throughout this period, even often including the lactation period. Literature suggests that at present there is not only a potential health hazard of chemicals during the second half of gestation, but during lactation as well, (e.g. PCPs; Schardein 1985). This is also important in relation to the increasing amounts of chemicals prescribed during lactation. The other important point Huisjes makes is that of the consequences for clinical practice when a drug, such as clonidine or ritodrine, is proven to be functionally teratogenic. Should the drug then be replaced by another one of which often nothing is known concerning functional teratology, and which may thus have even worse effects? Should we suspend the treatment and take the risk of the deleterious effects of the disease on the child and mother–child interaction?

These are important questions for which we do not have convincing answers as long as chemicals that have to be given sometimes during gestation have not been studied systematically for functional teratology in man. Only then can we make up the balance between the possible beneficial and detrimental effects of a compound. What we can conclude at present is, therefore, that studies on the functional teratogenicity of drugs used during the second half of gestation should be performed systematically in humans. In such studies the results obtained in animals can be used as guidelines of what to look for (Swaab *et al.* 1988). This requires a multidisciplinary type of research including both neuroscientists and clinicians, focusing on human research, since we believe that there is in fact only one good animal model for human development, and that is human.

Acknowledgement

We are grateful to Olga Pach for her secretarial assistance.

References

Ali, S. F., Holson, R. R., Pizzi, W. J., Newport, G. D., and Slikker, W. Jr. (1988). Neurochemical evaluation of rats prenatally exposed to the adrenergic agonists clonidine and lofexidine. *Neurotoxicology* **9**, 512–58.

Arduini, D., Rizzo, G., Dell Acqua, S., Mancuso, G., and Romanini, C. (1987). The effect of naloxane on fetal behavior near term. *American Journal of Obstetrics and Gynecology* **156**, 474–80.

Aubert, M. L. (1979). Ontogenese des fonctions hypothalamiques chez le foetus humain. *Journal de Physiologie (Paris)* **75**, 45–53.

Balázs, R., Hack, N., and Jørgensen, O. S. (1990). Selective stimulation of excitatory amino acid receptor subtypes and the survival of cerebellar granule cells in culture: effect of kainic acid. *Neuroscience* **37**, 251–8.

Benesova, O. (1989). Perinatal pharmacotheraphy and brain development. *International Journal of Prenatal and Perinatal Studies*, 417–24.

Benesova, O. and Pavlik, A. (1989). Perinatal treatment with glucocorticoids and the risk of maldevelopment of the brain. *Neuropharmacology* **28**, 197–8.

Bloch, B., Bugnon, C., Fellman, D., and Lenys, D. (1978). Immunocytochemical evidence that the same neurons in the human infundibular nucleus are stained with anti-endorphins and other related peptides. *Neuroscience Letters* **10**, 147–52.

Boer, G. J., Feenstra, M. G. P., Mirmiran, M., Swaab, D. F., and Van Haaren, F. (ed.) (1988). *Biochemical basis of functional neuroteratology. Progress in Brain Research*, Vol. 73. Elsevier Science Publishers, Amsterdam.

Boer, G. J., Feenstra, M. G. P., Erdtsieck-Ernste, B. H. W., Gorter J. A., and Mirmiran, M. (1990). Longlasting effects of early noradrenergic receptor occupation on brain noradrenaline turnover and on β-receptors. *Developmental Pharmacological Therapeutics* **15**, 224–33.

Boer, S. de, Mirmiran, M., Haaren, F. van, Louwerse, A., and Poll, N. E. van de. (1989). Neurobehavioral teratogenic effects of clomipramine and alpha-methyldopa. *Neurotoxicology and Toxicology* **11**, 77–84.

Boutroy, M. J., Gisonna, C. R., and Legagneur, M. (1988). Clonidine: placental transfer and neonatal adaption. *Early Human Development* **17**, 275–86.

Brooksbank, B. W. L., Martinez, M., Atkinson, D. J., and Balázs, R. (1978). Biochemical development of the human brain: I. Some parameters of the cholinergic system. *Developmental Neuroscience* **1**, 267–84.

Brooksbank, B. W. L., Atkinson, D. J., and Balázs, R. (1981). Biochemical development of the human brain: II. Some parameters of the GABAergic system. *Developmental Neuroscience* **4**, 188–200.

Bugnon, C., Bloch, B., and Fellman, D. (1977). Etude immunocytologique des neurons hypothalamiques à LH-RH chez le foetus humain. *Brain Research* **128**, 249–62.

Council on Environmental Quality (1981). Chemical hazards to human reproduction. Government Printing Office, Washington D. C.

Coyle, I. R., and Singer, G. (1975). The interaction effects of prenatal imipramine exosure and postnatal rearing condition on behavior and histology. *Psychopharmacology* **44**, 253–6.

Del Rio, J., Montero, D., and Ceballos, M. L. de. (1988). Long-lasting changes after perinatal exposure to antidepressants. In: Biochemical basis of functional neuroteratology (ed. G. J. Boer, M. G. P. Feenstra, M. Mirmiran, D. F. Swaab, and F. van Haaren). *Progress in Brain Research*, Vol. 73 pp. 173–88. Elsevier Science Publishers, Amsterdam.

Dinges, D. F., Davis. M. M., and Glass, P. (1980). Fetal exposure to narcotics: neonatal sleep as a measure of nervous system disturbances. *Science* **209**, 619–21.

Dobbing, J. and Sands, J. (1979). Comparative aspects of the brain growth spurt. *Early Human Development* **3**, 79–83.

Ducsay, C. A., Cook, M. J., Walsh, S. W., and Novy, N. J. (1983). Circadian patterns and dexamethasone-induced changes in uterine activity in pregnant rhesus monkeys. *American Journal of Obstetrics and Gynecology* **145**, 389–96.

Erdstieck-Ernste, B. H. W., Feenstra, M. G. P., Boer, G. J., and Van Galen, H. (1991). Chonic propanolol treatment in developing rats: acute and lasting effects on monoamines and beta-adrenergic receptors in the rat brain. *Research Bulletin* **26**, 731–7.

Eskes, T. K. A. B. and Finster, M. (ed.) (1983). *Drug therapy during pregnancy*. Butterworths, London.

Eskes, T. K. A. B., Nijdam, W., Buijs, M. J. R. M., and Rossum, J. M. van. (1983). Drug therapy during pregnancy: effects on mother, fetus and newborn. In: *Drug therapy during pregnancy* (ed. T. K. A. B. Eskes and M. Finster), pp. 1–8. Butterworths, London.

Feenstra, M. G. P., van Galen, H., and Boer, G. J. (1991). Early postnatal chonidine treatment results in altered regional catecholamine utilisation in adult rat brain. *Psychopharmacology*. In press.

Gorter, J. A., Mirmiran, M., Bos, N. P. A., and Werf, D. van der (1989). Hippocampal neuronal responsiveness to different neurotransmitters in the adult rat after neonatal interference with noradrenaline transmission. *Brain Research Bulletin* **23**, 293–7.

Gorter, J. A., Kamphuis, W., Huisman, E., Bos, N. P. A., and Mirmiran, M.

(1990). Neonatal clonidine treatment results in long-lasting changes in noradrenaline sensitivity and kindling epileptogenesis. *Brain Research* **535**, 62–6.

Hadders-Algra, M., Touwen, B. C. L., and Huisjes, H. J. (1986). Long-term follow-up of children prenatally exposed to ritodrine. *British Journal of Obstetrics and Gynaecology* **93**, 156–61.

Hilakivi, L. A., Taira, T., Hilvakivi, I., MacDonald, E., Tuomisto, L., and Hellevuo, K. (1988). Early postnatal treatment with propranolol affects development of brain amines and behavior. *Psychopharmacology* **96**, 353–9.

Huisjes, H. J. (1988). Problems in studying functional teratogenicity in man. In: Biochemical basis of functional neuroteratology (ed. G. J. Boer, M. G. P. Feenstra, M. Mirmiran, D. F. Swaab, and F. van Haaren), *Progress in Brain Research*, Vol. 73, pp. 51–67. Elsevier Science Publishers, Amsterdam.

Huisjes, H. J., Hadders-Algra, M., and Touwen, C. B. L. (1986). Is clonidine a behavioral teratogen in human? *Early Human Development* **13**, 1–6.

Hutchings, D. E. (1978). Behavioral teratology: embryonic and behavioral effects of drugs during pregnancy. In: *Studies on the development of behavior and the nervous system, early influences* (ed. G. Gotlieb), Vol. 4, p. 7. Academic Press, New York.

Hutchings, D. E., Feraru, E., Gorinson, H. S., and Golden, R. R. (1979). Effects of prenatal methadone on the rest-activity cycle of the pre-weanling rat. *Neurobehavioral Toxicology* **1**, 33–40.

Hyppä, M. (1972). Hypothalamic monoamines in human fetuses. *Neuroendocrinology* **9**, 257–66.

Lauder, J. M. and Bloom, F. E. (1974). Ontogeny of monoamine neurons in the locus coeruleus, raphe nuclei and substantia nigra of the rat. *Journal of Comparative Neurology* **155**, 469–81.

Livezey, G. T., Radulovacki, M., Isaac, L., and Marczynski, T. J. (1985). Prenatal exposure to diazepam results in enduring reductions in brain receptors and deep slow-wave sleep. *Brain Research* **334**, 361–5.

Masudi. N. A. and Gilmore, D. P. (1983). Biogenic amine levels in the mid-term human fetus. *Developmental Brain Research* **7**, 9–12.

Mirmiran, M. (1986). The role of the central monoaminergic system and rapid eye movement sleep in development. *Brain Development* **8**, 382–9.

Mirmiran, M. and Boer, S. de. (1988). Long-term effects of chemicals on developing brain and behavior. In: *Teratogens: chemicals which cause birth defects* (ed. V. Kolb-Myers), pp. 271–314. Elsevier Science Publishers, Amsterdam.

Mirmiran, M. and Swaab, D. F. (1987). Influence of drugs on brain neurotransmitters and behavioral states during development. *Developmental Pharmacological and Therapeutics* **10**, 377–84.

Mirmiran, M., Poll, N. E. van de, Corner, M. A., Oyen, H. G. van, and Bour, H. L. (1981). Suppression of active sleep by chronic treatment with chlorimipramine during early postnatal development: effects upon sleep and behavior in the rat. *Brain Research* **204**, 129–46.

Mirmiran, M., Scholtens, J., Poll, N. E. van de, Uylings, H. B. M., Gugten, J. van der, and Boer, G. J. (1983a). Effects of experimental suppression of active (REM) sleep during early development upon adult brain and behavior in the rat. *Developmental Brain Research* **7**, 277–86.

Mirmiran, M., Uylings, H. B. M., and Corner, M. A. (1983b). Pharmacological suppression of REM sleep prior to weaning counteracts the effectiveness of subsequent environmental enrichment on cortical growth in rats. *Developmental Brain Research* **7**, 102–5.

Mirmiran, M., Brenner, E., Gugten, J. van der, and Swaab, D. F. (1985). Neurochemical and electrophysiological disturbances during development mediate behavioral teratogenicity of medicines. *Neurobehavioral Toxicology and Teratology* **7**, 677–83.

Mirmiran, M., Feenstra, M. G. P., Dijcks, F. A., Bos, N. P. A., and Haaren, F. van. (1988). Functional deprivation of noradrenaline neurotransmission: effects of clonidine on brain development. In: Biochemical basis of functional neuroteratology (ed. G. J. Boer, M. G. P. Feenstra, M. Mirmiran, D. F. Swaab, and F. van Haaren. *Progress in Brain Research* Vol. 73 pp. 159–72. Elsevier Science Publishers, Amsterdam.

Mirmiran, M., Dijcks, F. A., Bos, N. P. A., Gorter, J. A., and Werf, d. van der (1990). Cortical neuron sensitivity to neurotransmitters following neonatal noradrenaline depletion. *International Journal of Developmental Neuroscience* **8**, 217–21.

Nelson, S. B., Schwartz, M. A., and Daniels, J. D. (1985). Clonidine and cortical plasticity: possible evidence for noradrenergic involvement. *Developmental Brain Research* **23**, 39–50.

Nobin, A. and Björklund, A. (1973). Topography of the monoamine neuron systems in the human brain as revealed in fetuses. *Acta Physiologica Scandinavica* (Suppl.) **388**, 1–40.

Nomura, Y., Tanaka, Y., and Segawa, T. (1978). Influences of sodium, ouabaine and tricyclic antidepressant drugs on L-[H]norepinephrine uptake into synaptosomal fractions of developing rat brain. *Japanese Journal of Pharmacology* **28**, 501–4.

Nomura, Y., Yotsumoto, I., and Nishimoto, Y. (1982). Ontogeny of influence of clonidine on high potassium-induced release of noradrenaline and specific (3H] clonidine binding in the rat brain cortex. *Developmental Neuroscience* **5**, 198–204.

Olson, L., Boréus, L. O., and Seiger, A. (1973). Histochemical demonstration and mapping of 5-hydroxytryptamine- and catecholamine-containing neuron systems in the human fetal brain. *Zeitschrift für die gesamte Anatomie* **139**, 259–82.

Paulin, C., Charnay, Y., Chayvialle, J. A., Danière, S., and Dubois, P. M. (1986). Ontogeny of substance P in the digestive tract, spinal cord and hypothalamus of the human fetus. *Regulatory Peptides* **14**, 145–53.

Pearson, J. (1983) Neurotransmitter immunocytochemistry in the study of human development, anatomy, and pathology. In: *Progress in neuropathology* (ed. H. M. Zimmerman), Vol. 5, pp. 41–97. Raven Press, New York.

Pearson, J., Brandeis, L., and Goldstein, M. (1980). Appearance of tyrosine hydroxylase immunoreactivity in the human embryo. *Developmental Neuroscience* **3**, 140–50.

Perry, B. D. (1988). Placental and blood element neurotransmitter receptor regulation in humans: potential models for studying neurochemical mechanisms underlying behavioral teratology. In: Biochemical basis of functional neuroteratology (ed. G. J. Boer, M. G. P. Feenstra, M. Mirmiran, D. F. Swaab, and F. van Haaren). *Progress in Brain Research*. Vol. 73 pp. 189–205. Elsevier Science Publishers, Amsterdam.

Perry, B. D., Pesarento, D. J., Kussie, P. H., O'Prichard, D. C., and Schnoll, S. H.

(1984). Prenatal exposure to drugs to abuse in humans: effects on placental neuro-transmitter receptors. *Neurobehavioral Toxicology and Teratology* **6**, 295–301.

Repressa, A., Tremblay, E., and Ben-Ari, Y. (1989). Transient increase of NMDA-binding sites in human hippocampus during development. *Neuroscience Letters* **99**, 61–6.

Riley, E. P. and Vorhees, C. V. (ed.) (1986). *Handbook of behavioral teratology*. Plenum Press, New York.

Schardein, J. L. (ed.) (1985). *Chemically induced brain defects*. Marcel Dekker Inc., New York.

Schlumpf, M. and Lichtensteiger, W. (1987). Benzodiazepine and muscarinic cholinergic binding sites in striatum and brainstem of the human fetus. *International Journal of Developmental Neuroscience* **5**, 283–7.

Schmand, B., Neuvel, J., Smolders-de Haas, H., Hoeks, J., Treffers, P. E., and Koppe, J. G. (1990). Psychological development of children who were treated antenatally with corticosteroids to prevent respiratory distress syndrome. *Pediatrics* **86**, 58–64.

Schulman, C. A. (1969). Alterations of the sleep cycle in heroin-addicted and suspect newborns. *Neuropädiatrie* **1**, 89–100.

Shimohira, M., Kohyama, J., Kawano, Y., Suzuki, H., Ogiso, M., and Iwakawa, Y. (1986). Effects of alpha-methyldopa administration during pregnancy on the development of the child's sleep. *Brain Development* **8**, 416–23.

Siler-Khodr, T. M. and Khodr, G. S. (1978). Studies in human fetal endocrinology. I. Luteinizing hormone-releasing factor content of the hypothalamus. *American Journal of Obstetrics and Gynecology* **130**, 795–800.

Sisson, T. R. C., Wickler, M., Tsai, P., and Rao, I. P. (1974). Effects of narcotic withdrawal on neonatal sleep patterns. *Pediatric Research* **8**, 451.

Smolders-de Haas, H., Neuvel, J., Schmand, B., Treffers, P. E., Koppe, J. G., and Hoeks, J. (1990). Physical development and medical history of children who were treated antenatally with corticosteroids to prevent respiratory distress syndrome: A 10- to 12-year follow-up. *Pediatrics* **86**, 65–70.

Swaab, D. F. and Mirmiran, M. (1984). Possible mechanisms underlying the teratogenic effects of medicines on the developing brain. In: *Neurobehavioral teratology* (ed. J. Yanai), p. 55. Elsevier Science Publishers, Amsterdam.

Swaab, D. F. and Mirmiran, M. (1988). Functional teratogenic effects on the developing brain. In: *Fetal and neonatal neurology and neurosurgery* (ed. M. I. Levene, M. J. Bennett, and J. Punt), pp. 258–64. Churchill Livingstone, Edinburgh.

Swaab, D. F., Boer, G. J., and Feenstra, M. G. P. (1988). Concept of functional neuroteratology and the importance of neurochemistry. In: Biochemical basis of functional neuroteratology (ed. G. J. Boer, M. G. P. Feenstra, M. Mirmiran, D. F. Swaab, and F. van Haaren). *Progress in Brain Research* Vol. 73 pp. 3–14. Elsevier Science Publishers, Amsterdam.

Tennyson, V. M., Gershon, P., Budininkas-Schoenenbeek, M., and Rothman, T. (1983). Effects of extended periods of reserpine and methyl-p-thyrosine treatment on the development of the putamen in the fetal rabbits. *International Journal of Developmental Neuroscience* **1**, 305–18.

Vogel, G., Neill, D., Hagler, M., and Kors, D. (1990). A new animal model of endogenous depression: a summary of present findings. *Neuroscience and Biobehavioral Reviews* **14**, 85–9.

Winters, A. J., Eskay, R. L., and Porter, J. C. (1974). Concentration and distribution of TRH and LRH in the human fetal brain. *Journal of Clinical Endocrinology and Metabolism* **39,** 960–3.

Yanai, J. (ed.) (1984). *Neurobehavioral teratology*. Elsevier Science Publishers, Amsterdam.

Part 3

Fetal behaviour and fetal psychology

11

Fetal psychology: an embryonic science

PETER G. HEPPER

Above all, we must be clear on this point, that the fundamental activities of mind, which are manifested only after birth, do not originate after birth

W. Preyer (1881). *The mind of the child*, p. xii.

The birth of a neonate marks for the parents and relations the start of a new period in their lives and perhaps to represent this the neonate is given the age of zero. For the neonate however, birth merely marks a transition from a prenatal environment to a new postnatal environment. Neonatal sensory abilities and behavioural capacities, although only directly observable after birth, are present before birth, and have their developmental origins in the nine months preceding birth. The prenatal period has, until recently, been ignored by researchers examining the development of behavioural abilities. Outside the scientific domain the origins of human behaviour and abilities have been the subject of much fascination and speculation, and given the lack of scientific examination, a multitude of differing views regarding the abilities of the fetus have been produced. These range from one extreme that the fetus may be considered as a well-formed invididual, linked to his mother physiologically and psychically, experiencing all aspects of his, and his mother's environment, and being profoundly affected by these experiences. At the other extreme the fetus has been viewed as a conglomeration of cells developing in isolation from environmental influences.

This chapter will review two aspects of fetal abilities, the sensory and learning competencies, which may be considered as part of a new discipline of fetal psychology. This review will not exhaustively detail all studies, but selected papers will be discussed to illustrate the developing individual's abilities. Because of limited space, I shall concentrate mainly on the human fetus; readers are referred to Smotherman and Robinson (1988), and Krasnegor *et al.* (1987), for reviews of research pertaining to animals.

Although there has been little scientific examination of the sensory abilities of the fetus it has long been argued that the fetus perceives aspects of his environment. Aristotle in *De Generatione Animalium* argued that the individual first acquired sensation during pregnancy and could thus experience various aspects of his environment. Suśruta, the great Indian medical scientist of the sixth century BC, proposed that the fetus becomes aware of his surroundings at about 12 weeks of age and actively searches for sensation. At 5 months the fetus wakes and acquires a mind, and has an intellect at 6 months (Suśruta 1954). There has been little doubt in the minds of many writers that prenatal experiences influence the development of the individual. Jacob influenced the colour of all lambs, goats, and cattle born in the herd he maintained to increase his holding of animals over that of Laban, by manipulating their prenatal environment (Genesis 31: 30–43). Empdocles, writing in approximately 480 BC, considered that the development of the embryo could be guided and interfered with by the mental state of the mother (Diels 1906). Caraka, the Indian embryologist, wrote before 1000 BC and argued that the fetus may be susceptible to the influence of the mother, and that psychological factors in the mother may cause mental disturbance in the fetus. The influence of the mother on the fetus and his development after birth was recognized by the Chinese over 1000 years ago, when 'prenatal clinics' were established to keep the mother tranquil, and thus to maintain the psychological health of the fetus (Ellis 1940). Speculations that the individual is affected by experiences in the womb have continued. Sir Kenelm Digby attempted to explain the phobia of King James to the sight of a naked sword as the result of influences experienced by the King whilst in the womb (Graham 1951). Today a variety of therapists offer services to overcome the effects of experiences acquired prenatally which are adversely affecting the individual after birth (Hepper 1989).

Whilst there have been many anecdotal observations of the fetal behaviour, scientific study has until the past decade been conspicuous by its absence. There have, however, been exceptions to this (Preyer 1885; Sontag 1966; Carmichael 1954).

Psychology: the neonate and the fetus

Psychology, although defined as the scientific study of behaviour and having its first psychological laboratory established over 100 years ago by Wilhelm Wundt in Leipzig, Germany, has, along with other disciplines, for example embryology, ignored behaviour during this earliest stage of development. Prior to the 1970s textbooks on developmental psychology often excluded the prenatal period totally. Even in those that did consider the prenatal period attention was focused on physical growth and development. Experiential effects were considered, but mainly with respect to the morphological changes induced by teratogens. The past 10 to 20 years have witnessed a change in the coverage given to the prenatal period and behaviour, although even now the perceptual environment and learning abilities of the fetus are only briefly mentioned, if at all. The recent sustained interest in this period may be attributed to a conceptual change regarding the origins of behaviour and it is instructive to examine the reasons behind this.

Obviously new technology has helped; real-time ultrasound has enabled direct observation of the fetus 'in action' and thus increased fetal accessibility. The increased interest in the fetal period may be attributed to a change in the views regarding the capabilities of the neonate. For a long time it was considered that the neonate was poorly developed. William James considered the neonate's world a 'blooming, buzzing confusion', and that the neonate was unable to control or adjust to it's environment. A few basic reflexes such as sucking and rooting were attributed to the neonate, but generally the neonate was considered unable to perceive, respond to, or learn, about the environment. The neonate was regarded as a physiological organism, and research concentrated on physiological aspects of development such as growth (Rau 1982). It is useful for those examining the abilities of the fetus to consider why the abilities of the neonate were underestimated for so long, if only to ensure that a similar underestimation of fetal abilities does not occur. This reappraisal of the neonate over the past 20 years has occurred not because of a sudden increase in neonatal abilities, but rather because scientists are now able to ask the right questions. Neonates are no longer looked at through adult eyes and expected to have adult abilities. Such viewpoints led to the neonate not matching up to adult standards, and consequently being regarded as incompetent. This error was further compounded by the fact that examination of the neonate proceeded apace, but used methodologies and paradigms best suited to adults or children.

Over the past 20 years researchers have adopted techniques appropriate to the neonate. This research has indicated that neonates possess a sophisticated perceptual and learning repertoire. They are capable of fine olfactory (Porter 1991), visual (Aslin 1985), and auditory (Fifer and Moon 1988) discriminations, and are capable of learning, for example imitation of facial expressions (Meltzoff and Moore 1983). These neonatal abilities have been further reinforced by examination of the premature infant (Allen and Capute 1986; Gekoski *et al.* 1984). The upshot of this research is that neonates are no longer regarded as incompetent and at the mercy of the environment, but have been shown to possess a diverse repertoire of behaviour enabling them to adjust and adapt to their environment.

With the recognition of the abilities of neonates and premature infants, it became obvious that these abilities did not suddenly manifest themselves at birth, but had been developed and refined during the preceding prenatal period. Researchers thus began the search for the developmental origins of behaviour in the prenatal period. It is worth emphasizing again, since this is perhaps the most crucial issue in the examination of the fetus, that a fetus lives in a very different environment from neonates, infants, and adults. Consequently the abilities of the fetus will be tailored to his environment, and methodologies used to investigate fetal abilities must be appropriate for the fetus, and not neonates or any other stage of development after birth. If this is not done fetal abilities will be underestimated, and errors made regarding neonatal capabilities will be repeated.

The sensory environment of the fetus

Perception and sensation

One question which should be addressed, is does the fetus perceive or sense its environment? A sense, for example, olfactory, visual, or auditory, is a system by which information from outside the nervous system is translated into neural activity, and thus gives the nervous system, especially the brain, information about the outside world. For example, for the visual sense light is converted by cells in the retina of the eyes into neural activity to provide information about its source. This information is a sensation, that is to say the basic information is provided by the senses. Perception on the other hand is the interpretation of these sensations based on previous experiences, which give meaning to the sensation. For example, reading these words, one is sensing patterns of light, dark, contours, and edges; these sensations are interpreted to give perception of letters and words, and then by further cognitive processes, meaning. Many perceptual abilities develop within the first months of neonatal life. For example, neonates show no preference for a picture of a face over a picture of a scrambled face, but by 3 months of age show a strong preference for the 'normal' face (Fantz and Nevis 1967). Furthermore observation of the visual scanning patterns of infants indicates that at one month areas of high contrast, for example, hair-line, are looked at, whereas at two months of age this is replaced by significant features of the face, for example the eyes (Haith *et al*. 1977). This suggests that by two months of age the stimuli presented by a face are regarded as a face and not a series of sensations, thus the infant now perceives rather than senses the face. Whilst many studies, as I shall review shortly, have demonstrated fetal responsiveness to various stimuli, they have not addressed the question of whether the fetus senses or perceives the environment. Throughout this section I shall refer to the sensory environment of the fetus and consider the fetus as sensing his environment rather than perceiving it.

Fetal sensory abilities

Because of the present lack of technology with which to record the neural activity of the various sensory systems in the womb directly, fetal sensory abilities are examined by observing a behavioural reaction to a stimulus. If the fetus overtly responds to the stimulus by a change in pattern of movement or fetal heart-rate (FHR), then it is likely that the fetus has sensed the stimulus. Of course it is important to use appropriate methodology to ensure that the response is due to the stimulus and is not a spontaneous occurrence occurring by chance after the stimulus was presented. Problems arise when the fetus does not respond; logically one can not say that the fetus does not sense the stimulus. Behavioural states have been demonstrated in the human fetus (Nijhuis 1986), and these can differentially influence responsiveness (Lecanuet *et al.* 1988). Non-responsiveness may therefore be due to the fetus being in a particular state. The fetus may sense the stimulus, but exhibit no observable response. We are continually bombarded by new stimuli much of which we show little response to. Likewise the fetus may sense the stimulus, but exhibit no response. Using fetal responsiveness as an indicator of sensation requires that the sensory apparatus is connected in some way to the motor apparatus, which elicits the response. A lack of response may be the result of under-developed motor responses, such that the fetus is unable to elicit the required response. Finally the lack of response may be due to an inability to sense the stimulus. It is thus important to remember that the lack of response to a particular stimulus need not be directly equated to a lack of sensory ability.

A second issue concerns the stimulus, in particular stimulus quality and stimulus reception. The stimulus presented to the fetus by the researcher may differ from that which is sensed by the fetus. This may be because the stimulus becomes altered *en route* to the fetus. For example, a sound stimulus presented externally to the fetus may have a very different quality after passing through the abdomen before reaching the fetal ear. The maternal abdomen will differentially attenuate different frequencies (Querleu *et al.* 1988). Thus the stimulus sensed by the fetus may be different to that which was presented. It should also be remembered that sensory reception of the stimulus may be mediated by a different modality or by different structures prenatally For example, the fetus responds to tactile information at approximately 8 weeks of gestational age (Hooker 1952), yet at this age the receptors used by adults to perceive tactile stimuli have yet to penetrate the basement layer of the skin (Humphrey 1966). Recently, my colleagues and I demonstrated responsiveness to sound at 16 weeks of gestational age, and possibly as early as 12 weeks (Hepper *et al.* 1991), prior to the completion of the auditory apparatus (Rubel 1985). It may be that the developing neural system and nerve plexus is responsive to stimulation prior to the formation of specific receptor cells, and stimulation early in gestation may be sensed by the undifferentiated neural system. Exactly what sensation this would provide remains an unanswered question. Thus it should be borne in mind that both the stimulus as it reaches the fetus, and its mechanism of sensation, may differ from that expected.

A final consideration is that of the relationship between fetal sensory abilities and the fetal sensory environment. It is important that the two are distinguished. The researcher may be able to present a diverse array of stimuli to the fetus and the fetus may respond, but the fact that the fetus responds does not necessarily mean that the fetus will experience such stimuli during the course of pregnancy. Similarly, stimuli that comprise the fetal environment are not restricted to those presented by the researcher and the fetal environment may be more diverse than that studied. In the following review both the fetal sensory abilities and its sensory environment will be discussed.

Cutaneous senses

Touch Some of the earliest studies examining fetal response to touch were performed by Hooker (1952). Using fetuses delivered and maintained in a warm water bath he found that at the end of the seventh week the fetus responded reflexively to touch on the lips. Responsiveness spreads to the cheeks and forehead. The fetus responds to touch on the palms of the hand at about 10.5 weeks, and to touch on the upper arms 3 to 5 days later. By 14 weeks the whole body, excluding the back and top of the head, are responsive to touch. Interestingly the initial response to touch on the cheek is to move away from the stimulus, thus fetuses stimulated on the right cheek turned their head to the left, away from the stimulus. Later on during pregnancy the fetus will turn its head towards the touch, and this is possibly the prenatal emergence of the 'rooting reflex,' which is important in breast feeding. More recently an attempt to provide tactile stimulation to the fetus whilst in the womb using a pressure jet of isotonic saline delivered during the active phase of labour has been reported (Baxi *et al.* 1988). Some responsiveness, as indicated by a change in FHR, was found although this was dependent on fetal capillary pH. The fetal environment will provide tactile stimulation. With growth the fetus becomes too large to float in the amniotic sac, and will come into contact with the uterine wall. Fetal activity, which commences at around 7 to 8 weeks of age (see Chapter 1 and Chapter 6) will also result in contact with the uterine wall. The fetus will touch himself, especially around the face region, which may be particularly sensitive to tactile stimulation (Hepper *et al.* 1990). Finally the umbilical cord will be constantly touching the fetus.

Temperature The temperature environment of the fetus is carefully controlled, and shows little variation, being maintained at 0.5–1.5°C above that of the mother (Walker 1969). This stability gives little reason to expect that the fetus will experience temperature stimulation during pregnancy. The fetus does respond to cold water stimulation. Cold water at 4°C on the face of the fetus during normal active labour elicited a change in FHR and this change appears to be independent of state (Timor-Tritsch 1986). Anecdotal reports from mothers indicate that more movements are felt when taking a hot bath; whether this reflects a response to temperature is unknown.

Pain It is difficult to assess pain sensation in the human fetus since pain is most commonly defined as a subjective phenomenon. FHR increases in response to such procedures as scalp blood sampling, and increases in FHR and movement have been observed after tactile stimulation during amniocentesis (Hill *et al.* 1979; Ron *et al.* 1976). These indicate that the fetus is responsive to stimuli which we may find painful. Physiologically the neural structures required for pain perception are well developed and active late in pregnancy, as are neurochemical systems associated with pain (Anand and Hickey 1987). There is now little doubt that pain-like responses are present in the neonate and the premature infant (Anand and Hickey 1987). However the question of pain sensation in the fetus has yet to be resolved. Given the problems of assessing whether the fetus can perceive pain, it is difficult to assess if the fetal environment contains painful stimuli. There is little chance of 'sharp' stimuli entering the fetal environment, but loud noises on the other hand can be clearly sensed by the fetus (Gagnon *et al.* 1987) and be 'painful' (Prechtl 1988).

Proprioception

The proprioceptive senses provide information about the body's position in space (vestibular sense), and the relation of bodily parts to each other (kinesthetic sense). Evidence pertaining to the kinesthetic sense is difficult to assess. Fetuses often lie in a preferred position; whether this reflects a response to kinesthetic stimulation is unknown. The vestibular sense is functioning from 25 weeks of age, since this is when the fetus exhibits a 'righting reflex' (Hooker 1952). Whether this is used to determine position prior to birth is unknown. Providing manual stimulation by rocking the fetus, either by shaking the uterus (Visser *et al.* 1983) or the head of the fetus (Issel 1983) had little effect on FHR during times of low FHR variability. Normal term fetuses exhibited no change in movement after shaking the womb (Richardson *et al.* 1981). There is no doubt that the fetus will be exposed to stimuli which stimulate the vestibular sense. The fetus does not float in the amniotic fluid as once thought (Reynolds 1962), but is susceptible to the influence of gravity. Also the motion of the mother (linear and angular acceleration) will be transmitted to the fetus. Thus the vestibular sense, if functioning, will be actively stimulated.

Vision

The fetus responds to light from 26 weeks of pregnancy. Light elicited increases in both FHR (Peleg and Goldman 1980) and movements (Polishuk *et al.* 1975). Whilst there is no doubt that the fetus can respond to light, the level of visual stimulation reaching the fetus during pregnancy is likely to be minimal. Sunbathing in a bikini during late pregnancy may provide enough stimulation for the fetus to sense. However the maternal skin will act as an effective filter, ensuring that the fetus experiences only a diffuse orange glow.

Chemosensation

Evidence is accumulating that the chemosensory environment of the fetus is rich and varied, and changes continually during pregnancy (Hepper 1990a). A variety of chemicals are present in the amniotic fluid; of these lactic and citric acids, fatty acids, uric acid, and amino acids are most likely to stimulate chemosensory receptors (Hepper 1990a). Preyer (1885) thought there could be no olfactory sensation whilst the nasal cavities were filled with amniotic fluid; however it is now known that odours dissolved in water can be sensed (Tucker 1963). Therefore both taste and olfactory receptors may be stimulated by chemicals in the amniotic fluid. Since both receptor types may be stimulated it is difficult to determine whether the response is the result of gustatory (taste) or olfactory (smell) stimulation, thus both are considered under the single heading of chemosensation. Fetuses appear to have a sweet tooth. De Snoo (1937) injected saccharin into the amniotic fluid along with a dye and observed an increased amount of dye in the mother's urine, significantly more than when the dye was injected alone. He concluded this was due to the fetus swallowing more amniotic fluid when it was sweetened. In contrast, a noxious tasting substance, Lipiodol (iodinated poppy-seed oil), led to a marked decrease in sucking when injected into the amniotic fluid (Liley 1972). Olfactory stimuli may also be perceived by diffusion from the fetal blood stream into the nasal capillary bed to stimulate the olfactory receptors (Maruniak *et al.* 1983). For example, after ingestion by the mother, garlic enters her blood stream, crosses the placenta, and enters the fetal blood stream, where it diffuses into the nasal capillary bed to stimulate the olfactory receptors and be perceived by the fetus (Hepper 1988*a*, 1990*a*). This may provide a further source of chemosensory stimulation for the fetus.

Audition

This is perhaps the most studied of all fetal abilities. The attention given to this sense reflects the ease at which auditory stimuli may be presented to the fetus. The plethora of studies on fetal audition has led to difficulties of comparison between the different studies since a variety of different techniques have been used. For example the fetus has been exposed to sounds produced by loudspeakers (Hepper and Shahidullah 1991), car horns (Peiper 1925), door buzzers (Ray 1932), vibro-acoustic stimulators (Gagnon 1989), and electric toothbrushes (Leader *et al*. 1984); sounds comprising a range of different frequencies (Madison *et al*. 1986; Lecanuet *et al*. 1989) and durations (Gelman *et al*. 1982; Goodlin and Schmidt 1972) have been used. Pure tones (Hepper and Shahidullah 1991), pink noise (Lecanuet *et al*. 1989), phonemes (Lecanuet *et al*. 1987), and music (Hepper 1988*b*) have been presented to the fetus. This sometimes bewildering array of stimuli makes it difficult to assess the auditory capabilities of the human fetus.

Until the late nineteenth century the neonate was regarded as deaf as well as dumb. In the mid 1920s two studies appeared which demonstrated that the fetus responded to sound. Peiper (1925) noted that the fetus responded to the sound of a car horn by increased movement. Forbes and Forbes (1927) presented a case study of a woman in her ninth month of pregnancy who noted an increase in movements on lying in a bath of warm water when the side of the metal bath was struck with a metal funnel. These early reports were the first to demonstrate a response to sound in the human fetus. Since this time fetal responsiveness to auditory stimuli has been repeatedly documented (Fifer and Moon 1988; Querleu *et al*. 1988). Originally it was thought that 'hearing' commences at approximately 24 weeks, but recent evidence indicates that the fetus may respond to sound earlier than this—at 16, and perhaps as early as 12, weeks of age (Hepper *et al*. 1991). Sound has been observed to elicit changes in FHR (Read and Miller 1977), eye blinks (Birnholz and Benacerraf 1983), and movements (Hepper and Shahidullah 1991). Recent studies have concentrated on observing responsiveness to a standardized vibro-acoustic stimulus (Gagnon 1989; see Chapter 15). The fetus appears to be responsive to intensity, higher intensity sounds generating a more marked response (Kisilevsky 1989). Responsiveness has been demonstrated to frequencies ranging from 83 Hz (Madison *et al*. 1986) to 5000 Hz (Lecanuet *et al*. 1989). It appears that the fetus first responds to frequencies around 250 Hz, and that the frequency range eliciting a response increases to 100 Hz, and then to 500 Hz, followed by higher frequencies (Hepper *et al*. 1991).

Having demonstrated that the fetus can hear in the womb the sound environment of the fetus should be considered. A number of studies have implanted microphones or hydrophones near the fetal head after rupture of the amniotic membranes and recorded the sound environment of the womb (Bench 1968; Henshall 1972). Major sources of sound appear to be the maternal heartbeat and vascular system, and borborygmi from the digestive system. Initially it was thought that these sounds would be so loud that external sounds would be masked (Walker *et al.* 1971), but recently it has been found that the frequency of these high amplitude sounds are too low (less than 32 Hz) to be sensed by the fetus (Querleu *et al.* 1989). It is likely therefore that external sounds can be heard by the fetus above the internal background noise. Voices other than the mother's emerge at approximately 8–12 dB above the background noise, and the mother's voice emerges at 24 dB above background (Querleu *et al.* 1988). The mother's voice appears louder to the fetus because her voice is also transmitted directly via vibrations through her body. External sounds have to pass through the maternal abdomen and through the amniotic fluid before reaching the fetus. This differentially attenuates the sound. Studies indicate attenuation of 2 dB at 250 Hz, 14 dB at 500 Hz, 20 dB at 1000 Hz, and 26 dB at 2000 Hz (Querleu *et al.* 1988). Thus the sounds sensed by the fetus will be different from those heard outside the womb. This is supported by the observation that neonates prefer the sound of their mother's voice when it is filtered to resemble that heard in the womb rather than an unfiltered 'normal' maternal voice (Fifer and Moon 1989). The quality of sounds reaching the fetus has yet to be determined. Animal studies, which recorded sounds from implanted microphones in the womb, have demonstrated that external voice sounds could be clearly understood from these recordings (Armitage *et al.* 1980; Vince *et al.* 1985). The quality of sound may be preserved further than was initially thought. Assessment of sound quality is made more difficult because the fetal ear is immersed in the amniotic fluid, and this may affect the quality of sound heard. Furthermore the auditory structures, such as the basilar membrane, are still developing during the latter stages of pregnancy (Rubel 1985), and thus the same sound presented at different gestational ages may be sensed differently by the fetus.

Fetal sensation

In 1962 an article appeared entitled 'Nature of fetal adaptation to the uterine environment: a problem of sensory deprivation' (Reynolds 1962). Research in recent years has clearly indicated that the fetus does not live in a featureless, stimulus-free, unchanging environment, but is exposed to a diverse and changing array of stimuli, which will stimulate most, if not all, of the fetal sensory modalities from early in pregnancy. The fetus is also capable of sensing his environment; from as early as eight weeks of age tactile stimulation elicits a response from the fetus. By 24 weeks and perhaps earlier, the fetus will have sensed cutaneous, chemosensory, proprioceptive, and auditory aspects of his environment. It should be noted that the fetus is not only sensing his environment by direct stimulation of his receptors by the stimuli. Information about his environment may also be acquired indirectly from the mother. In particular, information regarding circadian rhythms and day-length may be available to the fetus even though he is unable to perceive the visual stimuli required for this information directly (Reppert and Weaver 1988).

Animal studies have indicated that the circadian rhythms of the fetus are synchronized to those of their mother (Deguchi 1975; Weaver and Reppert 1987). In mammals a site on the anterior hypothalamus, the suprachiasmatic nuclei (SCN), is the circadian pacemaker generating behavioural and physiological rhythms (Moore 1983). After birth, light used to synchronize the SCN reaches this site by means of a monosynaptic retinohyothalamic pathway (Reppert and Weaver 1988). However, circadian rhythms have been found in prenatal and neonatal life before this neural pathway has innervated the SCN (Reppert and Schwartz 1983). The mother acts as a transducer between the environmental light information and the fetal brain, synchronizing her own and the fetal rhythms (Reppert and Weaver 1988). Melatonin appears crucial in the communication of information regarding day-length (Weaver and Reppert 1986), but the factors involved in the transmission of information regarding circadian phase to the fetus have yet to be fully determined; a number of different systems may be involved (Reppert and Weaver 1988). Thus, visual information, which is unlikely to be sensed by the fetus, may actually be sensed indirectly by the fetus after mediation by the mother. This strongly reinforces the view that the fetal environment is not one of sensory deprivation, but rather one of richness which variation, which will be sensed by the fetus.

Fetal learning

The first scientific study to demonstrate fetal learning was performed by Peiper in 1925. Peiper was interested in reports of fetal responses to sound during pregnancy, and examined the fetal response to 'a loud and shrill' motor car horn sounded within a few feet of the mother's abdomen during the later stages of pregnancy. He found that on initial presentation the fetus exhibited marked movements. On repeatedly presenting this stimulus, however, he found that the response exhibited by the fetus waned, until eventually the fetus no longer responded to the noise. Whilst Peiper performed the study to assess the auditory abilities of the fetus, and the study would be easy to criticize on methodological grounds, it does represent the first demonstration of learning, habituation, in the human fetus, and has since been replicated using modern technology and methodology (Hepper and Shahidullah 1992).

Learning can be defined as 'any relatively permanent change in the organism that results from past experience' (Bernstein *et al.* 1988), and is essential to human functioning, enabling the individual to acquire new skills and to adapt to his environment. Because learning is central to human functioning there has often been a certain reticence to accept that the fetus is able to learn, as if in some way learning would lose some of its importance if present in immature organisms. However there is now much evidence that learning before birth is present throughout the animal kingdom (see Hepper 1992) being documented in mammals (Hepper 1988*a*, 1990*a*; Smotherman 1982), birds (Shindler 1984), amphibians (Hepper and Waldman 1992), and even invertebrates (Isingrini *et al.* 1985). Neonates (Lipsitt 1986; Mayes 1989) and premature infants (Gekoski *et al.* 1984) are capable of learning, therefore it should not be surprising that the ability to learn is found in the fetus.

Habituation

Habituation can be defined as the decrement in response after repeated presentation of a stimulus (Thompson and Spencer 1966). Habituation is essential for the efficient functioning and survival of the organism, enabling it to ignore familiar stimuli and attend to new stimuli (Bornstein 1989). Individuals are faced with constant sensory stimulation, most of which is irrelevant. It is important to have a mechanism to disregard this and attend to important events in the environment. Habituation enables this to happen by decreasing responsiveness (attention) to familiar (repeated or constant) stimuli, but increasing responsiveness to novel stimuli. Habituation represents one of the simplest yet most essential learning processes the individual possesses, and underlies much of our functioning and development, present and future (Bornstein 1989; Hepper and Shahidullah 1992). Since the initial demonstration of habituation by Peiper (1925), a number of studies have reported habituation in the human fetus, for example habituation of body movements to a vibratory stimulus (Sontag and Wallace 1934; Leader *et al.* 1982*a*), and habituation of FHR to a pure tone (Goodlin and Lowe 1974) and pink noise (Granier-Deferre *et al.* 1985). Habituation has been demonstrated as early as 23 weeks of age and appears first in females (Leader *et al.* 1984).

One of the major problems in assessing studies of habituation is to determine whether the studies demonstrate habituation, adaptation, or motor fatigue (Hepper and Shahidullah 1992). When, after repeated presentation of a stimulus the individual stops responding, the response decrement may be the result of either adaptation, habituation, or motor fatigue. Adaptation occurs when the receptor cells or pathways become fatigued by repeated presentation of the stimulus and no longer respond. The response decrement may be the result of habituation, which has been proposed to result from more central factors, possibly self-generated transmission depression occurring somewhere in the pathway linking sensory receptors to the neurones controlling the response. The individual no longer responds, but the receptor cells are still able to respond if stimulated. Finally, the lack of response may be the result of fatigue in the response system; the muscle becomes tired and, despite receiving the appropriate signals, is unable to respond. Thus although able to sense the stimuli the individual is unable to respond. It is important that studies demonstrate habituation rather than either adaptation or response fatigue. Both adaptation and motor fatigue pose particular problems for fetal research given the immature state of the fetal physiological system, which may have a poor capacity for sustained responding. However appropriate methodology, in particular dishabituation, where the presentation of a novel stimulus elicits the response again, although rarely used, can distinguish between these different factors, and there is little doubt that the fetus can habituate in the womb (Hepper and Shahidullah 1992).

Classical conditioning

The first demonstration of what is today called classical conditioning was performed by Pavlov (1906) while working on the digestive system of dogs. Classical conditioning involves the pairing of an unconditioned stimulus (UCS), which elicits an unconditioned response (UCR), with the conditioned stimulus (CS), which is initially neutral and does not elicit the UCR, but after a number of pairings with the UCS, comes to elicit the conditioned response (CR). In Pavlov's demonstration meat powder was used as the UCS which when presented to the dog caused the dog to salivate, the UCR. A buzzer was used as the CS, which initially elicited no salivation; however after a number of pairings with the UCS, the meat powder, the buzzer alone elicited salivation (the CR).

A few studies have attempted to demonstrate classical conditioning in the human fetus. An initial study was reported by Ray (1932), when vibration, produced by an electric bell-striker hitting a wooden plate, was used as the CS and paired with a loud sound, the UCS. Although no data are reported, the last line of the paper reports that the subject of the experiment had 'so far, shown no ill-effects from her prenatal education' (Ray 1932, p. 177). Spelt (1948) repeated the experiment again using vibration from a doorbell as the CS and a loud sound from a wooden clapper as the UCS. He reported successful conditioning (i.e. the fetus responding to the vibration stimulus) during the last 2 months of pregnancy after approximately 15 to 20 pairings. It is interesting to note, given the use of acoustic-vibratory stimulation today (Gagnon 1989), that here it was used as a CS (i.e. a neutral stimulus eliciting no response). I have recently replicated Spelt's experiment using a 500 Hz auditory tone as the CS and a vibration (120 Hz) as the UCS, and found conditioning as early as 5.5 months of age (Hepper, submitted).

Feijoo (1975, 1981) classically conditioned 23 women using relaxation as the UCS paired with a sound (12 second burst of music) as the CS. Feijoo reports that before birth presentation of the sound stimulus reduced the latency for fetal movements to occur. After birth, fetuses that were stimulated between 22 and 36 weeks stopped crying, opened their eyes, and showed fewer clonic movements. Twenty-four pairings of the CS with the UCS were sufficient to induce these effects.

Instrumental or operant conditioning used by Thorndike (1898), but made popular by B. F. Skinner (1938) has not been demonstrated in the human fetus to my knowledge, although it has been documented in neonates (Rovee-Collier and Fagan 1981). Other studies examining fetal learning have not used a particular learning paradigm, but have exposed the fetus to a stimulus before birth and then observed his response after birth. These studies fall into three main areas.

Maternal voice

One of the most elegant series of studies examining the neonate's abilities are those examining response to his mother's voice (Fifer and Moon 1989). The possibility that the fetus hears voices in the womb has long been acknowledged, 'For behold, when the voice of your greeting came to my ears, the babe in my womb lept for joy'. (Luke 1:44). DeCasper and Fifer (1980) used the neonate's ability to suck to provide an indication of preference for his mother's voice. Sucking proceeds as a burst of sucks separated by an interval when no sucking occurs, and then a further burst of sucking, and so on. During a base-line period the mean time between sucking, the inter-burst interval, was calculated for each subject. Subjects were then placed into one of two conditions. In the first if the subject reduced the time between bursts of sucking below that of his mean he heard the voice of his mother through headphones; if he stopped sucking for longer than his mean interval he heard the voice of another woman. The second group underwent an identical procedure, but in reverse; in order to hear their mother's voice they had to increase the time between bursts of sucking, and reducing this produced the voice of another woman. The subjects were found to alter their sucking in order to receive the voice of their mother. This preference appears to be acquired before birth. Using a similar paradigm as above subjects were found to alter their sucking pattern to hear a story that had been read to them in the womb rather than an unfamiliar story (DeCasper and Spence 1986). Individuals show no preference for their father's voice (DeCasper and Prescott 1984), which may be due to masking of the lower frequency father's voice by internal sounds of the mother (Fifer and Moon 1989). It is possible that the mother's voice is also perceived by vibration resulting from the production of sounds transmitted through the mother's body. Recent work has examined the preference of neonates for the sound of their mother's voice as we would hear it, compared to the sound of the mother's voice filtered to sound as the fetus would hear it after passing through the mother's abdomen. It was found that the neonates preferred the sound of the mother's voice as the fetus would hear it (Fifer and Moon 1989). This result strongly suggests that the fetus perceives the sound of his mothers' voice whilst in the womb, and this prenatal auditory experience can influence postnatal auditory preferences.

Maternal heartbeat

Other research has examined the response of the neonate and the infant to the sound of maternal heartbeat. Salk (1960) proposed that the fetus imprints onto the sound of his mother's heartbeat and that this influences his response after birth. Initial studies by Salk (1960; 1962) examined the response of neonates between 1 and 4 days of age. One group was played a heartbeat sound at 72 beats/minute at 85 dB continually, whilst the control group were not played this sound. It was found that the group listening to the heartbeat sound showed a greater gain in weight than those not hearing the heartbeat over the first 4 days of life (+40 grams and −20 grams, respectively). There was no difference between the groups in the amount of food taken, but the control group cried more. Follow-up studies on infants 16 to 37 months of age, with one individual 50 months of age, indicated that those played the sound of a heartbeat at 72 beats/minute fell asleep faster than those played either a metronome at 72 beats/minute, or lullabies, or given no sound. Since this original report a number of studies have attempted to replicate the result with mixed success. Overall the weight of evidence seems to suggest that the maternal heartbeat sound does reduce arousal in neonates (Detterman 1978). It is questionable, however, whether this is the result of prenatal learning, imprinting of the maternal heartbeat, or the result of some genetic predisposition (Hepper 1989). There is little doubt that the maternal heartbeat sound is reinforcing for the neonate (DeCasper and Sigafoos 1983), but whether this reflects a learned or genetic preference has yet to be determined.

Music

The final series of studies has looked at the response of neonates to music played during their time in the womb. Hepper (1988b) demonstrated that neonates showed a response to the theme tunes of particular 'soap operas' watched by the mother during pregnancy. In this study two groups of neonates were examined for their response to the theme tune of the popular soap opera *Neighbours*. One group were born to mothers who watched the programme whilst pregnant, the other group born to mothers who had not watched the programme. Neonates born to the mothers who watched *Neighbours* stopped crying and adopted a 'quiet alert' behavioural state on hearing the tune, neonates of mothers who had not watched the programme showed no reaction to the tune. The reaction was specific to the theme tune; other tunes or the same tune played backwards elicited no response on the part of the neonate. Similar studies with similar results have also been reported (Feijoo 1981).

These studies demonstrate that the fetus can learn. The time at which the fetus can first learn has yet to be determined, but there is little doubt that the fetus can and does learn whilst in the womb. They also demonstrate that stimuli experienced by the fetus become preferred by their prenatal exposure and as such affect the individual's response to them after birth. The process by which these stimuli acquire their preferential quality is unknown, but is presumably related to increased familiarity caused by prenatal exposure. The ability to learn also has implications for other aspects of functioning. The fetus has the ability to associate events, as demonstrated by classical conditioning paradigms. Furthermore the retention of prenatal learning experiences indicates the presence, in some form, of a memory. Much more research is required before these abilities are fully understood.

Functions of fetal sensation and learning

The preceding pages have beyond doubt indicated that the fetal environment is one of diversity and change, and can be sensed by the fetus; furthermore, the fetus is capable of learning about his environment, and these prenatal experiences influence his behaviour after birth. Given that the fetus possesses these abilities, some consideration should be given to the function they may serve. It has been proposed that prenatal and birth experiences can profoundly influence later development and behaviour, to the extent of inducing a variety of psychiatric disorders in the individual later in life (Ridgway 1981). However there is little scientific validity to these claims and I shall not consider them here (Hepper 1989).

Neural development

One of the major tasks of the prenatal period is the development of the individual from a single cell to an organized and cohesive cellular structure with an integrated neural system. A role for early neural activity in the design of the nervous system is no longer in doubt (Greenough *et al.* 1987), and there is much evidence in the neuromuscular system that neural activity plays an important role in the development of this system (Purves and Lichtman 1985). The role of the sensory experiences in influencing future neural develoment is less well understood. However, it is likely that prenatal experiences are important for the development of sensory and sensorimotor systems. At a very general level activity promotes growth and dendritic branching of individual neurons, and thus sensation from the receptor cells may promote the development of the neural system. Post-natally there is much evidence that sensory experiences play a critical role in the development of central sensory processing systems. For example feature detectors within the visual system responsive to orientation require experience of these orientations after birth to be maintained (Hirsch and Spinelli 1970). It may be that prenatal sensory experiences play an important priming role in structuring this system, which is built up upon by postnatal experience. Furthermore, the fact that the fetus experiences sensation in a number of different modalities, and possibly at the same time, for example, the mother's voice may stimulate both auditory and cutaneous receptors, may play a role in the development of inter-modal neural connections.

As well as a role in tuning the neural system, prenatal sensory experience may serve as a 'running-in' period for the sensory systems. Some low level experience may be essential for the newly-developed systems to function before coping with the greater intensity of sensations experienced after birth. Thus sensory experience may play an important role in the development of the individual's sensory neural structure. There can be little doubt that learning experiences early in the individual's life, especially during the formation of the neural system, may have a permanent effect on it. Experiential effects may increase neural growth, either by increasing arborization and/or connections within the system (Wittrock 1980). These experiential effects may increase the child's ability to learn and maintain information. Thus prenatal sensory and learning experiences may, by enhancing neural development, provide the foundation for future learning abilities. A role for experience in shaping the developing neural system allows the incorporation of greater flexibility and plasticity in the structure of the nervous system, which may in turn enable more adaptivity to the environment on the part of the individual.

Communication

Communication forms a major role in all individual functioning, and the ability to use language is central to this. Exactly how language is learned has yet to be fully determined, but there is no doubt that experience with language in the early stages of life is essential for its acquisition. It is possible that this may commence in the womb. As I have previously discussed, the mother's voice and other voices can be clearly 'heard' by the fetus above the background level of noise. There is much evidence that the prosodic elements of speech (i.e. intonation, stress, and rhythm) are little affected by attenuation by the maternal abdomen and will thus be experienced 'intact' by the fetus. Infants pay attention to the prosodic elements of speech and this may have resulted from prenatal experience (Fifer and Moon 1989). Intrauterine auditory experience appears to convey rhythmic information to the fetus, and numerous studies have demonstrated the ease with which rhythmic auditory stimuli are learned by the fetus (Hepper 1988; Salk 1966). Social interactions after birth require turn-taking, based upon rhythmicity. For example, a conversation requires one person to talk, the other to listen, and then the roles are reversed. Rhythm, which is important for later social interactions, may be initially experienced in the womb.

Breast-feeding

Prenatal experiences are important for the initiation and maintenance of sucking in animals (Pedersen and Blass 1982), and the success of sucking may be influenced by manipulation of the chemosensory environment of the fetus via the dietary intake of the mother (Hepper 1990a). Recently, I examined the role of diet in the initiation of breast-feeding in the human neonate. Two groups of mothers were studied; one group of mothers had maintained a similar diet before and after birth, while the other group of mothers had dramatically changed their diet before and after the birth. This second group was composed of individuals who ate a very spicy diet prior to the birth, but a less spicy diet on admission to hospital. It was found that mothers who had maintained their diet were much more successful in initiating breast-feeding than the mothers who had changed their diet and that their infants took more food (Hepper, unpublished observations). This may be the result of prenatal familiarity with the maternal diet. The mother's milk contains information regarding her diet (Galef and Sherry 1973). Infants whose mothers ate the same diet before and after the birth experienced this diet both prenatally and in their mother's breast-milk. These individuals were thus familiar with the 'taste' of their mother's breast-milk and, therefore, show no hesitation in sucking. Infants whose mothers had a different diet before and after the birth will have had no prenatal experience of the 'taste' of their breast-milk and this may cause hesitation in feeding. Given the importance of successful breast-feeding for infant survival, although not so relevant today given the prevalence of bottle-feeding, it is to be expected that a mechanism to ensure that sucking is successfully initiated will exist.

Socialization and attachment

Prenatal learning may be important for the development of attachment and for social development of the individual. Conspecific preferences of a variety of animals are learned prenatally; ants, bees, wasps, amphibians, birds, and mammals, learn about their conspecifics prior to birth (Hepper 1992). Alterations in these experiences can profoundly affect later preferences (Hepper 1990a). One striking example of this is reported by Shindler (1984) where chick eggs were played the sound of a natural predator, a red-shouldered hawk. After birth when given a choice between the call of their mother and that of the hawk the chicks preferred the call of the hawk. There is little doubt that prenatal experiences are important in determining later preferences, and this is important in ensuring that these individuals learn about related individuals (Hepper 1986). In humans there is much evidence that neonates can recognize the voice (Fifer and Moon 1988), and odour (Porter 1991) of their mother, which may be the result of prenatal learning. This prenatal learning may promote the attachment of the individual. Secure attachment is essential for later postnatal social development (Ainsworth *et al.* 1978), and this attachment may be primed before birth (Hepper 1990a).

Clinical applications

Given that the individual can experience his environment, it should be considered whether this information is of use in the clinical management of the fetus. There is no doubt that the behaviour of the fetus can be used to assess his condition (Hepper 1990b). At a very general level the ability to learn implies that the fetus has a certain level of sensory competence, and associative and memory capabilities, with concomitant mediating neural structures. Assessment of fetal learning may be used to discover deficiencies, which in turn may be indicators of some disorder in the fetus. If learning is to be used to assess the condition of the fetus then information regarding abilities of the 'normal' population is required. Furthermore some correlation between any prenatal abnormalities in learning and postnatal behaviour or neural structure, must be demonstrated. Research on these aspects of development is only just commencing. However one technique, which looks promising and may well be used in the future, is that of habituation. Deficits in habituation performance have been reported after birth in hyperactive children (Hutt and Hutt 1964), schizophrenics (Gruzelier and Venables 1972), and Down's syndrome (Dustman and Callner 1979). Furthermore habituation performance during the first year of life is predictive of later cognitive functioning (Bornstein and Sigman 1986; Rose and Wallace 1985). Preliminary studies of the fetus have indicated habituation abnormalities in microcephalics, anencephalics, individuals with meconium staining, and low birth-weight individuals, (Leader *et al.* 1982*b*; Leader *et al.* 1984), but others have not reported these deficits (Bennett 1984). Transient maternal conditions such as smoking, reduction of oxygen, and the administration of drugs disrupt the normal habituation pattern (Leader and Bennett 1988; Leader and Baille 1988). Most recently habituation disorders have been found in fetuses diagnosed as trisomy 21 (Hepper and Shahidullah 1992). Furthermore, this study indicated that the severity of handicap was related to the decrement in habituation performance. Habituation may be used to assess the condition of the fetus and to enable the identification of the 'at-risk' individual.

Geniuses in the womb!!!

The ability of the fetus to learn and experience aspects of its environment has been taken to the extreme by the creation of 'Pre-Natal Universities', in which pregnant women enrol for a course of stimulation aimed to increase the development of their child. Ideas regarding stimulation of the fetus are not new. The Talmudic writings of second to sixth century Jews contain references to prenatal stimulation programmes. Recent years have seen much interest in the effects of early stimulation on later achievement, or 'hot-housing'. A general conclusion from studies examining early intensive education after birth is that stimulation can increase abilities, but not to the extent of producing geniuses (Howe 1988).

Programmes of fetal stimulation are relatively new and experimental evidence regarding their success is lacking. There is some evidence to suggest that prenatal stimulation enhances the neonates physical development and maturation (van de Carr *et al.* 1988). Graduates of the Pre-Natal University are reported to show greater physical and mental development than neonates who had not attended the 'University' (Warmsley and Margolis 1987). The principle behind these stimulation programmes is that prenatal stimulation can enhance neural development and, to a certain extent, prevent the neural cell die-off. There is evidence that stimulation can enhance nerve cell development (Wittrock 1980), and animal studies have indicated that programmes of enrichment do increase neural development in certain brain regions (Diamond 1988). These animal studies should be questioned, however, since it is not clear whether the results are due to the effect of enrichment or deprivation. Although there is much anecdotal evidence that such stimulation programmes work, scientific evidence is lacking. My own studies indicate that there may be some benefits resulting from prenatal stimulation, but this appears to be not the result of stimulation *per se*, but rather the result of increasing the interest of the mother in her pregnancy, which has 'knock-on' effects for development after birth (Hepper, unpublished observations).

Conclusions

As studies proceed there is now little doubt that the fetus does not face the problem of sensory deprivation, but experiences a rich diversity of sensations. Just as studies have indicated that the fetus possesses a sophisticated behavioural repertoire and behavioural states (see Chapter 3), there is now clear evidence that more psychological aspects of human functioning are present in the fetus (i.e. sensation and learning). Further work is required to elucidate the quality of these sensations and the development of learning abilities, but there can be little doubt that the origins of human abilities can be traced to the prenatal period. The functions of these experiences have yet to be fully determined, some speculations have been offered here, and future research will undoubtedly further reveal the importance of this period for later development. Fetal psychology, although in many respects an embryonic science, has drawn on its past 100 years of experience to assess that most complex of subjects, behaviour, and having learned from its previous mistakes in assessing neonatal abilities has started to unravel the origins of human behavioural abilities. Much work is still to be done, but there can be no doubt that the neonate arrives in the world with a behavioural repertoire that is structured, shaped, and refined by its experiences of the preceding nine months, which forms the foundation for the development of individual's future abilities.

Acknowledgements

I thank Professor Ken Brown, Dr Sara Shahidullah, and Fiona Hepper for their comments on this manuscript. I acknowledge the support of NATO, The British Council, and The Northern Ireland Mother and Baby Appeal, and thank Professor Ken Brown for providing facilities for this research.

References

Ainsworth, M. D. S., Blehar, M. C., Waters, E., and Wall, S. (1978). *Patterns of attachment*. Lawrence Erlbaum, Hillsdale.

Allen, M. C. and Capute, A. J. (1986). Assessment of early auditory and visual abilities of extremely premature infants. *Developmental Medicine and Child Neurology* **28**, 458–66.

Anand, K. J. S. and Hickey, P. R. (1987). Pain and its effects in the human neonate and fetus. *The New England Journal of Medicine* **317**, 1321–9.

Aristotle (1982). *De Generatione Animalium* (translation). Oxford University Press, Oxford.

Armitage, S. E., Baldwin, B. A., and Vince, M. A. (1980). The fetal sound environment of sheep. *Science* **208**, 1173–4.

Aslin, R. N. (1985). Oculomotor measures of visual development. In: *Measurement of audition and vision in the first year of postnatal life: a methodological overview* (ed. G. Gottlieb and N. A. Krasnegor), pp. 391–417. Ablex, Norwood.

Baxi, L. V., Randolph, P., and Miller, K. (1988). Fetal heart rate response to intrauterine saline solution flush. *American Journal of Obstetrics and Gynecology* **159**, 547–9.

Bench, R. J. (1968). Sound transmission to the human fetus through the maternal abdominal wall. *Journal of Genetic Psychology* **113**, 85–7.

Bennett, M. J. (1984). The assessment of fetal well-being. In: *Ultrasound in perinatal care* (ed. M. J. Bennett), pp. 117–26. Wiley, London.

Bernstein, D. A., Roy, E. J., Wickens, C. D., and Srull, T. K. (1988). *Psychology*. Houghton Mifflin, Boston.

Birnholz, J. C. and Benacerraf, B. R. (1983). The development of human fetal hearing. *Science* **222**, 516–18.

Bornstein, M. H. (1989). Stability in early mental development: From attention and information processing in infancy to learning and cognition in childhood. In: *Stability and continuity in mental development* (ed. M. H. Bornstein and N. A. Krasnegor), pp. 147–70. Lawrence Erlbaum, New Jersey.

Bornstein, M. H. and Sigman, M. D. (1986). Continuity in mental development from infancy. *Child Development* **57**, 251–74.

Carmichael, L. (1954). The onset and early development of behavior. In: *Manual of child psychology*. (2nd edn) (ed. L. Carmichael), pp. 60–185 J. Wiley, New York.

Carr, K. van de, Carr, R. van de, and Lehrer, M. (1988). Effects of prenatal intervention program. In: *Prenatal and perinatal psychology and medicine* (ed. P. Fedor-Freybergh and M. L. V. Vogel), pp. 489–96. Parthenon, Carnforth.

DeCasper, A. J. and Fifer, W. P. (1980). Of human bonding: newborns prefer their mothers' voices. *Science* **208**, 1174–6.

DeCasper, A. J. and Prescott, P. A. (1984). Human newborns' perception of male voices: preference, discrimination and reinforcing value. *Developmental Psychobiology* **17**, 481–91.

DeCasper, A. J. and Sigafoos, A. D. (1983). The intrauterine heartbeat: a potent reinforcer for neonates. *Infant Behavior and Development* **6**, 19–25.

DeCasper, A. J. and Spence, M. J. (1986). Prenatal maternal speech influences newborns' perception of speech sound. *Infant Behavior and Development* **9**, 133–50.

Deguchi, T. (1975). Ontogenesis of a biological clock for serotonin:acetyl coenzyme A N-acetyltransferase in the pineal gland of rat. *Proceedings of the National Academy of Sciences USA* **72**, 2914–20.

De Snoo, K. (1937). Das trinkende Kind im Uterus. *Monatsschr. Geburtsh Gynaekol* **105**, 88–97.

Detterman, D. K. (1978). The effect of heartbeat on neonatal crying. *Infant Behavior and Development* **1**, 36–48.

Diamond, M. C. 1988). *Enriching heredity*. The Free Press, New York.

Diels, H. (1906). *Fragmente der Vorsokratiker*, Weidmannsche Buchhandlung, Berlin.

Dustman, R. E. and Callner, D. A. (1979). Cortical evoked response and response decrement in non-retarded and Down's syndrome individuals. *American Journal of Mental Deficiency* **83**, 391–7.

Ellis, H. (1940). *Studies in the psychology of sex*. Random House, New York.

Fantz, R. L. and Nevis, S. (1967). Pattern preferences and perceptual cognitive development in early infancy. *Merrill-Palmer Quarterly* **13**, 77–108.

Feijoo, J. (1975). Ut conscientia Noscatue. *Cahier de Sophrologie* **13**, 14–20.

Feijoo, J. (1981). Le foetus Pierre et le loup . . . ou une approche originale de l'audition prenatale humaine. In: *L'aube des Sens* (ed. E. Herbinet and M. C. Busnel). Stock, Paris.

Fifer, W. P. and Moon, C. (1988). Auditory experience in the fetus. In: *Behavior of the fetus* (ed. W. P. Smotherman and S. R. Robinson), pp. 175–88. Caldwell, Telford.

Fifer, W. P. and Moon, C. (1989). Psychobiology of newborn auditory preferences. *Seminars in Perinatology* **13**, 430–3.

Forbes, H. S. and Forbes, H. B. (1927). Fetal sense reaction: hearing. *Journal of Comparative Psychology* **7**, 353–5.

Gagnon, R. (1989). Stimulation of human fetuses with sound and vibration. *Seminars in Perinatology* **13**, 393–402.

Gagnon, R., Hunse, C., Carmichael, L., Fellows, F., and Patrick, J. (1987). External vibratory acoustic stimulation near term: fetal heart rate and heart rate variability responses. *American Journal of Obstetrics and Gynecology* **156**, 323–7.

Galef, B. G. and Sherry, D. F. (1973). Mother's milk: a medium for transmission of cues reflecting the flavour of the mothers diet. *Journal of Comparative and Physiological Psychology* **83**, 374–8.

Gekoski, M. J., Fagan, J. W., and Pearlman, M. A. (1984). Early learning and memory in the preterm infants. *Infant Behavior and Development* **7**, 267–76.

Gelman, S. R., Wood, S., Spellacy, W. N., and Abrams, R. M. (1982). Fetal movements in response to sound stimulation. *American Journal of Obstetrics and Gynecology* **143**, 484–5.

Goodlin, R. C. and Schmidt, W. (1972). Human fetal arousal levels as indicated by heart rate recordings. *American Journal of Obstetrics and Gynecology* **114**, 613–21.

Goodlin, R. C. and Lowe, E. W. (1974). Multiphasic fetal monitoring. A preliminary evaluation. *American Journal of Obstetrics and Gynecology* **119**, 341–57.

Graham, H. (1951). *Eternal Eve, the history of gynecology and obstetrics*. Doubleday, New York.

Granier-Deferre, C., Lecanuet, J. P., Cohen, H., and Busnel, M. C. (1985). Feasibility of prenatal hearing test. *Acta Otolaryngologica (Stockholm)*, Supplement **421**, 93–101.

Greenough, W. T., Black, J. E., and Wallace, C. S. (1987). Experience and brain development. *Child Development* **58**, 539–59.

Gruzelier, J. H. and Venables, P. H. (1972). Skin conductance orienting activity in a heterogeneous sample of schizophrenics. *Journal of Nervous and Mental Disorders* **155**, 277–87.

Haith, M. M., Bergman, T., and Moore, M. J. (1977). Eye contact and face scanning in early infancy. *Science* **198**, 853–5.

Henshall, W. R. (1972). Intra-uterine sound levels. *American Journal of Obstetrics and Gynecology* **112**, 576–8.

Hepper, P. G. (1986). Kin recognition: functions and mechanisms. A review. *Biological Reviews of The Cambridge Philosophical Society* **61**, 63–93.

Hepper, P. G. (1988*a*). Adaptive fetal learning: Prenatal exposure to garlic affects postnatal preferences. *Animal Behaviour* **36**, 935–6.

Hepper, P. G. (1988*b*). Foetal 'soap' addiction. *The Lancet* (11th June), 1347–8.

Hepper, P. G. (1989). Foetal learning: implications for psychiatry? *British Journal of Psychiatry* **155**, 289–93.

Hepper, P. G. (1990*a*). Foetal olfaction. In: *Chemical signals in vertebrates V* (ed. D. W. Macdonald, D. Müller-Schwarze, and S. E. Natynczuk), pp. 282–8. Oxford University Press, Oxford.

Hepper, P. G. (1990*b*). Diagnosing handicap using the behaviour of the fetus. *Midwifery* **6**, 193–200.

Hepper, P. G. (ed.) (1992). Comparative prenatal learning and behaviour. *Quarterly Journal of Experimental Psychology* (special issue). In press.

Hepper, P. G. and Shahidullah, S. (1992). Habituation in normal and Down Syndrome fetuses. *Quarterly Journal of Experimental Psychology*. In press.

Hepper, P. G. and Waldman, B. (1992). Embryonic learning in an amphibian. *Quarterly Journal of Experimental Psychology*. In press.

Hepper, P. G., Shahidullah, S. and White, R. (1990). Fetal handedness? *Nature* **347**, 431.

Hepper, P. G., White, R., and Shahidullah, S. (1991). The development of fetal responsiveness to external auditory stimulation. *British Psychological Society Abstracts*, p. 30.

Hill, L. M., Platt, L. D., and Manning, F. A. (1979). Immediate effect of amniocentesis on fetal breathing and gross body movements. *American Journal of Obstetrics and Gynecology* **135**, 689–90.

Hirsch, H. V. B. and Spinelli, D. N. (1970). Visual experience modifies distribution of horizontally and vertically oriented receptive fields in cats. *Science* **168**, 869–71.

Hooker, D. (1952). *The prenatal origin of behavior*. University of Kansas Press, Kansas.

Howe, M. J. A. (1988). 'Hot-House' children. *The Psychologist* **1**, 356–8.

Humphrey, T. (1966). The development of trigeminal nerve fibers to the oral mucosa compared with their development to cutaneous surfaces. *Journal of Comparative Neurology* **126**, 91–108.

Hutt, S. J. and Hutt, C. (1964). Hyperactivity in a group of epileptic (and some non-epileptic) brain damaged children. *Epilepsia* **5**, 334–51.

Isingrini, M., Lenoir, A., and Jaisson, P. (1985). Preimaginal learning as a basis of colony-brood recognition in the ant, *Cataglyphis cursor*. *Proceedings of the National Academy of Sciences USA* **82**, 8545–7.

Issel, E. P. (1983). Fetal response to external mechanical stimuli. *Journal of Perinatal Medicine* **11**, 232–42.

James, W. (1890). *The principles of psychology*. Holt, New York.

Kisilevsky, B. S., Muir, D. W., and Low, J. A. (1989). Human fetal responses to sound as a function of stimulus intensity. *Obstetrics and Gynecology* **73**, 971–6.

Krasnegor, N. A., Blass, E. M., Hofer, M. A., and Smotherman, W. P. (1987). *Perinatal development. A psychobiological perspective*. Academic Press, London.

Leader, L. R. and Baille, P. (1988). The changes in fetal habituation patterns due to a decrease in inspired maternal oxygen. *British Journal of Obstetrics and Gynaecology* **95**, 664–8.

Leader, L. R. and Bennett, M. J. (1988). Fetal habituation. In: *Fetal and neonatal neurology and neurosurgery* (ed. M. I. Levene, M. J. Bennett, and J. Punt), pp. 59–70. Churchill Livingstone, Edinburgh.

Leader, L. R., Baille, P., Martin, B., and Vermeulen, E. (1982*a*). The assessment and significance of habituation to a repeated stimulus by the human foetus. *Early Human Development* **7**, 211–9.

Leader, L. R., Baille, P., Martin, B, and Vermeulen, E. (1982*b*). Foetal habituation in high risk pregnancies. *British Journal of Obstetrics and Gynaecology* **89**, 441–6.

Leader, L. R., Baille, P., Martin, B., Molteno, C., and Wynchank, S. (1984). Foetal responses to vibrotactile stimulation. A possible predictor of foetal and neonatal outcome. *Australian and New Zealand Journal of Obstetrics and Gynaecology* **24**, 251–6.

Lecanuet, J-P., Granier-Deferre, C., DeCasper, A. J., Maugeais, R., Andrieu, A-J., and Busnel, M. C. (1987). Perception et discrimination foetales de stimuli langagiers; mise en évidence à partir de la réactivité cardiaque; résultats préliminaires. *C. R. Comptes Rendus Hebdomadaires des seances, Academie des Sciences, Paris* **305**, 161–4.

Lecanuet, J. P., Granier-Deferre, C., and Busnel, M-C. (1988). Fetal cardiac and motor response to octave-band noises as a function of central frequency, intensity and heart rate variability. *Early Human Development* **18**, 81–93.

Lecanuet, J. P., Granier-Deferre, C., and Busnel, M.-C. (1989). Differential fetal auditory reactiveness as a function of stimulus charactersitics and state. *Seminars in Perinatology* **13**, 421–9.

Liley, A. W. (1972). The foetus as a personality. *Australian and New Zealand Journal of Psychiatry* **6**, 99–105.

Lipsitt, L. P. (1986). Learning in infancy: Cognitive development in babies. *The Journal of Pediatrics* **109**, 172–82.

Madison, L. S., Adubato, S. A., Madison, J. K., Nelson, R. M., Anderson, J. C., Erickson, J., Kuss, L. M., and Goodlin, R. C. (1986). Foetal response decrement: true habituation. *Developmental and Behavioral Pediatrics* **7**, 14–20.

Maruniak, J. A., Silver, W. L., and Moulton, D. G. (1983). Olfactory receptors respond to blood-borne odorants. *Brain Research* **265**, 312–6.

Mayes, L. C. (1989). Investigations of learning processes in infants. *Seminars in Perinatology* **13**, 437–49.

Meltzoff, A. and Moore, M. K. (1983). The origins of imitation in infancy: paradigm, phenomena and theories. *Advances in Infancy Research* **2**, 265–301.

Moore, R. Y. (1983). Organisation and function of a central nervous system circadian oscillator: the suprachiasmatic hypothalamic nucleus. *Federation Proceedings* **42**, 2783–9.

Nijhuis, J. G. (1986). Behavioural states: concomitants, clinical implications and the assessment of the condition of the nervous system. *European Journal of Obstetrics and Gynecology and Reproductive Biology* **21**, 301–8.

Pavlov, I. (1906). Scientific study of the so-called psychical processes in the higher animals. *The Lancet* **ii**, 911–15.

Pedersen, P. E. and Blass, E. M. (1982). Prenatal and post-natal determinants of the first suckling episode in albino rats. *Developmental Psychobiology* **15**, 349–55.

Peiper, A. (1925). Sinnesempfindungen des Kindes vor seiner geburt. *Monatsschrift fur Kinderheilkunde* **29**, 237–41.

Peleg, D. and Goldman, J. A. (1980). Fetal heart rate acceleration in response to light stimulation as a clinical measure of fetal well-being. A preliminary report. *Journal of Perinatal Medicine* **8**, 38–41.

Polishuk, W. Z., Laufer, N., and Sadovsky, E. (1975). Fetal reaction to external light. *Harefuah* **89**, 395–7.

Porter, R. H. (1991). Mutual mother-infant recognition in humans. In: *Kin recognition* (ed. P. G. Hepper), pp. 413–32. Cambridge University Press, Cambridge.

Prechtl, H. F. R. (1988). Developmental neurology of the fetus. *Clinical Obstetrics and Gynaecology* **2**, 21–36.

Preyer, W. (1881). *The mind of the child. Part 1. The senses and the will*. New York, Appleton.

Preyer, W. (1885). *Die spezielle physiologie des embryo*. Grieben, Leipzig.

Purves, D. and Lichtman, J. W. (1985). *Principles of neural development*. Sinauer Assoc., Sunderland MA.

Querleu, D., Renard, X., Versyp, F., Paris-Delrue, L., and Crepin, G. (1988). Fetal hearing. *European Journal of Obstetrics and Gynecology and Reproductive Biology* **29**, 191–212.

Querleu, D, Renard, X., Boutteville, C., and Crepin, G. (1989). Hearing by the human fetus? *Seminars in Perinatology* **13**, 409–20.

Rau, H. (1982). Frühe Kindheit. In: *Entwicklungspsychologie* (ed. R. Oerter and L. Montada), pp. 67–93. Urban & Schwarzenberg, Wien.

Ray, W. S. (1932). A preliminary report on a study of foetal conditioning. *Child Development* **3**, 175–7.

Read, J. and Miller, F. (1977). Fetal heart rate acceleration in response to acoustic stimulation as a measure of fetal well-being. *American Journal of Obstetrics and Gynecology* **129**, 512–7.

Reppert, S. M. and Schwartz, W. J. (1983). Maternal coordination of the fetal biological clock *in utero*. *Science* **220**, 969–71.

Reppert, S. M. and Weaver, D. R. (1988). Maternal transduction of light-dark information for the fetus. In: *Behavior of the Fetus* (ed. W. P. Smothermann and S. R. Robinson), pp. 119–39. Caldwell, Telford.

Reynolds, S. R. M. (1962). Nature of fetal adaptation to the uterine environment: a problem of sensory deprivation. *American Journal of Obstetrics and Gynecology* **83**, 800–8.

Richardson, B., Campbell, K., Carmichael, L., and Patrick, J. (1981). Effects of external physical stimulation on fetuses near term. *American Journal of Obstetrics and Gynecology* **139**, 344–52.

Ridgeway, R. (1981). Foetal memory: fact or fiction? *BMA News Review* (April), 13–18.

Ron, M., Yaffe, H., and Polishuk, W. Z. (1976). Fetal heart rate response to amniocentesis in cases of decreased fetal movements. *Obstetrics and Gynecology* **48**, 456–9.

Rose, S. A. and Wallace, I. F. (1985). Visual recognition memory: A predictor of later cognitive functioning in preterms. *Child Development* **56**, 843–52.

Rovee-Collier, C. K. and Fagen, J. W. (1981). The retrieval of memory in early infancy. *Advances in Infancy Research* **1**, 226–54.

Rubel, E. W. (1985). Auditory system development. In: *Measurement of audition and vision in the first year of postnatal life: a methodological overview* (ed. G. Gottlieb and N. A. Krasnegor). pp. 53–90. Ablex, Norwood.

Salk, L. (1960). The effects of the normal heartbeat sound on the behaviour of the newborn infant: Implications for mental health. *World Mental Health* **12**, 168–75.

Salk, L. (1962). Mothers' heartbeat as an imprinting stimulus. *Transactions of the New York Academy of Science* **24**, 753–63.

Shindler, K. M. (1984). A three year study of fetal auditory imprinting. *Journal of the Washington Academy of Science* **74**, 121–4.

Skinner, B. F. (1938). *The behaviour of organisms.* Appleton Century, New York.

Smotherman, W. P. (1982). Odor aversion learning by the rat fetus. *Physiology and Behavior* **29**, 769–71.

Smotherman, W. P. and Robinson, S. R. (1988). *The behavior of the fetus.* Telford, New Jersey.

Sontag, L. W. (1966). Implications of fetal behaviour and environment for adult personalities. *Annals of the New York Academy of Sciences* **134**, 782–6.

Sontag, L. W. and Wallace, R. F. (1934). Preliminary report of the Fels Fund. Study of fetal activity. *American Journal of Diseases of Children* **48**, 1050–7.

Spelt, D. K. (1948). The conditioning of the human fetus *in utero*. *Journal of Experimental Psychology* **38**, 338–46.

Suśruta, Suśrutasamhita (Sarirasthanam and Cikitsasthanam) (1954). Ambikadatta Sastri (ed.) Chowkhamba Sanskrit Series Office, Benares.

Thompson, R. F. and Spencer, W. A. (1966). Habituation: a model for the study of neuronal substrates of behavior. *Psychological Review* **73**, 16–43.

Thorndike, E. L. (1898). Animal intelligence: an experimental study of the associative processes in animals. *Psychological Review* (Monograph Supplement No. 8), 68–72.

Timor-Tritsch, I. E. (1986). The effect of external stimuli on fetal behaviour. *European Journal of Obstetrics and Gynecology and Reproductive Biology* **21**, 321–9

Tucker, D. (1963). Physical variables in the olfactory stimulation process. *Journal of General Physiology* **46**, 453–89.

Vince, M. A., Billing, B. A., Baldwin, B. A., Toner, J. N., and Weller, C. (1985). Maternal vocalisations and other sounds in the fetal lamb's sound environment. *Early Human Development* **11**, 179–190.

Visser, G. H. A., Zeelenberg, H. J., Vries, J. I. P. de, and Dawes, G. S. (1983). External physical stimulation of the human fetus during episodes of low heart rate variation. *American Journal of Obstetrics and Gynecology* **145**, 579–84.

Walker, D. (1969). Temperature of the human fetus. *Journal of Obstetrics and Gynaecology of the British Commonwealth* **76,** 503–11.

Walker, D., Grimwade, J., and Wood, C. (1971). Intrauterine noise: A component of the fetal environment. *American Journal of Obstetrics and Gynecology* **109,** 91–5.

Walmsley, J. and Margolis, J. (1987). *Hot house people*. Pan, London.

Weaver, D. R. and Reppert, S. M. (1986). Maternal melatonin communicates daylength to the fetus in Djungarian hamsters. *Endocrinology* **119,** 2861–3.

Weaver, D. R. and Reppert, S. M. (1987). Maternal-fetal communication of circadian phase in a precocious rodent, the spiny mouse. *American Journal of Physiology* **253,** E401–9.

Wittrock, M. C. (ed.) (1980). *The brain and psychology*. Academic, New York.

12

Maternal emotions during pregnancy and fetal and neonatal behaviour

B. R. H. VAN DEN BERGH

Introduction

The belief that the emotional state of the pregnant woman may affect the behaviour and development of the child she carries is apparently as old as the human race. It can be found in one form or another in every known society (Janssen 1967; MacFarlane 1977), and in our own culture it can be traced back to the Old (Genesis 30:37–39) and New (Luke 1:44) Testament, and to numerous Greek and medieval authors (Copans 1974; Ferreira 1965; Istvan 1986).

During the last decade prenatal emotional influences on the fetus have become the subject of scientific inquiry. The study of prenatal influences presents formidable methodological problems. Not only are there ethical and practical restraints on experimental research of this phenomenon in humans, but one also has to cope with maternal emotional, behavioural, biomedical, and sociodemographic factors, and with the complex psychophysiological interaction between mother and fetus (Istvan 1986; Joffe 1978).

In this chapter we review the literature relevant to prenatal emotional influences and present our longitudinal study on the influence of maternal emotions on fetal and neonatal behaviour. Finally, different mechanisms by which maternal emotions might exert their influence on fetal and neo-natal behaviour and development are discussed.

We review the literature with regard to prenatal emotional influences and to the different underlying mechanisms from the past 50 years. Although we will occasionally refer to infra-human research, this review is restricted in principle to studies on humans. Some of the earlier studies, and also some recent ones, may no longer have relevance in light of new insights on fetal behaviour and endocrine functioning. Yet, these studies have been included in our review just to show the ways in which research-ers, often guided by a certain fashion in their domain, have tried to disentangle the complex phenomenon of prenatal emotional influences. On the other hand, it is surprising to see how some of our predecessors already had a well-balanced view of prenatal behaviour, even though they were deprived of the sophisticated instruments of today.

Prenatal emotional influences—review of the literature (1940–1990)

The literature concerning prenatal emotional influences is extensive, diverse, and fragmented. The fetus in his intrauterine environment is relatively inaccessible and not observable in a direct way without the use of special equipment. Moreover, there is the constant need to consider and evaluate the mediating influence of the mother who provides the immediate environment for the fetus (Joffe 1978). This makes it difficult to gather direct evidence on prenatal emotional influences. Evidence was sought in all kinds of studies; they can be divided roughly into three different groups.

1. A first group of studies concentrated on the relationship between maternal emotions during pregnancy and the occurrence of pregnancy and delivery complications (Joffe 1969). Ferreira (1965, p. 109) states that all factors that interfere with the processes of pregnancy also interfere with the product of pregnancy (i.e. the fetus). Accordingly, all observations of the aetiological role of the emotional maternal state in disturbed pregnancy processes are relevant for the study of prenatal emotional influences on fetal behaviour.

2. In a second group of studies the relationship between maternal emotions during pregnancy and the occurrence of developmental irregularities in the child in the neonatal and postnatal period was studied. From the results of these studies inferences are made about prenatal emotional influences.

3. Thirdly, there is the group of studies in which prenatal emotional influences are studied in a more or less direct way, by observing the fetus in his intrauterine environment by means of special instruments.

We will consider only the second and third group of studies. The studies of the first group have been critically reviewed by several authors (Brown 1964; Carlson and LaBarba 1979; Ferreira 1965; Istvan 1986; James 1969; McDonald 1968; Stechler and Halton 1982; van den Bergh 1981, 1983, 1988, 1989). In general, the measures of obstetric outcome are found to be inconsistently related to indices of stress and anxiety. According to Istvan (1986) these findings seem to result from both a consistent commitment by investigators to a conventional correlational approach focusing on the use of self-report measures, and to disregard for the impact of important socio-demographic and biochemical factors on obstetric outcome. Although the results of the methodologically most acceptable studies (Chalmers 1983,

1984; Molfese *et al.* 1987*a*, 1987*b*; Norbeck and Tilden 1983; Rizzardo *et al.* 1985; Smilkstein *et al.* 1984) do support the notion of an overall relationship between maternal emotions during pregnancy and obstetric outcome, the first group of studies as a whole offers only marginal evidence for a relationship between prenatal emotional states of the mother and fetal behaviour or development.

The empirical efforts of the second group studying the influence of maternal emotions during pregnancy on neonatal behaviour and development are rather diverse. Maternal emotional stress has been associated with major morphological anomalies such as Down's syndrome, cleft lip and cleft palate (Drillien and Wilkinson 1964; Stott 1961), with several minor physical anomalies such as infantile pyloric stenosis (Dodge 1972) and gastric ulceration (Montagu 1962; Pugh *et al.* 1979), with physical handicaps (Stott 1957, 1973; Scott and Latchford 1976), and with an enhanced incidence of medical problems and mental handicaps in childhood (Stott 1957, 1973).

The influence of psychological stress on behavioural outcomes when there are no obvious morphological effects, is less clear (Farber *et al.* 1981). Sontag (1941, 1966) observed that infants of emotionally disturbed women tended to have high activity levels following birth. These infants are typically described as restless, irritable, poor sleepers, and prone to gastrointestinal difficulties, for example frequent vomiting, loose stools, excessive regurgitation (Carey 1968; Dodge 1972; Ferreira 1960; Sontag 1941; Turner 1956, Carlson and LaBarba 1979). According to Sontag (1941) the autonomic nervous systems of these infants show evidence of autonomic instability: they may show greater than average heart-rate changes, vasomotor instability, and changes in respiratory pattern. Ottinger and Simmons (1964) reported that, 2 to 4 days postpartum, infants of high-anxious pregnant women cried significantly more than infants of low-anxious pregnant women. Farber *et al.* (1981) observed that such babies showed a deviant behaviour on the Brazelton Neonatal Behaviour Assessment Scale, being less alert and responsive. In the study of Farber *et al.* (1981), the observed relationships were stronger for females. Chisholm *et al.* (1978) and Korner *et al.* (1980) found significant correlations between normotensive maternal blood pressures during pregnancy and neonatal irritability, which were measured by means of the Brazelton scale and an electronic activity monitor, respectively. Smith and Steinschneider (1975) reported that neonates of mothers with high heart-rates in late pregnancy cried more, took longer to fall asleep, and slept less than those of mothers with normal heart-rates. Davids *et al.* (1963) found that, compared to infants of low-anxious pregnant women, infants of high-anxious pregnant women scored significantly lower on the mental scale of the Bayley Scales of Infant Development. They also scored less on the motor scale, though this difference was only marginally significant. According to Vaughn *et al.* (1987) the babies of high-anxious pregnant women are perceived by their parents as babies with a difficult temperament. The authors used personality characteristics of women during pregnancy, and anxiety in particular, to predict babies' temperament scores, but failed to find empirical support for the idea of prenatal emotional influences.

Several authors (Carlson and LaBarba 1979; Copans 1974; Joffe 1969; Stechler and Halton 1982; Wolkind 1981) made a critical analysis of the methodology of the frequently cited studies of Ferreira (1960), Ottinger and Simmons (1964), Stott (1957, 1961, 1973), and Turner (1956), and found that the empirical support for a relation between maternal emotional state during pregnancy and postnatal behaviour of their offspring, as obtained in these studies, is rather weak.

We now turn to the third group of studies that tried to examine the effect of maternal emotions on fetal behaviour. It has been observed (presumably for the first time in 1867 by Whitehead) that mothers under severe emotional stress tend to have hyperactive fetuses (Ferreira 1965; McDonald 1968; Montagu 1962; Wolkind 1981). Sontag (1941) reported similar observations in eight cases in 1941. Other case reports showed that when the mother is anxious (Copher and Huber 1967) or emotionally upset (Eskes 1985) the fetus shows tachycardia. In 1980, during an earthquake in southern Italy, Ianniruberto and Tajani (1981) had the opportunity to examine with ultrasonography 28 panic-stricken women who were 18 to 36 weeks' pregnant. All fetuses showed intense hyperkinesia, which lasted from 2 to 8 hours, and their movements were numerous, disordered, and vigorous.

Sontag *et al.* (1969) and Zimmer *et al.* (1982) concluded from their study that far less intense maternal emotional conditions, for example listening to a favourite piece of music, can also affect fetal behaviour. Sontag *et al.* (1969) observed 17 women who were 36 to 40 weeks' pregnant and noted a gradual fetal heart-rate (FHR) acceleration (measured with 4 electrodes) following the onset of music; this reached a peak at about 2 minutes after the onset. The mother also recorded perceived fetal movements by pushing a small lever that activated an event pen. Yet, no significant changes in perceived fetal activity were observed as a function of stimulus onset. Zimmer *et al.* (1982) reported a significant decrease in fetal breathing movements and a trend towards an increase in body movements while their mothers ($n = 20$) were listening to their preferred type of music. A real-time ultrasound scanner was used for observation of fetal body and breathing movements. Talbert *et al.* (1982) subjected 40 women in late pregnancy to mild psychological stress (listening through headphones to a pre-coded sequence of words that included the sound of a crying baby). They observed that, after this particular stimulus, but also after internal stimuli such as recalling an alarming situation, maternal skin resistance and heart-rate declined and that coincidentally the FHR pattern changed, the most common changes being a change in beat-to-beat variability or a sudden fall in FHR followed by a recovery over-swing lasting about 1 minute, a so-called 'sigmoid blip'. In a study of the same group (Benson *et al.* 1987) it was observed that fetuses of anxious mothers showed pronounced FHR responses to the taped sound stimuli; this effect was not found for the fetuses of mothers with high hostility or depression scores. In both studies FHR was recorded with a phonocardiotachometer. Field *et al* (1985) compared a group of women ($n = 20$) who received video and verbal feedback during ultrasound examination with a no-feedback group ($n = 20$). Fetal movements were observed for four 2-minute episodes interspersed between ultrasound measurements for the assessments of gestational age at 17, 24, and 32 weeks of gestation. They concluded that the feedback appeared to reduce pregnancy anxiety and fetal activity. In a series of studies by Lederman *et al.* (1978, 1979, 1981) not only maternal anxiety and fetal behaviour, but also the possible mediating factors, such as the hormonal changes of cortisol, adrenaline, and noradrenaline were measured. These researchers found that maternal adrenaline, as measured at the onset of active labour, had a significantly positive correlation with concurrent maternal anxiety and that both were significantly correlated with the FHR pattern. Taken together, these findings indicate that fetuses of high-anxious women with high adrenaline levels experience abnormal FHR decelerations.

We may conclude that the studies of the third group offer only weak empirical support for prenatal emotional influences on fetal behaviour. A shortcoming that most of these studies share is their failure to study fetal behaviour in a standardized way (e.g. de Vries *et al.* 1982) and for a sufficiently long period. More specifically, no attempts have been made to control for fetal behavioural states. But because fetal behavioural states were only described in 1982 (Nijhuis *et al.* 1982), only studies conducted after this date can be criticized for this shortcoming.

Another criticism of the studies of the second and third group is that the influence of maternal emotions on fetal or neonatal behaviour was studied and not the relationship between fetal and neonatal behaviour. With the exception of the case study by Sontag (1941, 1966) the effects of prenatal emotional influences were not traced further to neonatal behaviour.

In the longitudinal study (van den Bergh 1989) presented below, we tried to overcome the shortcomings of the studies of the three groups mentioned above. The study is only briefly introduced. Our attention is directed mainly to the presentation of the results obtained on a sub-sample within this larger study in which the influence of maternal emotions during pregnancy on fetal and neonatal behaviour has been studied. Some other results of the follow-up study are also presented.

Longitudinal study of the effect of maternal emotions on fetal and neonatal behaviour

We studied the effect of maternal emotions during pregnancy and investigated the following two questions:

(1) Can the influence of maternal emotions upon fetal behaviour be established in the prenatal period, using real-time ultrasound echography and cardiography?

(2) Is the prenatal influence that is established in the prenatal period reflected in neonatal behaviour?

Another question, closely related to the second one, is whether significant correlations can be found between maternal emotions during pregnancy on the one hand, and neonatal and infant behaviour—for example neonatal neurological state and behavioural state organization, feeding behaviour, mother–infant interaction, and infant temperament—on the other.

With regard to the first question, a controlled study of 10 healthy near-term pregnant women (van den Bergh *et al*. 1989) revealed that acute emotions induced by showing a film of normal delivery had no effect on fetal behavioural state organization or on fetal motor activity. However, a significant correlation ($p < 0.01$) was found between anxiety (mean state anxiety), which occurs in women during echographic recording (120'), and mean motor activity level of the fetus. The present study has been conducted to corroborate this significant correlation on a larger sample and to study the influence of more chronic emotions during pregnancy on fetal (question 1) and neonatal (question 2) behaviour.

Methods

The longitudinal study was conducted on 70 healthy nulliparae, aged 18 to 30 years old, and with varying levels of anxiety, and their babies. Both mothers and infants were followed during a one-year period.

The emotional state of the mother was studied during each pregnancy trimester, and in the first, tenth, and twenty-eighth week after birth, using psychological tests. The State Trait Anxiety Inventory (STAI) (Spielberger *et al*. 1970) was the most important instrument and was administered on each occasion. This standardized questionnaire differentiates between an anxiety state (reflecting current tension or apprehension, and fluctuates) and an anxiety trait (of a characterological nature, i.e. a disposition or anxiety proneness). Other tests administered during pregnancy included a Pregnancy Anxiety Scale, a Pregnancy Symptom Checklist, a Life Event Scale, a Social Support Questionnaire, a Coping-list, and a Personality

Questionnaire. After birth, the women answered questionnaires regarding their experience of the birth process and the behaviour (feeding, sleeping) of the neonate. In the tenth and twenty-eighth week after the birth the women filled out questionnaires regarding their babies' temperament (Bates *et al* 1979; Carey 1970) and indicated the problems they had experienced with their baby.

To study the effect of maternal emotions on the fetus, the Trait anxiety scores (Spielberger *et al.* 1970) obtained during each pregnancy trimester were taken as a measure of the chronic anxiety of the women and were correlated with fetal behavioural measures. In order to have a measure of the situational anxiety the women also completed the State anxiety scale immediately before the fetal observations were started. Fetal observations were carried out at 36 to 37 weeks of pregnancy on a subgroup of 30 women with uneventful pregnancies and subsequent deliveries. Fetal behaviour (general movements, and eye, head, mouth, breathing, and limb movements) was continuously observed in a standardized way during a 2-hour period (16 to 18 hour) using two ultrasound units (Toshiba SAL 50A and SAL 10A). One real-time B-scanner was placed on the fetal face in a parasagittal position; the other was used to visualize the body movements. Both images were videotaped. Data on occurrence and duration of all the movements were encoded (on-line or off-line) with the use of event markers and were stored on a personal computer (Apple IIe) for statistical analysis. FHR was recorded using a HP 8040 cardiotocograph. On the fifth or sixth day after birth a comparable 2-hour observation of neonatal behaviour was carried out and analysed, using the same software specifically designed for this study.

Two operational measures were used for both fetal and neonatal behaviour. These measures will be designated as behavioural state organization (Nijhuis *et al.* 1982; Prechtl and O'Brien 1982) and motor activity, respectively.

Behavioural state organization was expressed as:

(1) percentage of observation time for coincidence or state 1F through 4F (in the fetus), or state 1 through 5 (in the neonate);
(2) mean duration of enclosed epochs of these coincidences or states.

Motor activity was expressed as:

(1) the percentage of time that general movements are present;
(2) the percentage of time that head movements are present;
(3) mean duration of a general movement.

Each of these three indices of fetal motor activity was expressed as a function of the entire recording period, and as a function of each of the types of coincidence (in the fetus) or state (in the neonate).

In the first and twenty-eighth week after birth the babies were also studied by means of standardized observations using the neonatal neurological examination introduced by Prechtl (1977), and the Bayley Scales of Infant Development (Bayley 1969). In the first and tenth week after birth, feeding behaviour (Daniëls and Casaer 1985) and mother–child interaction were observed during a feeding episode (Price 1983). Obstetric data were also gathered and Prechtl's optimality score was used in the analysis of these data.

Both multivariate (e.g. canonical correlation techniques, multiple regression, LISREL) and univariate analyses (e.g. Pearson correlations) were performed to analyse the results (van den Bergh 1989).

Results

To answer the first question, the maternal State anxiety scores (obtained before the fetal recordings; acute, situational anxiety) and the Trait anxiety scores (one for each pregnancy trimester; chronic anxiety) were correlated with the different fetal behavioural measures. Significant Pearson correlations are presented in Table 12.1.

Table 12.1 Overview of significant Pearson correlations between maternal anxiety and fetal behaviour

Fetal measure	State anxiety (before recording)	Trait anxiety Pregnancy trimester		
		First	Second	Third
Fetal behavioural states				
Percentage of periods 4F	0.38*	0.44**	0.49**	0.39*
Mean enclosed epochs 1F	—	−0.41*	−0.47**	—
Fetal motor activity				
Percentage of general movements:				
during entire recording	0.38*	—	0.33*	—
during periods 4F	0.47**	0.45**	0.44*	0.38*
Percentage of head movements:				
during entire recording	—	0.35*	0.35*	0.31*
during periods 4F	0.67***	0.51**	0.38*	0.49*
Mean duration of general movement:				
during entire recording	0.45**	0.44**	0.47**	0.35*
during periods of 2F	0.43**	0.36**	0.37*	—
during periods of 4F	0.37*	0.34*	0.48*	0.33*

Note: $n = 28$; $*p < 0.05$; $**p < 0.01$; $***p < 0.001$.

Positive significant correlations between maternal State anxiety and fetal motor activity were obtained ($r = 0.37$ to 0.67; $p < 0.05$ to 0.001), corroborating the results of the first study (van den Bergh *et al*. 1989). An additional significant correlation was found between State anxiety in the mother and fetal behavioural state organization ($r = 0.38$, $p < 0.05$).

For maternal Trait anxiety we also obtained significant positive correlations with fetal motor activity ($r = 0.33$ to 0.51; $p < 0.05$ to 0.01) and with fetal behavioural state organization ($r = 0.39$ to 0.49; $p < 0.05$ to 0.01).

To answer the second question comparable measures of fetal and neonatal behaviour relating to behavioural states and motor activity were correlated. Significant results are presented in Table 12.2. The finding that fetal head movements (rather than general movements) are correlated with neonatal head and general movements is the most consistent result across different states. Different Linear Structural Relations (LISREL) models on the combined effects of maternal anxiety and fetal behaviour on neonatal behaviour were tested. The models in which maternal anxiety had only an indirect effect on neonatal behaviour (i.e. by modifying fetal behaviour) produced the best fit to the data. In general, the results with regard to our two questions were corroborated by the LISREL models.

Pearson correlations between the maternal anxiety scores obtained during pregnancy and the different measures of neonatal and postnatal behaviour yielded interesting results. Compared to infants of low-anxious

Table 12.2 Overview of significant Pearson correlations between measures of fetal and neonatal behaviour in different behavioural states

Behavioural measure	Behavioural state			
	1F and 1	2F and 2	4F and 4	Total
Behavioural states				
Mean enclosed epoch	0.47*	—	—	—
Motor activity				
Percentage of general movement (GM)	0.34*	—	0.33*	—
Percentage of head movement (HM)	—	0.56**	0.40**	0.50**
Mean duration of GM	—	—	0.67***	—
Percentage GM (f) and percentage HM (n)	—	—	0.43*	—
Percentage HM (f) and percentage GM (n)	—	0.41*	0.40*	0.51**

Note the provision of cross-correlations between fetal (f) and neonatal (n) measures of general movements and head movements. $n = 27$. *$p < 0.05$; **$p < 0.01$; ***$p < 0.001$.

women, infants of high-anxious women cried more ($r = 0.29$; $p < 0.05$) and changed more frequently from one behavioural state to another ($r = 0.39$; $p < 0.005$) in the neonatal period. At 10 weeks these infants were more frequently diagnosed as infants with a difficult temperament $r = -0.35$; $p < 0.01$). Seven months after birth high-anxious women more frequently indicated the following behaviours of their children as being a problem for them: too active ($r = 0.39$; $p < 0.005$), being hungry ($r = 0.31$; $p < 0.05$), frequent crying ($r = 0.36$; $p < 0.05$), and having cramps ($r = 0.31$; $p < 0.05$). They also perceived their infants as having a difficult temperament ($r = 0.45$; $p < 0.001$). However, infants of high-anxious and low-anxious women obtained comparable scores for the neurological examination, the standardized observation of feeding behaviour, and the Bayley Scales of Infant Development.

Discussion and conclusion

With regard to Question 1, it may be concluded from our results that the influence of maternal emotions in the prenatal period has been established. Maternal emotions have a small, but significant effect on occurrence and duration of fetal movements. Fetuses of high-anxious women tend to be more active than fetuses of low-anxious women. This relationship has been established using both acute situational anxiety and more chronic anxiety as indices of maternal emotional state.

Regarding Question 2, we can say that the prenatal influence is reflected in neonatal behaviour. Indeed, our data seem to suggest a certain degree of continuity between fetal and neonatal behaviour. Active fetuses tend to have a high activity level after birth. We can also conclude that maternal emotions during pregnancy are correlated with neonatal and infant behaviour. These correlations indicate that children of high-anxious pregnant women have gastrointestinal problems, cry frequently, and are perceived as having a difficult temperament. They do not, however, have a deviant score on the neurological examination, the feeding observation, or on measures of mental and motor development.

Our results should be interpreted with caution. Although the correlations are significant, they are small in magnitude, and much of the variance remains unexplained. A clear explanation of the findings and the underlying mechanisms is (still) lacking.

We presume that the influence of maternal emotions on fetal behaviour is mediated by hormonal factors, but the exact physiological background is unclear (see below). A number of factors may also indirectly mediate the relation between maternal emotions and fetal behaviour. Anxiety can increase the use of substances like tobacco, alcohol, caffeine, and neuroleptics, and these substances in turn might influence fetal behaviour and development (Carlson and LaBarba 1979; Istvan 1986; Joffe 1969). Maternal physical activity, such as work, sports, and travelling (Lotgering *et al.* 1984; Steegers *et al.* 1988) and fatigue (Montagu 1962; Sontag 1962) can correlate with the maternal emotional state, and these physical conditions in turn exert their influence through the neuroendocrine system and can affect fetal behaviour. Finally, heredity can determine the level of fetal activity.

The findings on neonatal and postnatal behaviour can also be explained in different ways. One explanation holds that these behaviours reflect the prenatal influence of maternal anxiety during pregnancy and are mediated by maternal hormonal functioning (see below). A second interpretation could be that anxious women have more pregnancy and delivery complications and that these have an adverse effect on the infant's behaviour (Carlson and LaBarba 1976; Istvan 1986; Joffe 1969). A third possibility could be that anxious women have a negative perception of their child, a perception that causes bias when they are answering the questionnaires (Crockenberg and Acredolo 1983; Crockenberg and Smith 1982; Vaughn *et al.* 1987). Fourthly we could say that women who are anxious during pregnancy remain anxious after pregnancy (Davids 1971) and that their postnatal anxiety influences the behaviour of the child (Farber *et al.* 1981). A fifth factor can be heredity (Copans 1974; Sontag 1966). On the basis of our data we cannot test the plausibility of these different interpretations. Most probably they are all involved.

Discussion of possible underlying mechanisms

Most authors postulated that prenatal emotional influences are mediated by the maternal neuroendocrine system or by both the maternal and fetal hormonal systems. This can hardly surprise anyone for a number of reasons.

1. The assumption that hormonal changes are involved in the mechanism of transmission is implicit in the very use of terms such as 'stress' (Seley) or 'emotions' (Cannon).
2. There is no direct neural connection between mother and fetus, but hormones in the mother's blood can be transmitted across the placenta into the fetal circulatory system (Joffe 1978).

Ideally, an explanation of prenatal emotional influences on fetal and neonatal behaviour, based on the working of the neuroendocrine system, should be given at three different levels to correspond to three different questions. These questions are:

(1) what is the influence of maternal emotions on maternal homeostasis?
(2) how can (the changes in) maternal homeostasis or maternal psychophysiological functioning affect the fetus *in utero* and which fetal systems are involved in this particular type of transmission?

(3) how can the functioning of the fetal systems involved lead to the observed fetal or neonatal behaviour, or fetal/neonatal behavioural change?

Following a fashion in endocrinological research most researchers have used the working of either the sympatho-adrenomedullar (SA) system or the hypothalamo-pituitary-adrenocortical (HPA) system as a general explanatory framework for prenatal emotional influences on fetal and neonatal behaviour. For the most part, they have done so without making a clear distinction between the three levels of explanation mentioned above. Most interpretations of the results obtained in this particular body of literature are very general and of a speculative rather than a causal nature. On the one hand there is no full understanding of the principles governing endocrine regulation (Mason 1975*a*, 1975*b*), and on the other hand the knowledge of the mechanisms that control fetal behaviour is very limited (Dawes 1984*a*, 1984*b*, 1986; Prechtl 1981).

In this review, we:

(1) present the evidence that the studies of the second and third group (as defined earlier on in this chapter) offer for the role of mediating factors;

(2) briefly discuss the studies on the mechanisms that control fetal behaviour.

In the studies reviewed earlier the activation of the SA system was used to explain the relationship between more or less severe maternal emotions and the following fetal behaviours: high motor activity (Sontag 1941), fetal tachycardia (Eskes 1985), high FHR variability (Talbert *et al.* 1982), and FHR deceleration during labour (Lederman 1984). Sontag (1941, p. 1000) mentioned 'the increased adrenalin level in maternal and, therefore, the fetal blood' as a mediating factor. Eskes (1985) also points to the possibility of transplacental transport of catecholamines. Both of these authors thus suggest a direct effect of hormones on fetal behaviour. Finally, Talbert *et al.* (1982) and Lederman (1984) explain their findings as a secondary effect (i.e. as the result of the restriction of uterine blood flow under maternal sympathetic control).

Sontag (1941, 1962, 1966) found evidence for his explanation in the work of Jost, who reported that women who had the highest autonomic activity or the most labile functioning of the autonomous nervous system (ANS) (i.e. who showed the greatest change in skin conductance, respiration, and heart-rate in response to breath-holding for 20 seconds) had the most active fetuses (Joffe 1969; Myers and Myers 1979). If we keep in mind one of the basic assumptions in current theorizing on the SA system, that is that emotions (and other factors) exert their influence through the ANS, the results of Jost may be construed as evidence for Sontag's explanation. The findings of Jost are comparable with those of Richards *et al.* (1938) who found a correlation between fetal activity and the basal metabolic rate (BMR), and change in BMR of the mothers in the last 2 months of pregnancy. Talbert *et al.* (1982) and Lederman *et al.* (1984) found further evidence in experimental research on animals. In animals it has been shown that under psychological stress or after administration of cathecholamines, or after direct stimulation of the sympathetic nervous system, the utero-placental blood flow is reduced through vasoconstrictive properties of the cathecholamines, resulting in bradycardia and hypotension, hypoxia and asphyxia in the fetus (Myers and Myers 1979). However, the cardiovascular changes observed during pregnancy due to stress or anxiety have rarely been studied in man. Considerable caution must be exercised in generalizing animal findings to the situation in man because it is clear that there are species differences in uterine blood vessel reactivity (Myers and Myers 1979).

According to Joffe (1969), empirical evidence on the effects of emotional states on uterine contractions suggests a possible mechanism whereby maternal emotions might affect the fetus. He thought the effects are, in general, more likely to be hormonally rather than mechanically mediated. The studies by Kelly (1962*a*, 1962*b*) provided support for the theory that fear and anxiety can provoke increased myometrial activity, probably through the agency of adrenaline. Kaiser and Harris (1959) concluded that the effect of adrenaline depends entirely upon its concentration at the site of action. In high concentration it is oxytocic throughout the uterus, in low concentration it inhibits uterine activity. Sontag (cited in MacFarlane, 1977), and Bernard and Sontag (1947) suggested a mechanical mediation of prenatal emotional and environmental factors: the contractions of the uterus might increase the pressure in the fluid around the baby and this might make him move. Mulder and Visser (1987) observed that Braxton Hicks' contractions of 14 nulliparous women near term coincided with a specific clustering of body movements and breathing movements. Body movements, for example, showed a clustering in the ascending part of the contraction followed by a significant decrease during the descending part. The increase of body movements during the ascending part of the contraction suggests a stimulation of these movements by contractions. The mean duration of the FHR accelerations that occurred during contractions was longer than that of accelerations not associated with contractions. The latter fact might be due to compensatory FHR change induced by the transient reduction in feto-placental exchange during the contractions (Mulder and Visser 1987).

Sontag (1941, p. 1001) also suggested that the neonatal behaviour of babies whose mothers were anxious during pregnancy may result from the development of an irritable and hyperactive ANS, with poorly balanced adrenergic-cholinergic systems, in the prenatal period. Montagu (1962), and Smith and Steinschneider (1975), consider the possibility of 'calibration' or 'tuning' of the ANS by the level of stimulation *in utero*. In the fetus of an emotionally distressed mother, for example, the hypothalamus might have been exposed to higher amounts of adrenergic substances and an increased level of these substances will then be required to maintain normal operations after birth. According to Barrett (1982) direct research into such 'adaptation level' effects on the human fetal ANS remains a task for the future. Chisholm *et al.* (1978) also point to the possible role of catecholamines to explain the relationship between maternal blood pressure during pregnancy and neonatal irritability.

We refer to Joffe (1969, 1978) for a review of animal research of the hormonal mediation of the effects of prenatal stress on offspring behaviour, and present only the most important results of this research. Most of the research was conducted to test the hypothesis that the effects of prenatal stress were mediated by the maternal and fetal HPA system. Initially, however, experimenters concentrated on determining if the adrenal medullary hormones (adrenaline and noradrenaline) produced effects on offspring similar to the effects of prenatal stress (e.g. changes in open field activity, defaecation, performance in learning tasks such as mazes, or avoidance conditioning situations (Joffe 1978). The question of how hormones alter behaviour was raised. Joffe (1969, p. 109) hypothesized that exogenous adrenaline might have a direct effect on the fetus after crossing the placenta, it might alter the transport characteristics of the placenta or affect the hormone production in the placenta, or it might alter maternal and fetal endocrine activity, and very probably all, or most, of these responses might be involved. In 1978 Joffe (p. 123) concluded that adrenaline and noradrenaline experiments are unlikely to shed much light on the processes underlying the effects of prenatal stress. Adrenaline injections cause release of adrenocorticotropic hormone (ACTH) and an increase in the circulating level of corticosteroids, thus effects on the fetus could be the result of transfer of either adrenal medullary or cortical hormones.

With regard to the working of the HPA system it has been hypothesized that adrenal cortical hormones might alter the level of hormones circulating in the mother and hence in the fetus, and that these hormones might alter fetal brain function directly—assuming the fetal brain is sensitive to such effects in the prenatal period—or indirectly by altering the structure or function of the fetal adrenals. If these changes in adrenal functioning persist into the postnatal period they could presumably lead to effects on brain sensitivity at that age (Joffe 1969, 1978; Levine and Treiman 1969). Joffe (1978) analysed the results of these studies in a systematic fashion and showed that the effect of prenatal stress on offspring behaviour was probably not mediated by the maternal or fetal HPA systems.

Although the HPA system in humans has not been studied as a possible mediating factor in prenatal emotional influences, there is some evidence that the working of this system is important in controlling fetal behaviour. Nijhuis *et al.* (1982) established the existence of behavioural states in the human fetus in the last month of gestation. Besides ultradian cycles, the fetus also shows a circadian rhythm of general movements (Patrick *et al.* 1980*a*; Roberts *et al.* 1978), breathing movements (Patrick *et al.* 1982; Roberts *et al.* 1979), and FHR variability (Visser *et al.* 1982). Some of the diurnal rhythms are dependent on the mother because they are temporarily lost in the early neonatal period (Dawes 1986). Patrick *et al.* (1980*b*) showed that the diurnal FHR rhythm closely resembles the maternal plasma cortisol rhythm. Visser (1984) also suggested that the FHR might be influenced indirectly by maternal adrenal activity, and Arduini *et al.* (1986) suggested that maternal plasma cortisol could be involved in the alternation of fetal behavioural states. In an important double-blind study, the latter group of researchers showed that the inhibition of fetal and maternal adrenal glands (by administrating triamcinolone) could cause modifications of FHR and movement patterns. In the group with adrenal gland suppression the diurnal rhythm in FHR and fetal movements could no longer be found, and the ultradian patterns of FHR and fetal movements were modified (i.e. the 'active phase' was significantly longer and the 'quiet phase' was significantly shorter than in the group without suppression of adrenal glands). Among studies on human subjects this study seems to be the only one in which an aetiological relationship has been established between maternal endocrine functioning and fetal behaviour. However, the mechanisms through which the maternal and fetal adrenal glands affect fetal movements and FHR variability are still obscure (de Vries 1987; Visser 1984).

In animal studies it has been shown that prenatal stress affects the neurotransmitters of the fetal nervous systems (noradrenaline, dopamine, and serotonin) and it is possible that such neurochemical changes may underlie the reported behavioural deficits in the offspring of stressed female rats (Moyer *et al.* 1978; Peters 1984, 1986). The role of endorphins as a prenatal stress or anxiety stress-mediating factor has been suggested, also in man (Vaughn *et al.* 1987; Visser, personal communication 1985). The major role of the endorphins seems to be the modulation of pain sensitivity, and they also affect respiratory control in both the fetus and the neonate in ways not seen in the adult (Lagercrantz 1984). Endorphins increase in response to stressful perinatal events that involve pituitary activation, for example labour, neonatal and postpartum hypoxia, or general anesthesia (Golub *et al.* 1989). Endorphins may be produced by the maternal or fetal pituitary, or by the placenta (Golub *et al.* 1989).

What might be the conclusion of this discussion with regard to our longitudinal study in which we found a significant positive correlation between maternal anxiety during pregnancy and fetal behaviour? As the role of the HPA axis in controlling fetal behaviour has been experimentally verified in men, while the role of the SA system has not, it seems most plausible to involve the working of the HPA axis in the explanation of our findings. However, our results cannot be easily explained by increased maternal cortisol levels (corresponding with maternal anxiety state) since Arduini *et al.* (1986) found a negative correlation between cortisol levels and fetal activity. A further analysis of the results of Arduini *et al.* (1986) revealed an additional positive correlation between ACTH (which is also correlated with maternal anxiety) and fetal activity, and our results might be congruent with these data. Although no causal relationships have been established, the working of the SA system cannot be excluded as a mediating factor on the basis of these findings. Over the years, evidence has accumulated to suggest that stressors produce responses in a wide variety of endocrine systems and it is clear that besides cortisol, adrenaline and noradrenaline, other hormones such as prolactin, thyroxine, insulin, and testosterone also play an important role in responses to stressful stimuli (Mason 1975a, 1975b), and possibly in mediating the effect of maternal emotions on fetal and neonatal behaviour. As we did not measure hormones in our study we can neither exclude nor prove the mediating effect of any of these hormones. Moreover, neurotransmitters might also play a mediating role.

In this chapter we have reviewed the evidence regarding prenatal emotional influences on fetal and neonatal behaviour and discussed the possible underlying mechanisms. Although the evidence is weak due to our current failure to establish the causal relationships involved with a reasonable degree of certainty, this does not imply that these studies (including our longitudinal study) are unimportant. They certainly indicate that the fetus actively responds to his maternal environment, and that postnatal as well as prenatal behaviour may be influenced by maternal emotions during pregnancy.

References

Arduini, D., Rizzo, E., Parlati, E., Giorlandino, C., Valensise, H., Dell'acqua, S., and Romanini, C. (1986). Modification of ultradian and circadian rhythms of fetal heart rate after fetal-maternal adrenal gland suppression: A double blind study. *Prenatal Diagnosis* **6**, 409–17.

Barrett, J. H. W. (1982). Prenatal influences on adaptation in the newborn. In: *Psychobiology of the human newborn* (ed. P. Stratton), pp. 267–95. Wiley, Chichester.

Bates, J., Freeland, C., and Lounsburry, M. (1979). Measurement of infant difficultness. *Child Development* **50**, 794–803.

Bayley, N. (1969). *Manual for the Bayley Scales of Infant Development.* The Psychological Association, New York.

Benson, P. B., Little, B. C., Talbert, D. G., Dewhurst, J. Sir, and Priest, R. G. (1987). Foetal heart rate and maternal emotional state. *British Journal of Medical Psychology* **60**, 151–4.

Bergh, B. van den (1981). *Factoren die de prenatale ontwikkeling beïn-vloeden. Literatuurstudie aangaande factoren die het prenataal intra-uterien milieu bepalen en die te beschouwen zijn als prenatale determinanten van het postnataal gedrag.* Niet gepubliceerde licentiaatsverhandeling, Katholieke Universiteit Leuven.

Bergh, B. van den (1983). De psychische toestand van de zwangere en de prenatale ontwikkeling. Literatuurstudie en schets van een heuristisch model. *Tijdschrift voor Orthopedagogie, Kinderpsychiatrie en Klinische Kinderpsychologie* **8**, (1), 18–37.

Bergh, B van den (1988). The relationship between maternal emotionality during pregnancy and the behavioral development of the fetus and neonatus. In: *Prenatal and perinatal psychology and medicine* (ed. P. G. Fedor-Freybergh and M. L. V. Vogel), pp. 131–42. Parthenon: Carnforth, Lancs.

Bergh, B. van den (1989). De emotionele toestand van de (zwangere) vrouw, obstetrische complicaties en het gedrag en de ontwikkeling van de foetus en van het kind tot de leeftijd van zeven maanden. *Thesis*, Catholic University, Leuven, Belgium.

Bergh, B. R. H. van den, Mulder, E. J. H., Poelman-Weesjes, G., Bekedam, D. J., Visser, G. H. A., and Prechtl, H. F. R. (1989). The effect of (induced) maternal emotions on fetal behaviour: a controlled study. *Early Human Development* **9**, 9–19.

Bernard, J. and Sontag, L. W. (1947). Fetal reactivity to tonal stimulation. *The Journal of Genetic Psychology* **70**, 205–10.

Brown, L. B. (1964). Anxiety in pregnancy. *British Journal of Medical Psychology* **37**, 47–58.

Carey, W. B. (1968). Maternal anxiety and infantile colic: Is there a relationship? *Clinical Pediatrics* **7**, 590.

Carey, W. B. (1970). A simplified method for measuring infant temperament. *The Journal of Pediatrics* **77**, 188–94.

Carlson, B. and LaBarba, R. C. (1979). Maternal emotionality during pregnancy and reproductive outcome. *International Journal of Behavioral Development* **2**, 342–76.

Chalmers, B. (1983). Psychosocial factors and obstetric complications. *Psychological Medicine* **13**, 333–9.

Chalmers, B. (1984). Behavioural associations of pregnancy complications. *Journal of Psychosomatic Obstetrics and Gynaecology* **3**, 27–35.

Chisholm, J. S., Woodson, R. H., and Da Costa Woodson, F. M. (1978). Maternal blood pressure in pregnancy and newborn irritability. *Early Human Development* **2**, 171–8.

Copans, S. A. (1974). Human prenatal effects: Methodological problems and some suggested solutions. *Merrill-Palmer Quarterly* **20**, 43–52.

Copher, D. E. and Huber, C. P. (1967). Heart rate response of the human fetus to induced maternal hypoxia. *American Journal of Obstetrics and Gynecology* **98**, 320–35.

Crockenberg, S. B. and Acredolo, C. (1983). Infant temperament ratings: A function of infants, of mothers, or both? *Infant Behavior and Development* **6**, 61–72.

Crockenberg, S. B. and Smith, P. (1982). Antecedents of mother infant interaction and infant irritability in the first three months of life. *Infant Behavior and Development* **5**, 105–19.

Daniëls, H. and Casaer, P. (1985). Development of arm posture during bottle feeding in preterm infants. *Infant Behavior and Development* **8**, 241–4.

Davids, A. (1971). Consistency of maternal attitudes and personality characteristics during pregnancy and eight months after delivery. *American Journal of Orthopsychiatry* **33**, 291–2.

Davids, A., Holden, R. H., and Gray, G. (1963). Maternal anxiety during pregnancy and adequacy of mother and child adustment eight months following childbirth. *Child Development* **34**, 993–1002.

Dawes, G. S. (1984*a*). Fetal physiology and behaviour: changing direction. 1954–1983. *Journal of Developmental Physiology* **6**, 259–65.

Dawes, G. S. (1984*b*). The central control of fetal breathing and skeletal muscle movements. *Journal of Physiology* **346**, 1–18.

Dawes, G. S. (1986). The central nervous control of fetal behaviour. *European Journal of Obstetrics and Gynecology and Reproductive Biology* **21**, 341–6.

Dodge, J. A. (1972). Psychosomatic aspects of infantile pyloric stenosis. *Journal of Psychosomatic Research* **16**, 1–5.

Drillien, C. M. and Wilkinson, E. M. (1964). Emotional stress and mongoloid birth. *Developmental Medicine and Child Neurology* **6**, 140–3.

Eskes, T. K. A. B. (1985). Verloskundige consequenties van niet verwerkte rouw over een perinataal gestorven kind. *Nederlands Tijdschrift voor Geneeskunde* **129**, 433–6.

Farber, E. A., Vaughn, B., and Egeland, B. (1981). The relationship of prenatal maternal anxiety to infant behavior and mother-infant interactions during the first six months of life. *Early Human Development* **5**, 267–77.

Ferreira, A. J. (1960). The pregnant woman's emotional attitude and its reflection on the newborn. *American Journal of Orthopsychiatry* **30**, 553–61.

Ferreira, A. J. (1965). Emotional factors in prenatal environment. *The Journal of Nervous and Mental Disease* **141**, 108–18.

Field, T., Sandberg, D., Quetel, T. A., Garcia, R., and Rosario, M. (1985). Effects of ultrasound feedback on pregnancy anxiety, fetal activity and neonatal outcome. *Obstetrics and Gynecology* **66**, 525–8.

Golub, M. S., Eisele, J. H. Hwang, F. Y., and Arbabzadeh, H. (1989). Late-pregnant changes in peripheral plasma beta-endorphin in rhesus monkeys. *Gynecological and Obstetrical Investigations* **27**, 113–17.

Ianniruberto, A. and Tajani, E. (1981). Ultrasonographic study of fetal movements. *Seminars in Perinatology* **5**, 175–181.

Istvan, J. (1986). Stress, anxiety, and birth outcome: a critical review of the evidence. *Psychological Bulletin* **100**, 331–48.

James, W. H. (1969). The effect of maternal psychological stress on the fetus. *British Journal of Psychiatry* **115**, 811–25.

Janssen, M. C. (1967). *Zwangere en kraamvrouw in psychologisch perspectief.* Dekker & Van de Vegt, Nijmegen.

Joffe, J. M. (1969). *Prenatal determinants of behaviour* (International series of monographs in experimental psychology, Vol. 7). Pergamon Press, Oxford.

Joffe, J. M. (1978). Hormonal mediation of the effects of prenatal stress on offspring behavior. In: *Studies on the development of behavior and the nervous system* (Early influences, Vol. 4) (ed. G. Gottlieb), pp. 107–144. Academic Press, New York.

Kaiser, I. H. and Harris, J. S. (1959). The effect of adrenalin on the pregnant human uterus. *American Journal of Obstetrics and Gynecology* **59**, 775–84.

Kelly, J. V. (1962*a*). Effect of fear upon uterine motility. *American Journal of Obstetrics and Gynecology* **83**, 576–81.

Kelly, J. V. (1962*b*). Effect of hypnotically induced anxiety on uterine muscle. *American Journal of Obstetrics and Gynecology* **83**, 582–7.

Korner, A. F., Gabby, T., and Kraemer, H. C. (1980). Relation between prenatal maternal blood pressure and infant irritability. *Early Human Development* **4**, 35–9.

Lagercrantz, H. (1984). Classical and 'new' neurotransmitters during development: some examples from control of respiration. *Journal of Developmental Physiology* **6**, 195–205.

Lederman, R. P. (1984). *Psychosocial adaptation in pregnancy: assessment of seven dimensions of maternal development*. Prentice-Hall, Englewood Cliffs, NJ.

Lederman, R. P., Lederman, E., Work, B. A., and McCann, D. S. (1978). The relationship of maternal anxiety, plasma catecholamines, and plasma cortisol to progress in labor. *American Journal of Obstetrics and Gynecology* **132**, 495–500.

Lederman, R. P., Lederman, E., Work, B. A., and McCann, D. S. (1979). Relationship of psychological factors in pregnancy to progress in labor. *Nursing Research* **28**, 94–7.

Lederman, E., Lederman, R. P., Work, B. A., and McCann, D. S. (1981). Maternal psychological and physiological correlates of fetal-newborn health status. *American Journal of Obstetrics and Gynecology* **139**, 956–8.

Levine, S., and Treiman, L. J. (1969). Role of hormones in programming the central nervous system. In: *Foetal autonomy* (Ciba Foundation Symposium) (ed. G. E. W. Wolstenholme and M. O'Connor), pp. 271–285. J. and A. Churchill, London.

Lotgering, F. K., Gilbert, R. D., and Longo, L. D. (1984). The interactions of exercise and pregnancy: A review. *American Journal of Obstetrics and Gynecology* **149**, 560–8.

MacFarlane, A. (1977). *The psychology of childbirth*. Fontana Open Books, London.

Mason, J. W. (1975*a*). A historical view of the stress field: part 1. *Journal of Human Stress* **1**, (1) 6–12.

Mason, J. W. (1975*b*). A historical view of the stress field: part 2. *Journal of Human Stress* **1**, (3). 22–36.

McDonald, R. L. (1968). The role of emotional factors in obstetric complications. *Psychosomatic Medicine* **30**, 222 37.

Molfese, V. J., Bricker, M. C., Manion, L. G., Beadnell, B., Yaple, K., and Moires, K. A. (1987*a*). Anxiety, depression and stress in pregnancy: A multi-variate model of intra-partum risks and pregnancy outcomes. *Journal of Psychosomatic Obstetrics and Gynaecology* **7**, 77–92.

Molfese, V. J., Bricker, M. C., Manion, L., Yaple, K., and Beadnell, B. (1987*b*). Stress in pregnancy: the influence of psychological and social mediators in perinatal experiences. *Journal of Psychosomatic Obstetrics and Gynaecology* **6**, 33–42.

Montagu, A. (1962). *Prenatal influences*. Charles Thomas, Springfield, IL.

Moyer, J. A., Herrenkohl, L. R., and Jacobowitz, D. M. (1978). Stress during pregnancy: effect on catecholamines in discrete brain regions of offspring as adults. *Brain Research* **144,** 173–8.

Mulder, E. J. H. and Visser, G. H. A. (1987). Braxton Hicks' contraction and motor behavior in the near-term human fetus. *American Journal of Obstetrics and Gynecology* **156,** 543–9.

Myers, R. E. and Myers, S. E. (1979). Use of sedative, analgesic, and anesthetic drugs during labor and delivery: Bane or boon? *American Journal of Obstetrics and Gynecology* **133,** 83–104.

Nijhuis, J. G., Prechtl, H. F. R., Martin, C. B., and Bots, R. S. G. M. (1982). Are there behavioural states in the human fetus? *Early Human Development* **6,** 177–95.

Norbeck, J. S. and Tilden, V. P. (1983). Life stress, social support and emotional disequilibrium in complications of pregnancy: a prospective, multivariate study. *Journal of Health and Social Behavior* **24,** 30–46.

Ottinger, D. R. and Simmons, E. (1964). Behavior of human neonates and pre-natal maternal anxiety. *Psychological Reports* **14,** 391–4.

Packer, M. and Rosenblatt, D. (1979). Issues in the study of social behaviour in the first week of life. In: *The first year of life: psychological and medical implications of early experience* (ed. D. Schaffer and J. Dunn), pp. 7–35. Wiley, Chichester.

Patrick, J., Campbell, K., Carmichael, L., Natale, R., and Richardson, B. (1980*a*). Patterns of human fetal breathing during the last 10 weeks of pregnancy. *Obstetrics and Gynecology* **56,** 24–30.

Patrick, J., Challis, J., Campbell, K., Carmichael, L., Natale, R., and Richardson, B. (1980*b*). Circadian rhythms in maternal plasma-cortisol and estriol concentra-tions at 30 to 31, 34 to 35, and 38 to 39 weeks gestational age. *American Journal of Obstetrics and Gynecology* **136,** 325–34.

Patrick, J., Campbell, K., Carmichael, L., Natale, R., and Richardson, B. (1982). Patterns of gross fetal body movements over 24-hour observation intervals during the last 10 weeks of pregnancy. *American Journal of Obstetrics and Gynecology* **142,** 363–71.

Peters, D. A. V. (1984). Prenatal stress: effect on development of rat brain adrenergic receptors. *Pharmacology, Biochemistry and Behavior* **21,** 417–22.

Peters, D. A. V. (1986). Prenatal stress: effect on development of rat brain serotonergic neurons. *Pharmacology, Biochemistry and Behavior* **24,** 1377–82.

Prechtl, H. F. R. (1977). The neurological examination of the full-term newborn infant. *Clinics in Developmental Medicine*, No. 63. S.I.M.P. Heinemann, London.

Prechtl, H. F. R. (1981). The study of neural development as a perspective of clinical problems. In: Maturation and development: biological and psychological perspectives. *Clinics in Developmental Medicine*, No. 77/78 (ed. K. J. Connolly and H. F. R. Prechtl), pp. 198–215. S.I.M.P./Heinemann, London.

Prechtl, H. F. R. and O'Brien, M. J. (1982). Behavioural states of the full-term newborn: The emergence of a concept. In: *Psychobiology of the human newborn* (ed. P. Stratton), pp. 53–73, Wiley, Chichester.

Price, G. M. (1983). Sensitivity in mother-infant interaction: The AMIS scale. *Infant Behavior and Development* **6,** 353–60.

Pugh, R. J., Newton, R. W., and Piercy, D. M. (1979). Fatal bleeding from gastric ulceration during first day of life: possible association with social stress. *Archives of Diseases in Childhood* **54,** 146–7.

Richards, T. W., Newbery, N., and Fallgatter, R. (1938). Studies in fetal behavior: II. Activity of the human fetus *in utero* and its relation to other prenatal conditions, particularly the mother's basal metabolic rate. *Child Development* **9**, 69–77.

Rizzardo, R., Magni, G., Andreoli, C., Merlin, G., Andreoli, F., Fabbris, L., Martinotti, G., and Cosentino, M. (1985). Psychosocial aspects during pregnancy and obstetrical complications. *Journal of Psychosomatic Obstetrics and Gynaecology* **4**, 11–22.

Roberts, A. B., Little, D., and Campbell, S. (1978). 24-hour studies of fetal respiratory movements and fetal body movements: relationship to glucose, cathecholamine, oestriol, and cortisol levels. In: *Recent advances in ultrasound diagnosis* (ed. A. Kurjak), pp. 189–91. Excerpta Medica, Amsterdam.

Roberts, A. B., Little, D., Cooper, D., and Campbell, S. (1979). Normal patterns of fetal activity in the third trimester. *British Journal of Obstetrics and Gynaecology* **86**, 4–9.

Smilkstein, G., Helper-Lucas, A., Ashworth, C., Montano, D., and Pagel, M. (1984). Prediction of pregnancy complications: an application of the biopsychosocial model. *Social Science and Medicine* **4**, 315–21.

Smith, C. R. and Steinschneider, A. (1975). Differential effects of prenatal rhythmic stimulation on neonatal arousal states. *Child Development* **46**, 574–8.

Sontag, L. W. (1941). The significance of fetal environmental differences. *American Journal of Obstetrics and Gynecology* **42**, 996–1003.

Sontag, L. W. (1962). Effect of maternal emotions on fetal development. In: *Psychosomatics—obstetrics, gynecology and endocrinology* (ed. W. S. Kroger), pp. 8–14. Charles Thomas, Springfield, IL.

Sontag, L. W. (1966) Implications of fetal behavior and environment for adult personalities. *Annals of the New York Academy of Sciences* **134**, 782–6.

Sontag, L. W., Steele, W. G., and Mcwis, M. (1969). The fetal and maternal cardiac response to environmental stress. *Human Development* **12**, 1–9.

Spielberger, C. D., Gorsuch, R. L., and Lushene, R. E. (1970). *Manual for the State-Trait Anxiety Inventory (Self-Evaluation Questionnaire)*. Consulting Psychologists Press, Palo Alto, CA.

Stechler, G. and Halton, A. (1982). Prenatal influences on human development. In: *Handbook of developmental psychology* (ed. B. B. Wolman), pp. 177–89. Prentice-Hall, Englewood Cliffs, NJ.

Steegers, E. A. P., Buunk, G., Binkhorst, R. A., Jongsma, H. W., Wijn, P. F. F., and Hein, P. R. (1988). The influence of maternal excercise on the uteroplacental vascular bed resistance and the fetal heart rate during normal pregnancy. *European Journal of Obstetrics and Gynecology and Reproductive Biology* **27**, 21–6.

Stott, D. H. (1957). Physical and mental disturbances following a disturbed pregnancy. *The Lancet* (May 18), 1006–12.

Stott, D. H. (1961). Mongolism related to emotional shock in early pregnancy. *Vita Humana* **4**, 57–76.

Stott, D. H. (1973). Follow-up study from birth of the effects of prenatal stresses. *Developmental Medicine and Child Neurology* **15**, 770–87.

Stott, D. H. and Latchford, S. A. (1976). Prenatal antecedents of child health, development and behavior. *Journal of the American Academy of Child Psychiatry* **15**, 161–91.

Talbert, D. G., Benson, P., and Dewhurst, J. (1982). Fetal response to maternal anxiety: a factor in antepartum heart rate monitoring. *Journal of Obstetrics and Gynaecology* **3**, 34–8.

Turner, E. K. (1956). The syndrome in the infant resulting from maternal emotional tension during pregnancy. *The Medical Journal of Australia* **4**, 221–2.

Vaughn, B. E., Bradley, C. F., Joffe, L. S., Seifer, R., and Barglow, P. (1987). Maternal characteristics measured prenatally are predictive of ratings of temperament 'difficulty' on the Carey Temperament Questionnaire. *Developmental Psychology* **23**, 152–61.

Visser, G. H. A. (1984). Fetal behaviour and the cardiovascular system. *Journal of Developmental Physiology* **6**, 215–24.

Visser, G. H. A., Goodman, J. D. S., Levine, D. H., and Dawes, G. S. (1982). Diurnal and other cyclic variations in human fetal heart rate near term. *American Journal of Obstetrics and Gynecology* **142**, 535–44.

Vries, J. I. P. de, Visser, G. H. A., and Prechtl, H. F. R. (1982). The emergence of fetal behaviour: I. Qualitative aspects. *Early Human Development* **7**, 301–22.

Vries, J. I. P. de. (1987). Development of specific movement patterns in the human fetus. *Thesis*, University of Groningen, Groningen, The Netherlands.

Wolkind, S. (1981). Pre-natal emotional stress: effects on the foetus. In: *Pregnancy: a psychological and social study* (ed. S. Wolkind and E. Zajicek), pp. 177–94. Academic Press, London.

Zimmer, E. Z., Divon, M. Y., Vilensky, A., Sarna, Z, Peretz, B. A., and Paldi, E. (1982). Maternal exposure to music and fetal activity. *European Journal of Obstetrics and Gynecology and Reproductive Biology* **13**, 209–13.

Part 4

Fetal behaviour and the
assessment of fetal well-being

13
Growth retardation

DOMENICO ARDUINI, GIUSEPPE RIZZO, and CARLO ROMANINI

Introduction

Impaired fetal growth can be secondary to multiple and various aetiologies, including chromosomal aberrations, structural abnormalities, constitutionally low growth potentialities, or a variety of maternal and placental pathologies that can lead to a diminished supply of nutrients to the fetus across the placenta (so-called utero-placental insufficiency). Differentiating between these aetiologies is complex, but the recent introduction of non-invasive (i.e. high-resolution ultrasound imaging and Doppler ultrasonography), and invasive (i.e. cordocentesis) techniques has enabled differential diagnoses to be made in most cases (Nicolaides *et al.* 1986; Arduini and Rizzo 1988).

In clinical practice, it is important to monitor the fetal condition of fetuses with intrauterine growth-retardation (IUGR) secondary to utero-placental insufficiency as these fetuses are at increased risk of developing perinatal distress. In this chapter we will therefore restrict our interest to fetuses in which the growth retardation is likely to be secondary to utero-placental insufficiency. These fetuses show a temporal sequence of adaptive mechanisms concomitant with the progressive deterioration of fetal condition (Visser and Bekedam 1990). This sequence of events—which starts with haemodynamic changes that lead to preferential perfusion of vital organs such as the brain and heart with a concomitant deprivation of the splanchnic organs and extremities (i.e. the so-called brain-sparing effect)—is concluded by abnormal heart-rate patterns (such as late decelerations and reduced variability). Notwithstanding the large inter-fetal variability, the interval between the haemodynamic changes (easily detectable with Doppler recordings) and the heart-rate abnormalities is usually prolonged (several weeks). Since the abnormalities of fetal heart-rate (FHR) might already reflect brain damage (Dijxhoorn *et al.* 1987), it is of particular interest to study this period of fetal behaviour, which is believed to be indicative of the quality of the central nervous system (Prechtl 1985). In this chapter we will review the modifications of fetal behaviour present in IUGR fetuses during the time preceding the onset of FHR abnormal-

Fetal behaviour

ities. Different behavioural variables (i.e. FHR patterns, body movements, eye movements, and breathing movements) will be considered both
separately and in association.

Fetal heart-rate patterns

In healthy fetuses, from the late second trimester of gestation onward,
periods of fetal rest and activity cycles clearly alternate. These periods are
characterized by the presence of FHR patterns with low and high variability. These patterns resemble the patterns A and B used by Nijhuis *et al.*
(1982; see also Chapter 3) for the definition of behavioural states near
term. In healthy fetuses studied longitudinally from 28 weeks onwards we
confirmed the developmental changes in fetal behaviour and the existence
of behavioural states near term (Arduini *et al.* 1986).

   No significant differences were found when the distribution of FHR
patterns A and B of healthy fetuses was compared with the distribution in
two groups of IUGR fetuses, divided according to the severity of their
haemodynamic compromise, this was based on the presence or absence of
Doppler measured end-diastolic velocities in the fetal thoracic descending
aorta (Rizzo *et al.* 1987). The lack of differences makes it possible to
speculate that the alternation between FHR patterns A and B is already

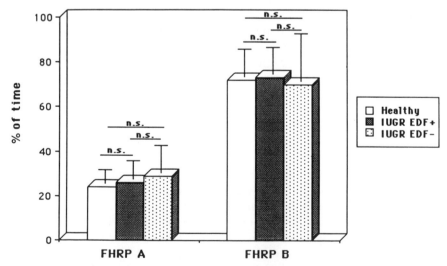

Fig. 13.1. Incidence (percentage of recording time) of fetal heart-rate (FHR)
patterns A and B in healthy and IUGR fetuses in relation to the presence or
absence of end-diastolic flow (EDF) in the descending thoracic aorta. (Redrawn
from Rizzo *et al.* 1987.)

established early in pregnancy and that it is not influenced by the progressive deterioration occurring in IUGR fetuses. Besides, when a quantitative analysis of FHR was performed by means of a computerized system, a progressive decrease of long-term FHR variations was seen in a longitudinal study of IUGR fetuses (Visser *et al.* 1990). However, the large inter-fetal differences in the reduction of variability limit the potential clinical application of this analysis.

Gross fetal body movements

Experimentally induced hypoxaemia causes a reduction or a cessation of movements in fetal sheep (Natale *et al.* 1981). In humans, a close association between sudden cessation of fetal body movements and subsequent intrauterine death has been reported (Pearson and Weaver 1976), but few data are available on the incidence of movements in IUGR fetuses in the time interval preceding fetal distress. In a quantitative comparison between either the number of movements or the percentage of time spent moving by IUGR fetuses and healthy fetuses of similar gestational age, there was only a slight reduction of these parameters for the IUGR fetuses (Fig. 13.2). These results are in agreement with those reported by Bekedam *et al.* (1987), who found that a noticeable decrease of fetal movements

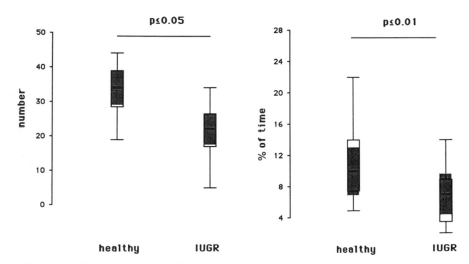

Fig. 13.2. Number and incidence (percentages of recording time) of gross fetal body movements in healthy and IUGR fetuses at 30 to 34 weeks of gestation. Boxes show interquartile ranges, bars indicate ranges, and the shaded areas show 95% confidence intervals.

is present only after the occurrence of late decelerations during FHR monitoring. This suggests that the decrease of fetal body movements is usually a late phenomenon in the series of events characterizing the fetal response to nutrient deprivation.

Qualitative assessment of fetal movements may be of greater importance, because qualitative changes of fetal movements seem to occur earlier. Body movements of IUGR fetuses have been described as 'weak' (Sadovsky *et al.* 1979) or 'slow and monotonous' (Bekedam *et al.* 1985) when compared to those of healthy fetuses. However, this qualitative analysis still requires the definition of inter-observer reproducibility and of inter-fetal variability before it can be applied clinically.

Fetal eye movements

In experimental animal models fetal hypoxia results in the arrest of fetal electro-ocular activity (Richardson *et al.* 1989). In the human, fetal eye movements are recorded using ultrasonic detection of lens movement, (Bots *et al.* 1981), and may be divided into the following three groups (Arduini *et al.* 1986) according to their frequency:

(1) rapid eye movements (REM) when there are more than six movements of the lens every minute;

(2) intermittent eye movements (IEM) when there are between one and six lens movements per minute;

(3) absent eye movements when there are no movements of the lens.

With advancing gestational age there is a progressive association of REM with FHR pattern B, and absence of eye movements with FHR pattern A, whereas the incidence of IEM significantly decreases (Arduini *et al.* 1986).

A significant decrease of the absolute number of eye movements is evident in IUGR fetuses (Arduini *et al.* 1988*a*). Furthermore, when the distribution of the different types of eye movements during the FHR patterns A and B was compared to that present in healthy fetuses at similar gestational ages a significant increase of IEM was noticed (Fig. 13.3), suggesting a delay in the development of eye motoricity in IUGR fetuses. However, these data on eye movements are based on cross-sectional recordings and do not, therefore, provide any information as to when these changes occur. Moreover, as all fetuses exhibited normal FHR tracings at the time of recording, it is possible to speculate that the changes in eye movements precede abnormalities in the FHR tracing.

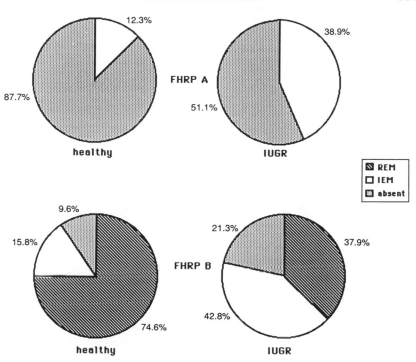

Fig. 13.3. Distribution of fetal eye movements during fetal heart-rate (FHR) patterns A and B in healthy and IUGR fetuses. Eye movements are classified as rapid eye movements (REM), intermittent eye movements (IEM), and absent. (From Arduini *et al.* 1988*b*.)

Fetal breathing movements

Hypoxaemia in fetal sheep results in decreased breathing movements, whereas hypercapnia increases their incidence (Natale *et al.* 981). In human IUGR fetuses the incidence of breathing movements remains within the reference limits when the FHR tracings are normal (Rizzo *et al.* 1987; van Vliet *et al.* 1985*a*). However, the mean duration of the episodes of breathing movements is significantly shortened (Fig. 13.4).

Applying the criteria of the biophysical profile (Manning *et al.* 1980), it has been shown that when FHR tracings become non-reactive, breathing movements seem to be the first variable to disappear, while body movements are compromised later (Ribbert *et al.* 1990). Furthermore, in this study, the absence of breathing movements was strongly associated with the presence of severe acidaemia.

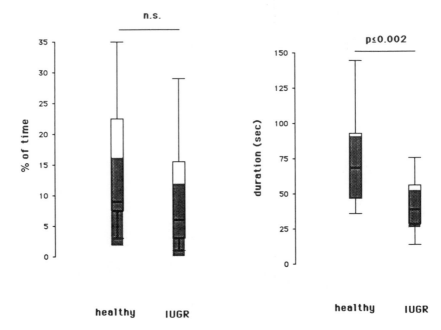

Fig. 13.4. Incidence (percentage of the recording time) and duration of fetal breathing movements in healthy and IUGR fetuses at 30 to 34 weeks of gestation. Boxes show interquartile ranges, bars indicate ranges, and shaded areas show 95% confidence intervals.

Fetal behavioural states

From 36 to 38 weeks onwards, the healthy human fetus exhibits well-regulated behavioural states with simultaneous changes of behavioural variables (i.e. FHR patterns, eye movements, and body movements) (Nijhuis *et al.* 1982; see also Chapter 3). The natural history of growth retardation does not usually allow these fetuses to reach this gestational age as they are usually delivered earlier due to the onset of fetal distress. However, IUGR fetuses reaching a gestational age greater than 36 weeks show evident disturbances in behavioural states (van Vliet *et al.* 1985*b*). Because these fetuses still had normal FHR records, it is likely that the impairment of fetal behavioural states precedes the occurrence of abnormal FHR tracings.

Before 36 weeks of gestation 'true' behavioural states do not exist, but it is sometimes possible to recognize periods of stable (i.e. lasting longer than three minutes) and recurrent associations (coincidence) between the behavioural variables, similar to those present during the behavioural states 1F to 4F. The incidence of these periods of coincidence, as well as the percentage of time spent by the fetus without coincidence of behavioural variables (i.e. percentage of time with no coincidence) can be calculated. This latter value, expressed as a function of gestational age, can be used as an index of the development of the fetal behavioural states (Arduini *et al.* 1991). Furthermore, by means of computerized systems (Rizzo *et al.* 1988), it is easy to analyse the transitional periods between two different periods of coincidence in terms of their duration and of their sequence of change of behavioural variables (Arduini *et al.* 1989).

Since both the percentage of time with 'no coincidence' and the characteristics of behavioural transitions change with gestation in healthy fetuses and are known, it is possible to compare the developmental trends of these parameters with those of IUGR fetuses at gestational ages earlier than 36 weeks.

Behavioural state coincidence

In healthy fetuses there is a progressive decrease of the percentage of time with no coincidence with advancing gestational age and an increased co-ordination between behavioural variables. This phenomenon is believed to be related to the development of the central nervous system (Prechtl 1985). In IUGR fetuses identified early in gestation by Doppler ultrasonography we found that the development of behavioural states was impaired and that this preceded the occurence of abnormal FHR tracings by weeks (Fig. 13.5). However, there is a large inter-fetal variability in the time interval

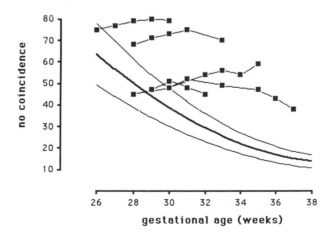

Fig. 13.5. Percentages time of 'no coincidence' in five IUGR fetuses diagnosed in early pregnancy by Doppler ultrasonography who later developed abnormal fetal heart-rate (FHR) tracings (late decelerations). Reference limits are shown as mean ± 2 SD (Arduini *et al.* 1991).

elapsing between abnormalities of behavioural state and the occurrence of abnormal FHR tracings. Furthermore, behavioural state analysis requires long recording times (preferably 2 hours or more), which seem to be incompatible with clinical practice, even when these procedures are restricted to selected fetuses.

Behavioural state transitions

In healthy fetuses there is a progressive decrease in the duration of behavioural state transitions from 28 weeks of gestation onwards (Arduini *et al.* 1991). With regard to the sequence of change of behavioural variables there is no prominent, leading variable whose appearance or disappearance heralds the transition until 34 weeks of gestation. Thereafter, body movements change first during transitions from coincidence 1F to 2F, whereas during transitions from 2F to 1F FHR patterns change first (Arduini *et al.* 1991).

In IUGR fetuses transitions lasted longer and the sequence of change of variables remained disorganized at similar gestational ages (Fig. 13.6) (Arduini *et al.* 1989). Furthermore, when transitions were evaluated longitudinally in IUGR fetuses, a progressive increase of durations, transitions became apparent, suggesting a potential role of their analysis in the monitoring of fetal condition (Fig. 13.7). It must be pointed out that a transition has usually occurred by 45.4 minutes of recording time (range 15 to 87 minutes); this time interval is compatible with clinical practice.

Effects of maternal hyperoxygenation

Maternal hyperoxygenation (see also Chapter 15) has been suggested as a potential therapy for severely IUGR fetuses (Nicolaides *et al.* 1987). During this treatment fetal pO_2 measured at cordocentesis increased significantly (Nicolaides *et al.* 1987) and the brain-sparing effect seemed to be abolished (Arduini *et al.* 1988*b*). Probably as a result of these modifications there are noticeable short-term changes of behaviour in IUGR fetuses during maternal hyperoxygenation. The incidence of gross body movements increases more than 250 per cent over base-line values, while breathing movements increase more than 75 per cent (Ruedrich *et al.* 1989). Similarly, long-term variability of FHR significantly increased during maternal hyperoxygenation, whereas no variations were present in the occurrence of FHR decelerations (Bekedam 1989). Up to now, few data are available on the long-term effects of this treatment. Visser and Bekedam (1990) reported their experience with a few IUGR fetuses; the initial increase of the behavioural variables was followed by a significant

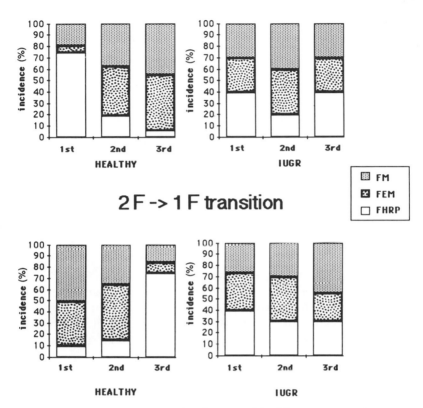

Fig. 13.6. Temporal sequence of the changes of fetal heart-rate (FHR) patterns, fetal eye movements (FEM), and fetal body movements (FM) during transitions from 1F to 2F and from 2F to 1F in healthy and IUGR fetuses. 1st, 2nd, and 3rd, the 1st, 2nd, or 3rd variable to change at a transition, e.g. FHR is the first variable to change at a transition from 1F to 2F in healthy fetuses in >70% of these transitions. In healthy fetuses, FEM is mostly the last variable to change from 'absent' to 'present' at a transition from 1F to 2F. (Redrawn from Arduini *et al.* 1989.)

decrease, and after seven days there were no noticeable differences compared to the pre-treatment values.

The discontinuation of maternal oxygen administration induces a rapid restoration of the brain-sparing effect (Arduini *et al.* 1988*b*) probably secondary to the concomitant decrease of fetal pO_2 levels. Similarly the incidences of both fetal body and breathing movements decrease to basal values, while the number of FHR decelerations significantly increases

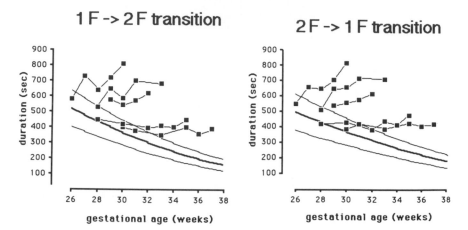

Fig. 13.7. Duration of transitions from 1F to 2F, and from 2F to 1F, in five IUGR fetuses diagnosed in early pregnancy by Doppler ultrasonography and who later developed abnormal fetal heart-rate (FHR) tracings (late decelerations). Reference limits are shown as mean ± 2 SD (Arduini *et al.* 1991).

(Bekedam 1989). This side-effect suggests that oxygen should be administered continuously without interruptions when used for chronic treatment. The significance of the analysis of fetal behaviour during maternal hyperoxygenation remains to be clarified, but preliminary results (Ruedrich *et al.* 1989) suggest that it may improve the diagnostic value of this procedure.

Concluding remarks

In fetal IUGR secondary to utero-placental insufficiency clear changes of fetal behaviour are present. The analysis of fetal movements alone seems to be of limited use as noticeable changes in their incidence are concomitant or subsequent to the appearance of abnormalities of FHR. Moreover, the simultaneous analysis of behavioural variables permits the identification of abnormalities in their integration, which are present in early gestation and may precede the onset of pathological cardiotocographic tracings by weeks. The restriction of behavioural analysis to transitional periods, thus reducing the required recording time makes this approach compatible with clinical practice. The potential applications of this analysis include the monitoring of the natural history of IUGR fetuses, and the assessment of the effects of possibly therapeutic intervention.

References

Arduini, D. and Rizzo, G. (1988). Differential diagnosis of small for gestational age fetuses by Doppler ultrasound. *Fetal Therapy* **3**, 31–6.

Arduini, D., Rizzo, G., Giorlandino, C., Dell'Acqua, S., Valensise, H., and Romanini C. (1986). The development of fetal behavioural states: a longitudinal study. *Prenatal Diagnosis* **6**, 117–24.

Arduini, D., Rizzo, G., Romanini, C., and Mancuso S. (1988a). Computerized analysis of fetal behavioural states in asymmetrical growth retarded fetuses. *Journal of Perinatal Medicine* **16**, 357–63.

Arduini, D., Rizzo, G., Mancuso, S., and Romanini, C. (1988b). Short-term effects of maternal oxygen administration on blood flow velocity waveforms in healthy and growth retarded fetuses. *American Journal Obstetrics and Gynecology* **159**, 1077–80.

Arduini D., Rizzo, G., Caforio, L., Boccolini, M. R., Romanini, C., and Mancuso, S. (1989). Behavioural state transitions in healthy and growth retarded fetuses. *Early Human Development* **19**, 155–62.

Arduini, D., Rizzo, G., Massacesi, M., Romanini, C., and Mancuso, S. (1991). Longitudinal assessment of behavioural transitions in healthy human fetuses during the last trimester of pregnancy. *Journal of Perinatal Medicine* **1**, 67–72.

Bekedam, D. J. (1989). Fetal heart rate and movement patterns in growth retardation. *Thesis*, University of Groningen.

Bekedam, D. J., Visser, G. H. A., Vries, J. J. de, and Prechtl, H. F. R. (1985). Motor behaviour in the growth retarded fetus. *Early Human Development* **12**, 155–65.

Bekedam, D. J., Visser, G. H. A., Mulder, E. J. H., and Poelmann-Weeijes, G. (1987). Heart rate variation and movement incidence in growth-retarded fetuses: the significance of antenatal late heart rate decelerations. *American Journal Obstetrics and Gynecology* **157**, 126–33.

Bots, R. S. G. M., Nijhuis, J. G., Martin, C. B. Jr., and Prechtl, H. F. R. (1981). Human fetal eye movements: election in utero by ultrasonography. *Early Human Development* **5**, 87–94.

Dijxhoorn, M. J., Visser, G. H. A., Touwen, B. C. L., and Huisjes, H. J. (1987). Apgar score, meconium and acidemia at birth in small for gestational age infants born at term, and their relation to neonatal neurological morbidity. *British Journal of Obstetrics and Gynaecology* **94**, 973–9.

Manning, F. A., Platt, L. D., and Sipos, L. (1980). Antepartum fetal evaluation: development of a fetal biophysical profile. *American Journal of Obstetrics and Gynecology* **136**, 787–95.

Natale, R., Clelow, F., and Dawes, G. S. (1981). Measurement of fetal forelimb movements in lambs in utero. *American Journal Obstetrics and Gynecology* **140**, 545–51.

Nicolaides, K. H., Soothill, P. W., Rodeck, C. H., and Campbell, S. (1986). Ultrasound-guided sampling of umbilical cord and placental blood to assess fetal well-being. *Lancet* **i**, 1065–7.

Nicolaides, K. H., Campbell, S., Bradley, R. J., Bilardo, C. M., Soothill, P. W., and Gibb, D. (1987). Maternal oxygen therapy for intrauterine growth retardation. *Lancet* **i,** 942–5.

Nijhuis, J. G., Prechtl, H. F. R., Martin, Jr. C. B., and Bots, R. S. G. M. (1982). Are there behavioural states in the human fetuses? *Early Human Development* **6,** 177–95.

Pearson, J. F. and Weaver, J. B. (1976). Fetal activity and fetal well-being: an evaluation. *British Medical Journal* **i,** 1305–7.

Prechtl, H. F. R. (1985), Ultrasound studies of fetal behaviour *Early Human Development* **12,** 91–8.

Ribbert, L. S. M., Snijders, R. J. M., Nicolaides, K. H., and Visser, G. H. A. (1990). Relationship of fetal biophysical profile and blood gas values at cordocentesis in severely growth retarded fetuses. *American Journal of Obstetrics and Gynecology* **163,** 569–71.

Richardson, B. S., Rurak, D., and Patrick, I. E. (1989). Cerebral oxidative metabolism during sustained hypoxemia in fetal sheep. *Journal of Developmental Physiology* **11,** 37–43.

Rizzo, G., Arduini, D., Romanini, C., and Mancuso S. (1987). Fetal behaviour in growth retardation: its relationship to fetal blood flow. *Prenatal Diagnosis* **7,** 229–38.

Rizzo, G., Arduini, D., Romanini, C., and Mancuso, S. (1988). Computer-assisted analysis of fetal behavioural states. *Prenatal Diagnosis* **8,** 479–84.

Ruedrich, D. A., Devoe, L. D., and Searle N. (1989). Effects of maternal hyperoxia on the biophysical assessment of fetuses with suspected intrauterine growth retardation. *American Journal of Obstetrics and Gynecology* **161,** 188–92.

Sadovsky, E., Laufer N., and Allen, J. W. (1979). The incidence of different types of fetal movements during pregnancy. *British Journal of Obstetrics and Gynaecology* **86,** 10–14.

Visser, G. H. A. and Bekedam, D. J. (1990). Serial observations on adaptation in the human fetus. In: *Fetal autonomy and adaptation* (ed. G. S. Dawes, F. Borruto, A. Zacutti and A. Zacutti, Jr.), pp. 67–80. Wiley, Chichester.

Visser, G. H. A., Bekedam, D. J., and Ribbert, L. S. M. (1990). Changes in antepartum heart rate patterns with progressive deterioration of the fetal condition. *International Journal of Biomedical Computers* **25,** 239–46.

Vliet, M. A. T. van, Martin, C. B. Jr., Nijhuis, J. G., and Prechtl, H. F. R. (1985*a*). The relationship between fetal activity and behavioural states and fetal breathing movements in normal and growth retarded fetuses. *American Journal of Obstetrics and Gynecology* **153,** 582–8.

Vliet, M. A. T. van, Martin, C. B. Jr., Nijhuis, J. G., and Prechtl, H. F. R. (1985*b*). Behavioural states in growth retarded fetuses. *Early Human Development* **12,** 183–97.

14
Diabetic pregnancy
E. J. H. MULDER

Introduction

Maternal type-1 (insulin-dependent) diabetes mellitus (IDDM) is associated with several embryonic and fetal developmental disorders. These include an increased incidence of structural malformations (Mills 1982; Mills et al. 1988), early growth delay (Mulder and Visser 1991a; Pedersen and Mølsted-Pedersen 1979, 1981; Pedersen et al. 1984), late macrosomia (Small et al. 1987; Visser et al. 1984), and disturbances in the functional development of the placenta (Laurini et al. 1987; Pedersen et al. 1986) and of fetal organ systems, such as the liver (Cuckle et al. 1989), lungs (Bourbon and Farrell 1985), kidneys (Cowett and Schwartz 1982) and central nervous system (CNS) (Dierker et al. 1982; Hassan et al. 1986; Schulte et al. 1969a,b,c).

Among the spectrum of fetal malformations in IDDM pregnancy, the CNS is often affected, and the rate of neural tube defects has been reported to be 3 to 20 times higher than that in the general population (Mills 1982; Milunsky et al. 1982). It may therefore be postulated that the functional development of the fetal CNS is also different in IDDM pregnancy, even when gross structural malformations are absent. Indicative of this are some signs of impaired development, demonstrable after birth. For instance, the behaviour of otherwise healthy infants of IDDM mothers has been found to be markedly different from that of controls in the first week after birth (Yogman et al. 1982), and disturbances have been found in the organization of neonatal behavioural states (Schulte et al. 1969b). Moreover, reports on follow-up studies have mentioned low intellectual performance (Churchill et al. 1969), and a moderate (Stehbens et al. 1977) or high (Bibergeil et al. 1975; Yssing 1975) incidence of cerebral dysfunction. However, these results suggesting delayed or disturbed functional development of the CNS have largely been obtained in an era in which maternal glucose control during pregnancy was poor (i.e data from 1946 to 1966 was analysed by Yssing (1975)).

Nowadays, intensified conventional insulin therapy and treatment by continuous subcutaneous insulin infusion (CSII), in combination with HbA1c determinations and blood glucose self-monitoring, have been shown to be an efficient way of achieving and maintaining tight glucose control (Van Ballegooie *et al*. 1985).

The general aim of the studies summarized below, was to investigate whether advanced treatment of IDDM women with CSII positively influences the functional development of the fetal nervous system. For this purpose, we studied longitudinally the emergence and rate of occurrence of specific fetal movement patterns in the first trimester, and the development of behavioural states in the third trimester and neonatal period. The study design and analyses of the data were identical to those employed in the first and third trimesters of normal pregnancy, as described by De Vries (see Chapter 1) and Nijhuis (see Chapter 3), respectively. The results of the behavioural studies on IDDM pregnancy were related to the quality of maternal blood glucose control. Since IDDM is essentially a condition affecting glycaemic control, a review of the literature on the subject of maternal blood glucose concentration and some aspects of fetal behaviour is also presented.

Fetal behaviour in normal pregnancy

Recent research has shown the normal repertoire of human fetal behaviour to comprise a set of distinct movement patterns. For each pattern, the age of first appearance in early development has been established. Reports have appeared on developmental trends in the occurrence of these various movements during the first 20 weeks of pregnancy. Similarly, figures on the variability, range of occurrence, and the intervals at which they are generated by the CNS have been published (see Chapter 1). During further development, the temporal patterning of several movements undergoes change, resulting in rest–activity cycles, which finally develop into true behavioural states (see Chapter 3). The fetal states reflect a certain degree of maturity or integrity of the fetal brain and are homologous with those seen in the neonate. These phenomena provide us with the most detailed information on fetal CNS functioning at different stages of development.

Effect of maternal blood glucose level on fetal movements and fetal heart-rate pattern

Before presenting our data on fetal behaviour in IDDM pregnancy, the possible effects of maternal blood glucose concentration on each of the three state variables (i.e. fetal heart-rate (FHR) pattern, fetal body movements, and fetal eye movements) are discussed separately. The effects of glucose on fetal breathing movements are included. The data reported in the literature relate to both normal and IDDM pregnancies.

Fetal body movements

There is controversy with respect to the fetal response to alterations in the maternal glucose levels that occur during normal pregnancy. The majority of reports state that increased maternal glucose levels, either induced naturally by a meal, or induced by an oral or intravenous glucose load, do not influence the incidence of fetal body movements (Bocking *et al.* 1982; Natale *et al.* 1983; Patrick *et al.* 1982). Some authors, however, found an increase in fetal body movements after an oral (Aladjem *et al.* 1979; Miller *et al.* 1978) or intravenous glucose bolus (Aladjem *et al.* 1979; Gelman *et al.* 1980). Others on the other hand found decreased body activity after meals (Roberts *et al.* 1979) or during the first hour of a 3-hour period of a glucose infusion producing a sustained mild maternal hyperglycaemia of about 7 mmol/litre, which was achieved by clamping (Edelberg *et al.* 1987).

In two studies performed on pregnancy in IDDM, no change in the incidence of fetal body movements was found in relation to maternal glucose concentrations (Roberts *et al.* 1980; Wladimiroff and Roodenburg 1982). The study by Holden *et al.* (1984) carried out on near-term fetuses of women with well-controlled IDDM is of interest. Using the glucose clamp technique, they showed that there was no difference in the occurrence of body movements and associated FHR accelerations between periods of maternal normoglycaemia (i.e. 3.3 to 7.8 mmol/litre) and periods of hyperglycaemia (i.e. greater than 7.8 mmol/litre). In contrast, under conditions of hypoglycaemia (i.e. less than 3.3 mmol/litre) a significant increase in body movements associated with FHR accelerations was observed. However, it has also been reported that the incidence of body movements is unaffected during maternal hypoglycaemia (Stangenberg *et al.* 1983).

Fetal eye movements

Reports on the possible effect of glucose on the occurrence of fetal eye movements are non-existent.

Fetal heart-rate pattern

Fetal body movements are closely associated with FHR accelerations in the third trimester of normal pregnancy (Timor-Tritsch *et al.* 1978; van Woerden *et al.* 1989). Few reports are available for IDDM pregnancy.

Sorokin *et al.* (1982) compared the amplitude and duration of FHR
accelerations monitored at 36 to 38 weeks in IDDM and normal pregnancies, and found no significant differences. The previously mentioned
study by Holden *et al.* (1984) also indicated that neither IDDM *per se*, nor
alterations in the maternal glucose level seem to disrupt the association
between fetal body movements and FHR accelerations. Whether these
factors influence FHR or its base-line variability, is largely unknown. The
induction of hypoglycaemia in IDDM women during the last trimester of
pregnancy resulted in a transient decrease in FHR variation, while FHR
remained unaltered (Stangenberg *et al.* 1983).

In two case reports, FHR changes (i.e. tachycardia with late decelerations) were described, which occurred during diabetic ketoacidosis under
hyperglycaemic (i.e. greater than 20 mmol/litre) conditions. The administration of insulin to the mother immediately abolished the late decelerations, but the raised FHR persisted for six hours (Hughes 1987; LoBue and
Goodlin 1978).

Fetal breathing movements

Numerous studies on normal pregnancy have demonstrated that raising
the maternal blood glucose level 1.5 to 3 times either naturally or
artificially, results in an increased incidence of breathing movements
(Adamson *et al.* 1983; Bocking *et al.* 1982; Harper *et al.* 1987; Natale *et al.*
1978; Patrick *et al.* 1978; de Vries *et al.* 1987). This effect of hyperglycaemia can be seen from 20 weeks of gestation onwards (de Vries *et al.*
1987), but probably originates at an earlier stage (i.e. 16 weeks, unpublished data). Hyperglycaemia does not change the generation pattern of
breathing movements in normal pregnancy (Adamson *et al.* 1983). It is
unknown whether hypoglycaemia affects the occurrence of breathing
movements.

The effect of hyperglycaemia on fetal breathing movements has also
been studied in IDDM pregnancies, but with conflicting results. Roberts *et
al.* (1980) saw a significantly increased breathing incidence after breakfast
and lunch, whereas in the study by Wladimiroff and Roodenburg (1982)
there were significantly less breathing movements immediately after lunch
and dinner than in controls. After breakfast, the incidence of breathing
movements was similar in the IDDM and control group. No correlation
with maternal glucose concentration was found.

To the author's knowledge, no reports have appeared on the effects of
artificially induced hyperglycaemia or hypoglycaemia on fetal breathing
movements in IDDM pregnancy.

Fetal behaviour in IDDM pregnancy

First trimester

All of the types of motor activity observed in the embryos and fetuses of women with generally well-controlled IDDM (i.e. by CSII) could be classified in accordance with the movement patterns of normal fetuses (Mulder and Visser 1991*b*). However, with the exception of breathing movements, there was a one to two week delay in the first appearance of all movement patterns, which normally emerge during the first 12 weeks of pregnancy (Fig. 14.1). Breathing movements were observed for the first time at an earlier age than in the control fetuses. This early emergence was even more striking when the generally smaller fetal size was taken into account.

When the emergence of frequently occurring movement patterns (the uppermost seven in Fig. 14.1) was plotted against fetal crown–rump length

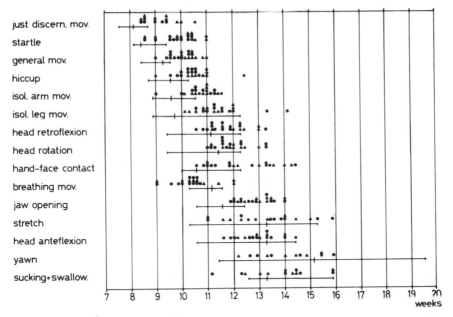

Fig. 14.1. First occurrence of specific fetal movement patterns in women with insulin-dependent diabetes melitus. Each symbol represents an individual. ● = preconceptional start of CSII; ▲ = start of CSII after conception. Ages at observation are given in full weeks and days. Data on the control group are shown as medians and ranges. CSII, continuous subcutaneous insulin infusion. (Reproduced with permission from Mulder and Visser 1991*b*.)

(CRL), which is usually smaller in IDDM pregnancy[1], there was still a general delay in comparison with the control group. The delay in motor development therefore does not run completely parallel with the delay in growth. This indicates the possible existence of a specific IDDM-related influence on the functional development of the embryonic and fetal nervous system. Hyperglycaemia, for example, may be responsible, as the delay in the emergence of fetal general movements was most profound in the women whose peri-conceptional glucose control was poor (Mulder and Visser 1991b).

The developmental trends in the occurrence of all movement patterns, except startles, were similar to those seen in the control fetuses (Mulder *et al.* 1991). Due to delayed emergence, fetal movements occurred less frequently before 9 weeks of gestation, but after 12 weeks the overall incidence (total motor output) was higher than in the control group. The latter was mainly due to an increase in the incidence of fetal breathing movements (Fig. 14.2). Breathing movements were generated differently by the CNS in the fetuses of women with IDDM at the end of the first trimester. They occurred with longer intervals between two consecutive breaths, resulting in a slower rate. No relationship was found between the incidence of breathing movements at 12 to 16 weeks and the maternal blood glucose levels measured immediately prior to the recording.

The temporal patterning of other movements, such as general movements and hiccups, did not differ between fetuses of the IDDM and control groups (Mulder *et al.* 1991).

Third trimester

The emergence of behavioural states in the fetuses of women with IDDM, was disturbed in comparison to control fetuses (Mulder *et al.* 1987, 1990). A low occurrence of FHR pattern A and coincidence 1F (C1F) appeared to be a common feature in IDDM pregnancy, and has been found throughout the third trimester [2] (Fig. 14.3a). It appeared that FHR pattern A was almost exclusively absent in the recordings from the fetuses who were macrosomic at birth (Table 14.1). On the other hand, the fetuses of IDDM women showed more of FHR pattern B, but had a similar incidence of coincidence 2F (C2F) as controls (Fig. 14.3b). This was due to a large

[1] Pedersen and Mølsted-Pedersen (1979) first made the observation that many embryos and fetuses of IDDM women are smaller than controls as judged by the CRL between 7 and 14 weeks of pregnancy. This phenomenon, called early growth delay, has been found in cross-sectional studies (Pedersen and Mølsted-Pedersen 1979, 1981; Tchobroutsky *et al.* (1985) and in a longitudinal study (Mulder and Visser 1991a).
[2] During 2-hour observations made between 32 and 38 weeks of gestation we did not see any FHR pattern A period in 8 of 47 (i.e. 17 per cent) recordings in the IDDM group, compared to 6 out of 98 (i.e. 6 per cent) control recordings.

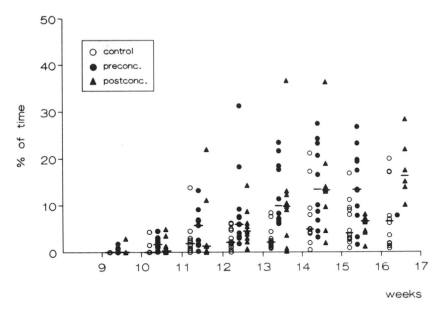

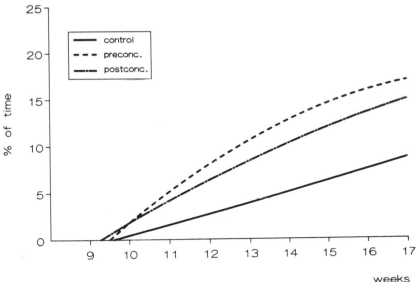

Fig. 14.2. Percentage of time during which breathing movements occurred in fetuses of women with insulin-dependent diabetes mellitus in the pre-conceptional and post-conceptional continuous subcutaneous insulin infusion (CSII) sub-groups during the first trimester of pregnancy as compared to control values, and the corresponding curves of best fit. (Reproduced with permission from Mulder *et al.* 1991.)

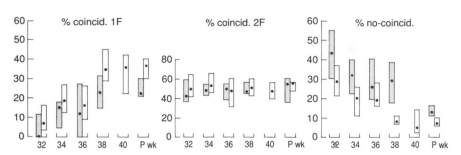

Fig. 14.3. Developmental course of coincidence 1F and 2F, and of no-coincidence for the fetuses and neonates of women with IDDM (shaded bars) compared to control values (unshaded bars). The median and interquartile range are given for each age studied. P = polygraphical recording in the first week after birth at 40 weeks post-menstrual age on average. (Reproduced with permission from Mulder *et al.* 1987.)

Table 14.1 Distribution of eight recordings without fetal heart-rate (FHR) pattern A among a total of 47 recordings from fetuses of mothers with IDDM in relation to fetal birth-weight centiles

| | Birth-weight centile | | | | |
	<25	25–50	50–75	75–90	>90
Number of fetuses (n = 17)	2	4	3	3	5
Number of recordings without FHR pattern A	0/6	0/12	0/9	2/7	6/13

number of asynchronous transitions into or out of C1F episodes, and to frequent interruption of the expected concordant association between the state 2F parameters. A high proportion of no-coincidence (Fig. 14.3c) and a rare occurrence of true behavioural states were the result. The criteria of behavioural states were met, for example, in only three out of the ten fetuses studied at 38 weeks of pregnancy (Mulder *et al.* 1990).

These results suggest delayed and/or disturbed development of fetal brain function in IDDM pregnancies. The same conclusion was drawn by others (Dierker *et al.* 1982) who investigated active and quiet periods of fetal motility (based on body movements and long-term FHR variation only). They found that the doubling of the duration of these periods which takes place between 28 and 40 weeks in normal fetuses, did not occur in the IDDM group.

In our series, the incidence of no-coincidence was especially high in the fetuses with a history of growth delay during early gestation, demonstrating the impact of early developmental disturbances on later development (Mulder 1990, pp. 134–9). This finding is in line with that of Bloch Petersen *et al.* (1988) who reported impaired psychomotor development at four years of age in the infants of mothers with IDDM who showed intrauterine growth delay during early pregnancy. Mention was made of impairments in personal–social development, gross motor development, and language and speech development in particular.

The generation of fetal general movements did not differ between the fetuses of the IDDM and control groups (Mulder *et al.* 1990), as also described for the first trimester (Mulder *et al.* 1991).

In contrast, the analysis of breathing movements at 38 weeks of pregnancy revealed altered neural regulation in the fetuses of IDDM women. As described for the first trimester, breathing movements were more numerous, but occurred at a considerably slower rate than in the control fetuses (Mulder *et al.* 1990). Apparently, IDDM has an effect on fetal breathing and the influence is present from the emergence of these movements onwards.

In normal pregnancy, fetal breathing activity is related to maternal plasma glucose concentration (Adamson *et al.* 1983; Bocking *et al.* 1982; de Vries *et al.* 1987). However, the underlying mechanism in IDDM pregnancy might be different, since no clear relationship was found between the breathing incidence and the glucose level either in the first (Mulder *et al.* 1991) or in the third trimester (Wladimiroff and Roodenburg 1982). Moreover, glucose has no effect on the breath-to-breath interval in non-IDDM pregnancy and, hence, does not alter the rate of breathing (Adamson *et al.* 1983).

Fetal breathing movements consume significant amounts of oxygen and glucose. It can be speculated that the increased incidence of fetal breathing found throughout IDDM pregnancy might be a compensatory mechanism for reducing excessive quantities of delivered energy substrate. The fact that third trimester fetuses of IDDM women, especially the macrosomic ones, spend less time in coincidence 1F ('quiet sleep') and have longer activity cycles than control fetuses might serve a similar purpose. Thus, maybe an excess of glucose is initially diminished by maximizing the movement incidence and, if hyperglycaemia persists or exceeds a certain level, fetal accretion mechanisms are activated, which stimulate fetal over growth (Mulder 1990, pp. 144–5). If true, fetal movements may have functional significance in three distinct ways. Firstly, some movement patterns are of importance to the instantaneous survival or behavioural and morphological development of the fetus. Secondly, other movements prepare the fetus by practice and exercise for his or her postnatal life. Thirdly, as moving costs energy, fetal motility may regulate the flow of energy (Mulder 1990, p. 144).

Infants of women with IDDM

Poor organization of behavioural states, as reflected by a high incidence of no-coincidence (Fig. 14.3), was also present at one week after birth in neonates of mothers with IDDM and must, therefore, be considered as a sequel of long-term exposure to the non-optimal intrauterine environment (Mulder *et al*. 1990).

The electroencephalogram (EEG) patterns of the neonates of IDDM women were generally judged to be quite immature. Moreover, periodic breathing occurred much more often during state 2 in the neonates of the IDDM group than in controls (on average 14 per cent and 2 per cent, respectively). The higher incidence of periodic breathing reflects less stable control of the respiratory system. This is probably due to immaturity of the neural mechanism underlying respiration, as suggested by the fact that the amount of periodic breathing decreased with age in control infants, but not in those of IDDM mothers (Mulder *et al*. 1990).

The poor behavioural state organization in the IDDM group, both before and after birth, resembles more immature patterns. The observed immature EEG patterns and the high incidence of periodic breathing in the neonates of IDDM mothers, corroborate this conclusion.

Still other evidence of delayed cerebral maturation are the increased levels of alpha-melanocyte-stimulating hormone (α-MSH) found in the cord blood of neonates of IDDM women (Hassan *et al*. 1986). The protein α-MSH is produced by the pars intermedia of the fetal pituitary which regresses with increasing age during normal third trimester development. The higher levels of α-MSH may therefore reflect a delay in the regression of the pars intermedia.

The observations made over 20 years ago by Schulte *et al*. (1969*a,b,c*), are in accordance with the former results. They studied behavioural states in the neonates of IDDM mothers and found several immature characteristics of sleep (Schulte *et al*. 1969*b*). Their EEG patterns resembled those of less mature normal infants (i.e. of 36 weeks or younger) (Schulte *et al*. 1969*a*). The neurological condition of the neonates of IDDM mothers was often judged as hyperexcitable (Schulte *et al*. 1969*c*). Others, investigating neonates of IDDM mothers during the first week of life, found marked differences in behaviour compared to that of control infants. In the neonates of IDDM mothers, there was a higher incidence of neurological disorders, which were mainly caused by hypotonia, and which correlated with hypoglycaemia (Priestly 1972). Furthermore, neonates of IDDM mothers scored lower on the Brazelton scale on days 3, 5, and 7, comprising items on motor performance, sensory orientation, and autonomic stability (Yogman *et al*. 1982).

Controversy exists as to whether these neonatal differences persist and influence later development. In our series, later development appeared to be favourable. A follow-up study was carried out on 40 infants of IDDM mothers, including a number of the infants studied *in utero* (Holwerda-Kuipers and Visser 1986). The children were investigated at various ages between 10 months and 4.5 years of age using a set of different psychological tests appropriate for the age at examination (e.g. Bayley-test between 10 and 30 months of age). Assessment was made of the level of mental, speech, motor, temperament, and behavioural development. These aspects of neuropsychological development did not differ between the study group and a group of matched controls. When a sub-group of the children of IDDM mothers with a high birth-weight was analysed separately, one difference was found: there was a delay in motor development in comparison to the control infants with a high or normal birth-weight. It therefore seems that generally, the children of IDDM mothers develop successfully after birth. This is in line with the conclusion drawn by others who found no impairment of the intellectual status of such children at 5 years of age (Persson and Gentz 1984), 7 years of age (Cummins and Norrish 1980), or at other ages (Hadden *et al.* 1984). Nevertheless, infants with a history of early embryonic/fetal growth delay (Bloch Petersen *et al.* 1988; Mulder 1990, pp. 134–9) or those who are macrosomic at birth (Holwerda-Kuipers and Visser 1986) continue to run an increased risk of neurological dysfunction.

Studies on neurological and psychomotor development in infants born to IDDM mothers which were carried out before 1980, generally indicate a poor prognosis for these infants. Long-term effects on the development of these children were shown, and were reflected by low intellectual performance at the age of 4 years (Churchill *et al.* 1969) and by a moderate (Stehbens *et al.* 1977) or high incidence (Bibergeil *et al.* 1975; Yssing 1975) of cerebral dysfunction. The improvements made during the past decennium may be due to better blood glucose control during pregnancy and/or to better obstetrical and neonatal management.

Epilogue

The data presented in this chapter demonstrate that the functional development of the fetal CNS during IDDM pregnancy differs from that observed in normal pregnancy. The development of CNS-related functions shows delayed and/or disturbed characteristics. Indicative of this are the delayed emergence of movement patterns in the first trimester of pregnancy, the delayed emergence of behavioural states in the third trimester, and after birth, the continuity of poor behavioural state organization, immature EEG patterns, and a high incidence of periodic breathing. Evidence of delayed functional development of other fetal organ systems (i.e. the lung, liver, and placenta) is in accordance with these findings of delayed cerebral maturation in fetuses and neonates of IDDM women. Of special interest is the observation that embryos and fetuses who were smaller than normal during early IDDM pregnancy exhibit the poorest organization of behavioural states near term.

What really happens during the peri-conceptional period and during early IDDM pregnancy remains largely obscure. Although hyperglycaemia is a likely disturbance-causing factor, the structural (CRL) (Mulder and Visser 1991a) and functional development of the embryos and fetuses were still affected when the circulating maternal blood glucose levels were (near) normal before conception. Thus, tight glucose control of the mother is no guarantee that developmental disorders will be prevented. It must be realized that during IDDM pregnancy, a degree of glucose control which approaches that of the finely regulated daily glucose levels normally present in the non-IDDM pregnant woman, is only rarely achieved. It might be that particularly the minute-to-minute fluctuations in blood glucose affect embryonic/fetal cells, rather than sustained high glucose concentrations. Moreover, the glycosylation of haemoglobin as a measure of the quality of glycaemic control over the near past, may not reveal true episodes of hyperglycaemia. In addition, adequate glucose control is not necessarily identical to adequate 'metabolic' control and it may well be that other disturbances (for example of amino acids, free fatty acids, etc.) persist despite (near) normoglycaemia. Nevertheless, good glucose control set up well in advance of conception is recommended by everyone, as it is virtually the only remedy at the moment.

Acknowledgement

The author is most grateful to Professor Dr G. H. A. Visser and Dr R. H. Stigter for critically reading the manuscript.

References

Adamson, S. L., Bocking, A., Cousin, A. J., Rapoport, I., and Patrick, J. E. (1983). Ultrasonic measurement of rate and depth of human fetal breathing: Effect of glucose. *American Journal of Obstetrics and Gynecology* **147**, 288–95.

Aladjem, S., Feria, A., Rest, J., Gull, K., and O'Connor, M. (1979). Effect of maternal glucose load on fetal activity. *American Journal of Obstetrics and Gynecology* **134**, 276–80.

Ballegooie, E. van, Visser, G. H. A., and Laurini, R. N. (1985). Continuous subcutaneous insulin infusion (CSII) in pregnancy. *Netherlands Journal of Medicine* **28**, (Suppl. 1), 3–6.

Bibergeil, H., Gödel, E., and Amendt, P. (1975). Diabetes and pregnancy: Early and late prognoses of children of diabetic mothers. In: *Early diabetes in early life* (ed. R. A. Camerini-Davalos and H. S. Cole), pp. 427–34. Academic Press, New York.

Bloch Petersen, M., Pedersen, S. A., Greisen, G., Pedersen, J. F., and Mølsted-Pedersen, L. (1988). Early growth delay in diabetic pregnancy: relation to psychomotor development at age 4. *British Medical Journal* **296**, 598–600.

Bocking, A., Adamson, S. L., Cousin, A., Campbell, K., Carmichael, L., Natale, R., and Patrick, J. (1982). Effects of intravenous glucose injections on human fetal breathing movements and gross fetal body movements at 38 to 40 weeks' gestational age. *American Journal of Obstetrics and Gynecology* **142**, 606–11.

Bourbon, J. R. and Farrell, P. M. (1985). Fetal lung development in the diabetic pregnancy. *Pediatric Research*, **19**, 253–67.

Churchill, J. A., Berendes, H. W., and Nemore, J. (1969). Neuropsychological deficits in children of diabetic mothers. *American Journal of Obstetrics and Gynecology* **105**, 257–68.

Cowett, R. M. and Schwartz, R. (1982). The infant of the diabetic mother. *Pediatric Clinics of North America* **29**, 1213–31.

Cuckle, H. S., Wald, N. J., and Hughes, D. R. (1989). Cord serum alpha-fetoprotein and maternal insulin-dependent diabetes mellitus. *British Journal of Obstetrics and Gynaecology* **96**, 1450–2.

Cummins, M. and Norrish, M. (1980). Follow-up of children of diabetic mothers. *Archives of Diseases in Childhood* **55**, 259–64.

Dierker, L. J., Pillay, S., Sorokin, Y., and Rosen, M. G. (1982). The change in fetal activity periods in diabetic and nondiabetic pregnancies. *American Journal of Obstetrics and Gynecology* **143**, 181–5.

Edelberg, S. C., Dierker, L. J., Kalhan, S., and Rosen, M. G. (1987). Decreased fetal movements with sustained maternal hyperglycemia using the glucose clamp technique. *American Journal of Obstetrics and Gynecology* **156**, 1101–5.

Gelman, S. R., Spellacy, W. N., Wood, S., Birk, S. A., and Buhi, W. C. (1980). Fetal movements and ultrasound: Effect of maternal intravenous glucose administration. *American Journal of Obstetrics and Gynecology* **137**, 459–61.

Hadden, D. R., Byrne, E., Trotter, I., Harley, J. M. G., McClure, G., and McAuley, R. R. (1984). Physical and psychological health of children of type 1 (insulin-dependent) diabetic mothers. *Diabetologia* **26**, 250–4.

Harper, M. A., Meis, P. J., Rose, J. C., Swain, M., Burns, J., and Kardon, B. (1987). Human fetal breathing response to intravenous glucose is directly related to gestational age. *American Journal of Obstetrics and Gynecology* **157**, 1403–5.

Hassan, M. M., Bottoms, S. F., Evans, M. I., Dombrowski, M. P., Mariona, F. G., and Mukherjee, A. B. (1986). Fetal α-melanocyte-stimulating hormone levels: No correlation with late fetal growth but increased with diabetes mellitus. *American Journal of Obstetrics and Gynecology* **154**, 428–30.

Holden, K. P., Jovanovic, L., Druzin, M. L., and Peterson, C. M. (1984). Increased fetal activity with low maternal blood glucose levels in pregnancies complicated by diabetes. *American Journal of Perinatology* **1**, 161–4.

Holwerda-Kuipers, J. and Visser, G. H. A. (1986). Psychological development of infants of women with type-1 diabetes. In: *Proceedings of the 27th meeting of the Dutch Federation of Medical Scientific Societies*, April 1986, Abstract 171. Groningen, The Netherlands.

Hughes, A. B. (1987). Fetal heart rate changes during diabetic ketosis. *Acta Obstetrica et Gynecologica Scandinavica* **66**, 71–3.

Laurini, R. N., Visser, G. H. A., Ballegooie, E. van, and Schoots, C. J. F. (1987). Morphological findings in placentas of insulin-dependent diabetic patients treated with continuous subcutaneous insulin infusion (CSII). *Placenta* **8**, 153–165.

LoBue, C. and Goodlin, R. C. (1978). Treatment of fetal distress during diabetic keto-acidosis. *Journal of Reproductive Medicine* **20**, 101–4.

Miller, F. C., Skiba, H., and Klapholz, H. (1978). The effect of maternal blood sugar levels on fetal activity. *Obstetrics and Gynecology* **52**, 662–5.

Mills, J. L. (1982). Malformations in infants of diabetic mothers. *Teratology* **25**, 385–94.

Mills, J. L., Knopp, R. H., Simpson, J. L., Jovanovic-Peterson L., Metzger, B. E., Holmes, L. B. *et al.* (1988). Lack of relation of increased malformation rates in infants of diabetic mothers to glycemic control during organogenesis. *New England Journal of Medicine* **318**, 671–6.

Milunsky, A., Alpert, E., Kitzmiller, J. L., Younger, M. D., and Neff, R. K. (1982). Prenatal diagnosis of neural tube defects. VIII. The importance of serum alpha-fetoprotein screening in diabetic pregnant women. *American Journal of Obstetrics and Gynecology* **142**, 1030–2.

Mulder, E. J. H. (1990). Fetal behaviour: studies on normal and diabetic pregnancy. *Thesis*, University of Groningen, The Netherlands.

Mulder, E. J. H. and Visser, G. H. A. (1991*a*). Growth and motor development in fetuses of women with type-1 diabetes. I. Early growth patterns. *Early Human Development* **25**, 91–106.

Mulder, E. J. H. and Visser, G. H. A. (1991*b*). Growth and motor development in fetuses of women with type-1 diabetes. II. Emergence of specific movement patterns. *Early Human Development* **25**, 107–15.

Mulder, E. J. H., Visser, G. H. A., Bekedam, D. J., and Prechtl, H. F. R. (1987). Emergence of behavioural states in fetuses of type-1 diabetic women. *Early Human Development* **15**, 231–52.

Mulder, E. J. H., O'Brien, M. J., Lems, Y. L., Visser, G. H. A., and Prechtl, H. F. R. (1990). Body and breathing movements in near-term fetuses and newborn infants of type-1 diabetic women. *Early Human Development* **24**, 131–52.

Mulder, E. J. H., Visser, G. H. A., Morssink, L. P., and De Vries, J. I. P. (1991). Growth and motor development in fetuses of women with type-1 diabetes. III. First trimester quantity of fetal movement patterns. *Early Human Development* **25**, 117–33.

Natale, R., Patrick, J., and Richardson, B. (1978). Effects of human maternal venous plasma glucose concentrations on fetal breathing movements. *American Journal of Obstetrics and Gynecology* **132**, 36–41.

Natale, R., Richardson, B., and Patrick, J. (1983). The effect of maternal hyperglycemia on gross body movements in human fetuses at 32–34 weeks' gestation. *Early Human Development* **8**, 13–20.

Patrick, J., Natale, R., and Richardson, B. (1978). Patterns of human fetal breathing activity at 34 to 35 weeks' gestational age. *American Journal of Obstetrics and Gynecology* **132**, 507–13.

Patrick, J., Campbell, K., Carmichael, L., Natale, R., and Richardson, B. (1982). Patterns of gross fetal body movements over 24-hour observation intervals during the last 10 weeks of pregnancy. *American Journal of Obstetrics and Gynecology* **142**, 363–71.

Pedersen J. F. and Mølsted-Pedersen, L. (1979). Early growth retardation in diabetic pregnancy. *British Medical Journal* **1**, 18–19.

Pedersen, J. F. and Mølsted-Pedersen, L. (1981). Early fetal growth delay detected by ultrasound marks increased risk of congenital malformation in diabetic pregnancy. *British Medical Journal* **283**, 269–71.

Pedersen, J. F., Mølsted-Pedersen, L., and Mortensen, H. B. (1984). Fetal growth delay and maternal hemoglobin Alc in early diabetic pregnancy. *Obstetrics and Gynecology* **64**, 351–2.

Pedersen, J. F., Mølsted-Pedersen, L., and Lebech, P. E. (1986). Is the early growth delay in the diabetic pregnancy accompanied by a delay in placental development? *Acta Obstetrica et Gynecologica Scandinavica* **65**, 675–7.

Persson, B. and Gentz, J. (1984). Follow-up of children of insulin-dependent and gestational diabetic mothers. Neuropsychological outcome. *Acta Paediatrica Scandinavica* **73**, 349–58.

Priestly, B. L. (1972). Neurological assessment of infants of diabetic mothers in the first week of life. *Pediatrics* **50**, 578–83.

Roberts, A. B., Little, D., Cooper, D., and Campbell, S. (1979). Normal patterns of fetal activity in the third trimester. *British Journal of Obstetrics and Gynaecology* **86**, 4–9.

Roberts, A. B., Stubbs, S. M., Mooney, R., Cooper, D., Brudenell, J. M., and Campbell, S. (1980). Fetal activity in pregnancies complicated by maternal diabetes mellitus. *British Journal of Obstetrics and Gynaecology* **87**, 485–9.

Schulte, F. J., Michaelis, R., Nolte, R., Albert, G., Parl, U., and Lasson, U. (1969*a*). Brain and behavioural maturation in newborn infants of diabetic mothers. Part I: Nerve conduction and EEG patterns. *Neuropädiatrie* **1**, 24–35.

Schulte, F. J., Lasson, U., Parl, U., Nolte, R., and Jürgens, U. (1969*b*). Brain and behavioural maturation in newborn infants of diabetic mothers. Part II: Sleep cycles. *Neuropädiatrie* **1**, 36–43.

Schulte, F. J., Albert, G., and Michaelis, R. (1969*c*). Brain and behavioural maturation in newborn infants of diabetic mothers. Part III. Motor behaviour. *Neuropädiatrie* **1**, 44–55.

Small, M., Cameron, A., Lunan, B., and MacCuish, A. C. (1987). Macrosomia in pregnancy complicated by insulin-dependent diabetes mellitus. *Diabetes Care* **10**, 594–9.

Sorokin, Y., Dierker, L. J., Chik, L., Kollar, L. L., and Rosen, M. G. (1982). Fetal heart rate accelerations in low-risk and diabetic pregnancies during active behavioral periods. *American Journal of Obstetrics and Gynecology* **143**, 224–5.

Stangenberg, M., Persson, B., Stånge, L., and Carlström, K. (1983). Insulin-induced hypoglycemia in pregnant diabetics. *Acta Obstetrica et Gynecologica Scandinavica* **62**, 249–52.

Stehbens, J. A., Baker, G. L., and Kitchell, M. (1977). Outcome at ages 1, 3, and 5 years of children born to diabetic women. *American Journal of Obstetrics and Gynecology* **127**, 408–13.

Tchobroutsky, C., Breart, G. L., Rambaud, D. C., and Henrion, R. (1985).

Correlation between fetal defects and early growth delay observed by ultrasound. *Lancet* **i**, 706–7.

Timor-Tritsch, I. E., Dierker, L. J., Zador, I., Hertz, R. H., and Rosen, M. G. (1978). Fetal movements associated with fetal heart rate accelerations and decelerations. *American Journal of Obstetrics and Gynecology* **131**, 276–80.

Visser, G. H. A., Van Ballegooie, E., and Sluiter, W. J. (1984). Macrosomia despite well-controlled diabetic pregnancy. *Lancet* **i**, 284–5.

Vries, J. I. P. de, Visser, G. H. A., Mulder, E. J. H., and Prechtl, H. F. R. (1987). Diurnal and other variations in fetal movement and heart rate patterns at 20–22 weeks. *Early Human Development* **15**, 333–48.

Wladimiroff, J. W. and Roodenburg, P. J. (1982). Human fetal breathing and gross body activity relative to maternal meals during insulin-dependent pregnancy. *Acta Obstetrica et Gynecologica Scandinavica* **61**, 65–8.

Woerden, E. E. van (1989). Fetal heart rate and movements; their relationship within behavioural states 1F and 2F. *Thesis*, Free University, Amsterdam, The Netherlands.

Yogman, M. W., Cole, P., Als, H., and Lester, B. M. (1982). Behavior of newborns of diabetic mothers. *Infant Behaviour and Development* **5**, 331–40.

Yssing, M. (1975). Long-term prognosis of children born to mothers diabetic when pregnant. In: *Early diabetes in early life* (ed. R. A. Camerini-Davalos and H. S. Cole), pp. 575–86. Academic Press, New York.

15
Fetal behaviour in relation to stimulation
ROBERT GAGNON

Introduction

It is recognized by clinicians that the presence of fetal heart-rate (FHR) accelerations with fetal body movements (state 2F or active sleep state) is an indicator of fetal health. These observations, along with the demonstration of rest–activity cycles in the human fetus, have provided the physiological basis for antepartum FHR testing (Brown and Patrick 1981). The behavioural response of the neonate to stimuli is an essential part of the neurological examination of the new-born infant to measure the integrity and function of the central nervous system (Prechtl 1974). Different sensory channels, such as auditory, vibro-tactile, or olfactory, have been used to elicit a response (Hutt *et al*. 1969; Lenard *et al*. 1968). Fetal behavioural activity remains unchanged during stimulation using an external source of light (Polishuk *et al*. 1975), external manipulation of the fetus (Richardson *et al*. 1981; Visser *et al*. 1983; Druzin *et al*. 1985), and maternal ingestion of glucose (Bocking *et al*. 1982). However, significant alterations in fetal behaviour have been reported following external sound and vibration (Gagnon *et al*. 1987*a*).

Neonatal responses to external stimulation

In order to provide a better understanding of the fetal behavioural responses to stimulation, a brief overview of the neonatal responses to different stimuli is essential. Studies using stimulation of peripheral sensory receptors in neonates face four major problems:

(1) choice of an event to be termed a 'reproducible response';

(2) determination of whether the occurrence of this response is causally related to the stimulus;

(3) accurate measurement of the response;

(4) analysis of the effect of behavioural states at the time of stimulus on

the occurrence, magnitude, and temporal course of the response (Prechtl 1974).

The well co-ordinated behaviours of the infant, such as startles, head-turning, and sucking, have all been successfully used as indices of response to stimulation. Proprioceptive (vibratory) reflexes, such as ankle clonus and the Moro reflex, are well elicited during regular sleep (state 1) and during quiet wakefulness (state 3). These reflexes are weak or absent during state 2 (rapid eye movements (REM) present). Nociceptive (pain-elicited) reflexes, such as the Babinski reflex, can be obtained in any behavioural state (Prechtl 1974). Table 15.1 summarizes the pattern of the responses to various stimuli in relation to the different neonatal behavioural states (Prechtl 1974).

Hutt *et al.* (1969) reported that broadband acoustic signals (such as square-wave pulses) at an intensity above 90 dB sound pressure level (SPL) applied during quiet sleep state (state 1) generally produced a 'startle reflex', followed by a period of state 2 or by waking (state 4). The same authors recorded the electromyographic (EMG) activity from six sites: the right and left biceps brachii, the right and left triceps, and the right and left quadriceps. Pure-tone sine wave at frequencies between 70 and 2000 Hz were applied at 40 cm from one ear. The same experiments were repeated using square-wave stimuli at the same frequencies. The probability of obtaining EMG responses was highest (i.e. 93 per cent) at low frequency (i.e. 125 Hz) when using square-wave stimulus, whereas with sine wave it was only 65 per cent. The probability of an EMG response decreased rapidly with increasing frequency, being only 35 per cent at 2000 Hz. Similarly, an increase in heart rate was seen only when using a square-wave, low-frequency (125 Hz) stimulation. Therefore, in term healthy neonates, the types of stimulus used in addition to the behavioural states are important determinants to the correct evaluation of fetal heart-rate and movement responses.

Maturation of fetal sensory receptors

The embryonic human ear develops from an ectodermal thickening, the auditory placode (Altmann 1950). As the placode invaginates into surrounding mesenchyme, a pit develops that assumes a vesicular shape and is termed the otocyst. In the 4- to 5-week-old embryo, the otocyst divides into two lobes; one lobe becomes the cochlea and the other the labyrinth. At 6 months, both the organ of Corti and the tunnel of Corti are present in all turns of the cochlea. Peripheral vibration-sensitive endings include Meissner's and Pacinian corpuscles, which transmit vibro-tactile stimuli, and have been described in the hands of human fetuses at 24 weeks of

Table 15.1 Response to stimulation in different states (Adapted with permission from Prechtl 1974)

	State 1	State 2	State 3
Proprioceptive reflexes			
Knee jerk	+ + +	±	+ +
Biceps jerk	+ + +	±	+ +
Lip jerk	+ + +	±	+ +
Ankle clonus	+ + +	−	−
Moro tap	+ + +	−	+ +
Moro head drop	+ + +	−	+ +
Exteroceptive skin reflexes			
Tactile			
Rooting	−	−	+ +
Palmar grasp	−	+	+ +
Plantar grasp	−	+ +	+ +
Lip protrusion	−	+ + +	+ +
Finger reflex	±	+	+ +
Toe reflex	−	+	+ +
Tibial reflex	±	+ +	+ +
Fibular reflex	±	+ +	+ +
Axillary reflex	±	+ +	+ +
Pressure			
Babkin	−	+	+ +
Palmomental	−	+ +	+ +
Nociceptive			
Babinski reflex	+ +	+ + +	+ + +
Abdominal reflex	+ +	+ + +	+ + +
Thigh	+ +	+ + +	+ + +
Pubic	+ +	+ + +	+ + +
Inguinal	+ + +	+ + +	+ + +
Auditory response			
Auditory orienting	±	+ +	+ + +
Visual response			
Visual pursuit	−	−	+ +
Vestibular response			
Vestibulo-ocular	−	+ +	+ + +

gestation (Bradley and Mistretta 1975). By about the 25th week of intrauterine life, the cochlea and peripheral sensory end organs have reached their normal development.

Fetal behavioural responses to sound and vibration

The intrauterine sound environment

In contrast to the neonate who is exposed to different stimuli of known and measurable intensities, the human fetus is surrounded by the amniotic cavity. Until recently, it was not technically feasible to measure the fetal sound environment during the application of external acoustic stimulation on the surface of the maternal abdomen. We measured the intrauterine background noise in 10 women in active labour using a miniaturized hydrophone placed transcervically at the level of the fetal neck under ultrasonographic guidance (Benzaquen *et al.* 1990). In eight women no cardiovascular sound was audible and the intrauterine noise consisted predominantly of low-frequency (i.e. less than 100 Hz) noise with intensities between 60 and 85 dB. In only two women were maternal cardiovascular sounds audible during uterine relaxation, but they disappeared during uterine contraction. Maternal bowel sounds and maternal vocalization featured well above the intrauterine background noise (Fig. 15.1).

Vibratory acoustic stimulation (VAS) using an electronic artificial larynx (EAL; Western Electric, Model 5C, New York) is now widely used in the assessment of fetal health. Significant alterations in fetal behaviour have been reported following stimulation with the EAL (Visser *et al.* 1989). The device produces a broadband noise at a fundamental frequency of 87 Hz, with multiple harmonics up to 15 000 Hz (Gagnon 1989). The surface of the instrument vibrates at all frequencies between 10 and 15 000 Hz, and maximum vibration occurs at 450 Hz. Figure 15.2 is an example of intrauterine sound spectrum recorded during external stimulation with the EAL. It consists of a fundamental frequency of 87 Hz with multiple harmonics up to 20 000 Hz at intensities between 90 and 100 dB. Although it has been previously suggested that frequencies above 3000 Hz would be attenuated by at least 70 dB (Walker *et al.* 1971), it is not the case during stimulation with the EAL when coupling between the vibrating surface of the instrument and maternal soft tissues provides optimal transmission of frequencies up to at least 20 000 Hz (Gagnon *et al.* 1990*a*).

Fetal heart-rate response

FHR is easy to measure and for this reason is widely used in the assessment of fetal health. Four different patterns (1F to 4F) have been described in

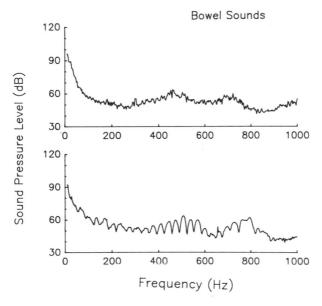

Fig. 15.1. Recording of typical intrauterine background noise recorded during audible low-pitched (upper) and high-pitched (lower) bowel sounds (2×10^{-5} newtons/m^2). (Reprinted with permission from Benzaquen *et al.* 1990.)

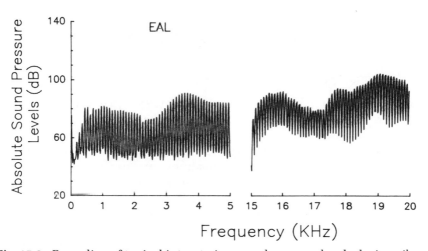

Fig. 15.2. Recording of typical intrauterine sound pressure levels during vibratory acoustic stimulation applied on the surface of the maternal abdomen. Frequencies between 5000 and 15 000 Hz have not been included due to lack of space. (2×10^{-5} newtons/m^2.)

relation to the four different fetal behavioural states (Nijhuis *et al*. 1982). With the development of antenatal FHR monitoring, Read and Miller (1977) were the first to suggest the use of FHR response to a pure-tone external sound stimulation to assess fetal health. A wide variety of acoustic stimuli have been used since, at different frequencies, SPLs, and durations (Davey *et al*. 1984; Kuhlman and Depp 1988; Querleu *et al*. 1984; Read and Miller 1977; Serafini *et al*. 1984; Trudinger and Boylan 1980). External stimulation with the EAL has produced the most reliable FHR response and this method has disseminated rapidly into clinical practice.

We conducted studies to determine more systematically the effect of a 5-second VAS on human FHR. Eighty-three healthy pregnant women between 26 and 40 weeks of gestation were studied. Computerized FHR analysis was used to fit a base-line to the FHR record, and to automatically detect FHR accelerations above the base-line (Dawes *et al*. 1985). A 1-hour control period was followed by application of the EAL over the fetal head for 5 seconds. Control groups received a similar stimulus on the maternal hand.

The FHR response to VAS was dependent on gestational age. There was a prolonged increase in the basal FHR in healthy fetuses after 30 weeks (Gagnon *et al*. 1987*a*). This fetal tachycardia was prolonged for up to 1 hour following the 5-second stimulus in some healthy, term fetuses (Gagnon *et al*. 1987*b*). It is important that neither maternal heart-rate nor blood pressure were influenced by the stimulation. Between 26 and 30 weeks of gestation, FHR response to EAL consisted of a single, prolonged FHR acceleration. Conversely, in fetuses more than 33 weeks' gestation, there was a delayed increase in the number of FHR accelerations between 10 and 20 minutes following the stimulus (Gagnon *et al*. 1987*a,b*).

Fetal breathing and body movements

It was originally reported by Gelman *et al*. (1982) that fetal movements increased following acoustic stimulation applied on the surface of the maternal abdomen over a period of 1 minute. We pursued these observations by measuring fetal breathing and body movements before and after a 5-second VAS performed under the conditions mentioned above in healthy selected women volunteers between 26 and 40 weeks of gestation (Gagnon *et al*. 1986, 1987*a*). In fetuses aged between 33 and 40 weeks, there was an increase in gross fetal body movements which began 10 minutes after the stimulus and persisted for up to 1 hour. However, in fetuses between 26 and 32 weeks' gestation, gross fetal body movements were not altered by the stimulus.

Fetal breathing activity was altered only in fetuses aged between 36 and 40 weeks (Gagnon *et al*. 1986, 1987*a*). Following stimulation with EAL, the incidence of fetal breathing movements immediately decreased, and examination of histograms of breath-to-breath intervals indicated that breathing activity became more irregular for a period of up to 1 hour following VAS. Fetal breathing movements were not altered by EAL stimulation in fetuses of 26 to 35 weeks' gestational age.

Fetal behavioural states

Visser *et al.* (1989) reported on a small number (n = 9) of healthy pregnant women at term; following stimulation with the EAL there was a switch from fetal state 1F to state 2F in four women, and to state 4F in three women. The fetal tachycardia persisted in the absence of fetal movement for 1.5 hour in one fetus. Devoe *et al.* (1990) examined the occurrence of behavioural state 30 minutes before and after a 3-second stimulus with EAL in 28 fetuses near term. The four fetuses in state 1F before the stimulus switched to state 4F, and 11 out of 16 in state 2F switched to state 4F. Importantly, 26 out of 28 fetuses exhibited FHR accelerations immediately following the stimulus. These observations demonstrated definitive alterations of human fetal behavioural states. Also, the pre-stimulus behavioural state was important in predicting FHR responses to VAS, this response being more consistent when the stimulus was applied in state 1F rather than in state 2F. More recently, Spencer *et al.* (1991) compared FHR response to vibro-acoustic stimulation applied during an episode of low FHR variability (i.e. amplitude less than 10 beats per minute) or high FHR variability (i.e. amplitude greater than 10 beats per minute). Their observations, in contrast to Devoe *et al.* (1990), suggested no difference in FHR response to VAS applied during the two different fetal states of activity.

It is important to note that under normal basal conditions, the human fetus experiences spontaneous transitions from state 1F to state 2F, and then to state 4F (Nijhuis *et al.* 1982; Prechtl 1974). This is in contrast to the transitions from state 1F to state 4F that are described following vibro-acoustic stimulation. This should make us even more careful regarding the use of such a strong stimulus in clinical practice.

Concerns regarding possible adverse effects of loud noise on human fetal development have recently led us to study the effects of low-frequency vibration (100 Hz, square wave) as a stimulus applied on the surface of the maternal abdomen in late human gestation during state 1F (Gagnon *et al.* 1989a, 1989b). The transition time from the stimulus to the onset of state 2F was three minutes compared to 23 minutes following a sham stimulus. Figure 15.3 illustrates a typical shift in human fetal behavioural states following vibratory stimulation. These changes in fetal behavioural states persisted for 20 minutes and were associated with a sustained increase in

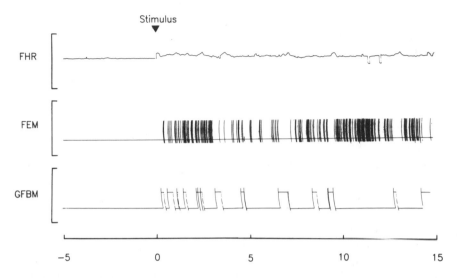

Fig. 15.3. Recording of a typical transition from state 1F (quiet sleep state) to state 2F (rapid eye movement sleep state) after a five-second external vibratory stimulation (arrow) in a healthy term human fetus. (FHR, fetal heart rate; FEM, fetal eye movements; GFBM, gross fetal body movements.) (Reprinted with permission from Gagnon *et al.* 1989*b*.)

long-term FHR variability, the number of FHR accelerations, and fetal body movements. This response was similar to data from neonates reported by Hutt *et al.* (1969). It remains to be determined if this vibratory stimulus might be clinically useful in assessing fetal health.

Vibratory acoustic stimulation in growth-retarded fetuses

Between 32 and 40 weeks gestational age

In order to determine responses to VAS in growth-retarded human fetuses, we recruited a group of 17 pregnant women of 33 to 40 weeks' gestation who subsequently delivered a baby with a birth-weight less than the third percentile (Gagnon *et al.* 1988*a*). Twenty-five healthy pregnant women with normally-grown infants matched for gestational age were used as controls. The umbilical cord arterial blood gas values demonstrated that the 17 growth-retarded fetuses were not acidaemic at birth, but had a slightly lower pO_2 (i.e. 3 mm Hg less) than normally grown controls. Studies were conducted as mentioned above.

Prior to VAS, the growth-retarded fetuses demonstrated a 40 per cent decrease in the incidence of gross fetal body movements and a 25 per cent decrease in long-term FHR variability. Following stimulation, FHR and fetal activity patterns in the growth-retarded fetuses were similar to those in the normally-grown fetuses (Gagnon *et al.* 1988*a*). These data suggested that fetal responses to EAL could not be used to differentiate the late-onset (i.e. occurring after 32 weeks) severely growth-retarded human fetus from normally-grown fetuses.

Less than 32 weeks of gestational age

We recruited nine pregnant volunteers prior to 32 weeks' gestation who delivered infants on average at 32.8 weeks gestation, all of whom were less than the third percentile in weight (Gagnon *et al.* 1989*c*). All infants survived the neonatal period and none exhibited congenital anomalies. Only one had a low umbilical artery pH (7.04) at birth. Infants were matched with a control group of normally-grown fetuses of the same gestational age.

Before stimulation the nine growth-retarded fetuses exhibited diminished FHR variability, FHR accelerations, and fetal movements compared to the control fetuses. We did not demonstrate any significant effect of VAS on either the FHR or fetal movement patterns in the growth-retarded fetuses. The data suggested that in this small group of growth-retarded fetuses there might be a delay in the maturation of fetal sensory receptors or brain stem function.

Animal studies

Glucose utilization in the fetal central auditory structures is higher than in other cerebral structures in the fetal lamb under normal laboratory sound conditions (Abrams *et al.* 1984). Using broadband external sound stimulation of 105 to 120 dB, Abrams *et al.* (1987*a*) reported an increase in glucose utilization of auditory related and unrelated cerebral structures in the fetal lamb. In contrast, bilateral cochlear ablation results in a global decrease in local cerebral glucose utilization of both grey and white matter of all auditory and non-auditory pathways (Abrams *et al.* 1987*b*). These observations suggest that the function of auditory pathways may play a role in the normal function and development of the fetal brain.

More recently Fletcher *et al.* (1988) determined the effect of external VAS in the fetal lamb. Their data demonstrated that VAS produced a change in electrocortical activity, which is a direct measure of behavioural activity, from high-voltage to low-voltage for 89 per cent of the time. These changes in electrocortical activity were associated with a significant increase in fetal nuchal muscle activity. These observations suggested a state of wakefulness in the fetal lamb following VAS similar to that seen in human fetuses.

Fetal behavioural activity during maternal hypocapnia and hypercapnia

Connors *et al.* (1989) have studied the fetal behavioural responses to alterations in maternal end-tidal pCO_2 between 24 and 40 weeks' gestation. The incidence of breathing movements correlated significantly with maternal end-tidal pCO_2, increasing with maternal breathing of 2 per cent and 4 per cent carbon dioxide, and decreasing with maternal hyperventilation, for each of the gestational age groups studied. However, the slope of this fetal response was higher at 28 to 40 weeks than at 24 to 26 weeks' gestational age. This indicated that although the carbon dioxide level is an important stimulus for the generation of respiratory movements, there was evidence of a developmental change in the sensitivity to CO_2. The same authors also reported no change in FHR and fetal body movements during maternal hypocapnia and hypercapnia, indicating that changes in the incidence of fetal breathing activity were relatively independent of changes in fetal behavioural states.

Fetal behavioural activity during maternal hyperoxia

Maternal administration of oxygen has been suggested as a therapeutic approach to hypoxic growth-retarded fetuses (Nicolaides *et al.* 1987), and as a diagnostic test to discriminate growth-retarded from normally-grown fetuses (Arduini *et al.* 1988; Ruedrich *et al.* 1989).

We examined the effect of continuous maternal oxygen administration— sufficient to double maternal transcutaneous pO_2 from 79 mm Hg on average to 158 mm Hg—in 13 pregnant women who subsequently delivered infants with a birth-weight less than the third percentile (Gagnon *et al.* 1990*b*). Each study was duplicated on two half-days under the same experimental conditions, the only difference being that women randomly received either oxygen (FiO_2 50 per cent) or room air (Fig. 15.4). All studies started during an episode of fetal quietness (i.e. low FHR variability and no gross fetal body movements). During the 2 hours of maternal hyperoxia, the fetuses made breathing movements for 33.5 per cent ± 4.5 per cent of the time, which was significantly higher than when room air was administered (18.4 per cent ± 3.3 per cent; p = 0.024). Gross fetal body movements, FHR accelerations, and FHR variability increased significantly

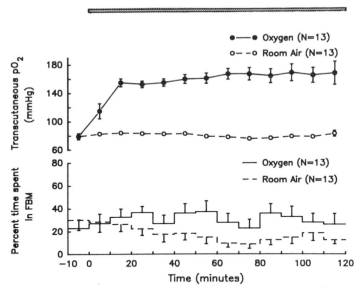

Fig. 15.4. Mean maternal transcutaneous pO_2 (mm Hg) ± SEM plotted in 10-minute intervals before and after maternal administration of oxygen or room air (top). Mean incidence of fetal breathing movements (bottom) was also plotted on the same time scale. Horizontal bar indicates the time during which oxygen or room air was administered. (Reprinted with permission from Gagnon *et al.* 1990*b*.)

with increasing observation time, but were not significantly altered by maternal hyperoxia or room air administration. Our data are in agreement with those recently reported by deVleeschouwer *et al.* (1989), and do not support the concept that ultrasonographic observation of fetal behavioural activity during maternal hyperoxia could be used to differentiate fetuses with intrauterine growth-retardation from normally-grown fetuses as recently suggested (Ruedrich *et al.* 1989). We believe that this effect of maternal hyperoxia on fetal breathing activity is independent of fetal behavioural activity, and is due to increased fetal pCO_2 and not due to fetal hyperoxia *per se*.

Intercostal-to-phrenic inhibitory reflex

Prolonged apnoeas usually occur during state 2 (active sleep) in the neonate when paradoxical breathing is more frequent. The inward movement of the thoracic wall causes spreading of the caudal ribs which may elicit an intercostal-to-phrenic inhibitory reflex leading to apnoea. Tas *et al.* (1990)

used continuous ultrasonographic observation of the fetal chest and FHR
to identify the presence of fetal breathing movements and the different
fetal behavioural states.

Fetal apnoea followed external compression of the fetal chest in both
state 1F and state 2F. These observations indicated that an intercostal-to-
phrenic inhibitory reflex is already present *in utero* and is relatively independent of fetal behavioural states.

Clinical significance

Fetal behaviour in response to stimulation

The classic work of Prechtl (1974) demonstrated that the clustering of
variables such as body movements, heart-rate variability, and eye movements could define five separate states of activity during neonatal life. An
underlying assumption in the measurement of fetal behavioural states is
that they may reflect fetal cortical function. It is assumed that fetal cortical
function might be an important marker of fetal hypoxia and, therefore,
useful in the assessment of fetal health. Unfortunately, it is not clear yet
if this assumption is valid. Recent data have demonstrated that certain
hypoxic conditions that result in diminished breathing and rapid eye movement activity in the fetal lamb have different time courses of effect on these
measurements. Bocking *et al.* (1988) induced fetal hypoxaemia in sheep by
reducing maternal uterine blood flow over a period of 48 hours. Under the
conditions of their experiment, fetal rapid eye activity returned hours
before the return of fetal breathing movements, and electrocortical activity
was not altered throughout the time fetal hypoxaemia was maintained.
Therefore, under normal conditions, the clustering of variables such as
rapid eye movements, fetal breathing activity, body movements, and FHR
changes can be used as a reasonable indicator of fetal electrocortical
activity. However, under conditions of different gestational ages, hypoxia
and other stimuli such as sound, vibration, hypocapnia, hypercapnia,
maternal hyperoxia, and biophysical variables are dissociated from each
other in time. It is against this background that the clinical significance of
changes in human fetal behavioural activity following different external
stimuli must be considered.

Using fetal stimulation for antenatal surveillance

The literature regarding the effectiveness and predictive value of antepartum fetal assessment usually relates the results of a given test to intrapartum
fetal distress (i.e. the 5-minute Apgar score) and the occurrence of unex-

pected intrauterine fetal death within 1 week of a normal test as primary outcome parameters.

Although it has been shown that external VAS produces remarkable changes in FHR and fetal movement patterns, FHR response to VAS has been the most widely investigated indicator of fetal health. From currently available data (Davey *et al.* 1984; Querleu *et al.* 1984; Read and Miller 1977; Serafini *et al.* 1984; Trudinger and Boylan 1980; Smith *et al.* 1988), the following conclusions can be made.

1. The increasing experience with VAS stimulation shows that the positive predictive value for fetal distress during labour is probably below 15 per cent and that the negative predictive value is above 90 per cent. These observations suggest that fetal acoustic stimulation tests, like non-stress testing, indicate fetal health at the time of the test only and can not predict events associated with fetal distress during labour or a low Apgar score.

2. The risk of intrauterine fetal death within 7 days of a 'reactive' fetal VAS can not be determined because too few patients have been studied. However, data suggest that this risk, which is 1.9/1000, is probably not higher than that following a spontaneously reactive non-stress test, which is 1.6/1000 (Smith *et al.* 1988).

3. The definition and nomenclature of an adequate FHR response to VAS based on physiological studies remain to be determined. From previous studies, FHR response to VAS can be affected by gestational age (Gagnon *et al.* 1987*a*), pre-stimulation base-line (Gagnon *et al.* 1988*b*), labour (Luz *et al.* 1980), and rupture of membranes (Richards *et al.* 1988).

If clinicians wish to use VAS to assess fetal health criteria for reactivity, one FHR acceleration of at least 10 beats per minute for at least 15 seconds and/or an increase in the FHR base-line of at least 10 beats per minute for at least two minutes would be adequate criteria after 30 weeks' gestation, based on data obtained in healthy fetuses (Davey *et al.* 1984; Gagnon *et al.* 1987*a*,*b*; Gagnon *et al.* 1988*b*). However, no controlled clinical trials that suggest any clinical benefit as measured by improved perinatal outcome from the use of EAL in routine antenatal surveillance have yet been published.

Regarding the role of maternal hyperoxia for fetal therapy in pregnancies complicated by intrauterine growth-retardation, no randomized clinical trial has been published to prove or suggest any benefit in term of fetal outcome.

Using fetal stimulation for intrapartum surveillance

The metabolic status of the human fetus can be assessed during labour using fetal scalp sampling to measure fetal pH. It has been suggested that FHR response to EAL can predict fetal acidosis during labour. Intrapartum studies evaluating the relationship between FHR response to acoustic stimulation and fetal scalp pH were all conducted using the EAL as the external source, and used the same criteria for an adequate FHR response (i.e. a FHR acceleration of at least 15 beats per minute for 15 seconds at least). Currently available data (Edersheim *et al.* 1987; Polzin *et al.* 1988; Smith *et al.* 1986; DiGiovanni and Zuidema 1989; Irion *et al.* 1989) suggest the following.

1. The presence of a FHR acceleration following VAS during labour is associated with a fetal scalp pH greater than 7.20 97 per cent of the time. However, occasionally a normal FHR response can be seen in a fetus with significant metabolic acidosis.

2. The absence of a FHR acceleration following VAS during labour is a poor predictor of significant fetal metabolic acidosis (i.e. it has a positive predictive value of 20 per cent for a pH smaller ($<$) than 7.20, and should be followed by fetal scalp sampling to confirm the metabolic status of the fetus. If fetal scalp sampling can not be done, the usual criteria of fetal distress using FHR patterns should be used to decide if immediate delivery is indicated or not.

Conclusion

At present, assessment of fetal health is based on observation of normal fetal behaviour. The methods are time-consuming, labour-intensive, and prone to error in interpretation because of the periodicities in fetal activity. The purpose of this chapter was to review briefly the normal physiology of human fetal behavioural activity under conditions that could change the fetal intrauterine environment and could alter the spontaneous patterns in fetal behavioural activity. Although external fetal stimulation with an external source of sound and vibration can reproducibly alter fetal biophysical variables used to assess fetal health, it is prudent to conclude that the routine use of fetal stimulation in obstetric care should be withheld until clear evidence of its safety and benefit are established.

Acknowledgements

This work was supported by the Physicians' Services Incorporated Foundation, Medical Research Council of Canada, and The Variety Club of Ontario. R.G. is a Canadian Medical Research Council scholar.

References

Abrams, R. M., Ito, M., Frisinger, J. E., Patlak C. S., Pettigrew, K. O., and Kennedy, C. (1984). Local cerebral glucose utilization in fetal and neonatal sheep. *American Journal of Physiology* **246**, R608–18.

Abrams, R. M., Hutchison, A. A., Gerhardt, F. J., Evans, S. L., and Pendergast, J. (1987a). Local cerebral glucose utilization in fetal sheep exposed to noise. *American Journal of Obstetrics and Gynecology* **157**, 456–60.

Abrams, R. M., Hutchison, A. A., McTiernan, M. J., and Merwin, G. E. (1987b). Effects of cochlear ablation on local cerebral glucose utilization in fetal sheep. *American Journal of Obstetrics and Gynecology* **157**, 1438–42.

Altmann, E. (1950). Normal development of the ear and its 2 mechanics. *Archives in Otolaryngology* **52**, 725–30.

Arduini, D., Rizzo, G., Mancuso, S., and Romanini, C. (1988). Short-term effects of maternal oxygen administration on blood flow velocity waveforms in healthy and growth-retarded fetuses. *American Journal of Obstetrics and Gynecology* **159**, 1077–80.

Benzaquen, S., Gagnon, R., Hunse, C., and Foreman, J. (1990). The intrauterine sound environment of the human fetus during labor. *American Journal of Obstetrics and Gynecology* **163**, 484–90.

Bocking, A. D., Adamson, L., Cousin, A., Campbell, K., Carmichael, L., Natale, R., and Patrick, J. (1982). Effects of intravenous glucose injection on human fetal breathing movements and gross fetal body movements at 38 to 40 weeks' gestational age. *American Journal of Obstetrics and Gynecology* **142**, 606–11.

Bocking, A. D., Gagnon, R., Milne, K. M., and White, S. E. (1988). Behavioral activity during prolonged hypoxemia in fetal sheep. *Journal of Applied Physiology* **65**, 2420–6.

Bradley, R. M. and Mistretta, C. M. (1975). Fetal sensory receptors. *Physiology Reviews* **55**, 352–82.

Brown, R. and Patrick, J. (1981). The nonstress test: how long is enough? *American Journal of Obstetrics and Gynecology* **141**, 646–51.

Connors, G., Hunse, C., Carmichael, L., Natale, R., and Richardson, B. (1989). Control of fetal breathing in the human fetus between 24 and 34 weeks' gestation. *American Journal of Obstetrics and Gynecology* **160**, 932–7.

Davey, D. A., Dommisse, J., Macnab, M., and Dacre, D. (1984). The value of an auditory stimulatory test in antenatal fetal cardiotocograph. *European Journal of Obstetrics and Gynecology and Reproductive Biology* **18**, 273–7.

Dawes, G. S., Redman, C. W. G., and Smith, J. H. (1985). Improvements in the registration and analysis of fetal heart rate records at the bedside. *British Journal of Obstetrics and Gynaecology* **92**, 317–25.

deVleeschouwer, M. H. M., Palstra, I. Y. G. M., Tas, B. A. P. J., Mulders, L. G. M., and Nijhuis, J. G. (1989). The influence of oxygen administration on fetal behaviour and doppler flow profiles in normal and growth retarded fetuses. *Proceedings, 16th annual meeting of the Society for the Study of Fetal Physiology* July 2–4. Reading, UK.

Devoe, L. D., Murray, C., Faircloth, D., and Ramos, E. (1990). Vibroacoustic stimulation and fetal behavioral state in normal term human pregnancy. *American Journal of Obstetrics and Gynecology* **163**, 1156–61.

DiGiovanni, L. M. and Zuidema, L. J. (1989). Fetal vibroacoustic stimulation as a predictor of fetal acid-base status in labor. *Proceedings, 9th annual meeting of the Society of Perinatal Obstetricians* Feb. 1–4. New Orleans, Louisiana.

Druzin, M. L., Gratacos, J., Paul, R. H., Broussard. P., McCart, D., and Smith, M. (1985). Antepartum fetal heart rate testing XII. The effect of manual manipulation of the fetus on the nonstress test. *American Journal of Obstetrics and Gynecology* **151,** 61–4.

Edersheim, T. G., Hutson, J. M., Druzin, M. L., and Kogut, E. A. (1987). Fetal heart rate response to vibratory acoustic stimulation predicts fetal pH in labor. *American Journal of Obstetrics and Gynecology* **157,** 1557–60.

Fletcher, D. J., Hanson, M. A., Moore, P. J., and Parkes, M. J. (1988). Stimulation of the sheep fetus in utero by sound. *Journal of Physiology* **409,** 42P.

Gagnon, R. (1989). Stimulation of human fetuses with sound and vibration. *Seminars in Perinatology* **13,** 393–402.

Gagnon, R., Hunse, C., Carmichael, L., Fellows, F., and Patrick, J. (1986). Effects of vibratory acoustic stimulation on human fetal breathing and gross fetal body movements near term. *American Journal of Obstetrics and Gynecology* **155,** 1227–30.

Gagnon, R., Hunse, C., Carmichael, L., Fellows, F., and Patrick. J. (1987*a*). Human fetal responses to vibratory acoustic stimulation from twenty-six weeks to term. *American Journal of Obstetrics and Gynecology* **157,** 1375–81.

Gagnon, R., Hunse, C., Carmichael, L., Fellows, F., and Patrick J. (1987*b*). External vibratory acoustic stimulation near term: fetal heart rate and heart rate variability reponses. *American Journal of Obstetrics and Gynecology* **156,** 323–7.

Gagnon, R., Hunse,C., Fellows, F., Carmichael, L., and Patrick. J. (1988*a*). Fetal heart rate and activity patterns in growth-retarded fetuses: changes after vibratory acoustic stimulation. *American Journal of Obstetrics and Gynecology* **158,** 265–71.

Gagnon, R., Hunse, C., and Patrick, J. (1988*b*). Fetal responses to vibratory acoustic stimulation: Influence of basal heart rate. *American Journal of Obstetrics and Gynecology* **159,** 835–9.

Gagnon, R., Foreman, J., Hunse, C., and Patrick, J. (1989*a*). Effects of low-frequency vibration on human term fetuses. *American Journal of Obstetrics and Gynecology* **161,** 1479–85.

Gagnon, R., Hunse, C., and Foreman, J. (1989*b*). Human fetal behavioral states after vibratory stimulation. *American Journal of Obstetrics and Gynecology* **161,** 1470–6.

Gagnon, R., Hunse, C., Carmichael, L., and Patrick, J. (1989*c*) Vibratory acoustic stimulation in the 26- to 32-week, small-for-gestational-age fetus. *American Journal of Obstetrics and Gynecology* **160,** 160–5.

Gagnon, R., Benzaquen, S., Hunse, C., and Foreman J. (1990*a*). Vibroacoustic stimulation near term: quantification of the transmission of sound and vibration across maternal soft tissues. *Proceedings, 10th annual meeting of the Society of Perinatal Obstetricians* Jan. 23–27. Houston, Texas.

Gagnon, R., Hunse, C., and Vijan, S. (1990*b*). The effect of maternal hyperoxia on behavioral activity in growth-retarded human fetuses. *American Journal of Obstetrics and Gynecology* **163,** 1897–9.

Gelman, S. R., Wood, S., Spellacy, W. N., and Abrams, R. M. (1982). Fetal movements in response to sound stimulation. *American Journal of Obstetrics and Gynecology* **143,** 484–5.

Grimwade, J. G., Walker, D. W., Bartlett, Gordon, S., and Wood, G. (1971). Human fetal heart rate change and movement in response to sound and vibration. *American Journal of Obstetrics and Gynecology* **109**, 86–90.

Hutt, S. J., Lenard, H. G., and Prechtl, H. F. R. (1969). Psychophysiological studies in newborn infants. *Advances in Child Development* **4**, 127–50.

Irion, O., Stuckelberger, P., and Extermann, P. H. (1989). Intrapartum fetal heart rate reactivity (spontaneous or induced): does it correlate with normal fetal acid-base status? *Proceedings, 9th annual meeting of the Society of Perinatal Obstetricians* Feb. 1–4. New Orleans, Louisiana.

Kuhlman, K. A. and Depp, R. (1988). Acoustic stimulation testing. *Obstetrics and Gynecology Clinics in North America* **15**, 303–13.

Lenard, H. G., Bermuth, L., and Prechtl, H. F. R. (1968). Reflexes and their relationship to behavioural state in the newborn. *Acta Paediatrica Scandinavica* **3**, 177–85.

Luz, N. P., Lima, C. P., Luz, S. H., and Feldens, V. L. (1980). Auditory evoked responses of the human fetus. I. Behaviour during progress of labor. *Acta Obstetrica et Gynecologica Scandinavica* **59**, 395–404.

Nicolaides, K. H., Campbell, S., Bradley, R. J., Bilardo, C. M., Soothill, P. W., and Gibb, D. (1987). Maternal oxygen therapy for intra-uterine growth retardation. *Lancet* **i**, 942–7.

Nijhuis, J. G., Prechtl, H. F. R., Martin, C. B. Jr, and Bots, R. S. G. M. (1982). Are there behavioural states in the human fetus? *Early Human Development* **6**, 177–95.

Polishuk, W. Z., Laufer, N., and Sadovsky, E. (1975). Fetal responses to external light stimulus. *Harefuah* **89**, 395–7.

Polzin, G. B., Blakemore, K. J., Petrie, R., and Amon, E. (1988). Fetal vibro-acoustic stimulation: magnitude and duration of fetal heart rate accelerations as a marker of fetal health. *Obstetrics and Gynecology* **72**, 621–6.

Prechtl, H. F. R. (1974). The behavioural states of the newborn infant (a review). *Brain Research* **76**, 185–212.

Querleu, D., Boutteville, C., and Renard, X. (1984). Evaluation diagnostique de la souffrance foetale pendant la grossesse au moyen d'un test de stimulation sonore. *Journal de Gynecologie et Obstetrique en Biologie de la Reproduction* **13**, 789–96.

Read, J. A. and Miller, F. C. (1977). Fetal heart rate acceleration in response to acoustic stimulation as a measure of fetal well-being. *American Journal of Obstetrics and Gynecology* **129**, 512–17.

Richards, D. S., Cefalo, R. C., Thorpe, J. M., Salley, M., and Rose, D. (1988). Determinants of fetal heart rate response to vibroacoustic stimulation in labor. *Obstetrics and Gynecology* **71**, 535–40.

Richardson, B., Campbell, K., Carmichael, L., and Patrick, J. (1981). Effects of external physical stimulation on fetuses near term. *American Journal of Obstetrics and Gynecology* **39**, 344–52.

Ruedrich, D. A., Devoe, L. D., and Searle, N. (1989). Effects of maternal hyperoxia on the biophysical assessment of fetuses with suspected intrauterine growth retardation. *American Journal of Obstetrics and Gynecology* **161**, 188–92.

Serafini, P., Lindsay, M. B. J., Nagey, D. A., Pupkin, M. J., Tseng, P., and Crenshaw, C. J. (1984). Antepartum fetal heart rate response to sound stimulation: the acoustic stimulation test. *American Journal of Obstetrics and Gynecology* **148**, 41–5.

Smith, C. V., Nguyen, H. N., Phelan, J. P., and Paul, R. H. (1986). Intrapartum assessment of fetal well-being: a comparison of fetal acoustic stimulation with acid-base determinations. *American Journal of Obstetrics and Gynecology* **155,** 726–8.

Smith, C. V., Phelan, J. P., Nguyen, H. N., and Paul, R. H. (1988). Continuing experience with the fetal acoustic stimulation test. *Journal of Reproductive Medicine* **33,** 365–8.

Spencer, J. A. D., Deans, A., Nicolaides, P., and Arulkumaran, S. (1991). Fetal heart rate response to vibroacoustic stimulation during low and high heart rate variability episodes in late pregnancy. *American Journal of Obstetrics and Gynecology.* **165,** 86–96.

Tas, B. A. P. J., Nijhuis, J. G., Lucas, A. J., and Folgering, H. T. M. (1990). The intercostal-to-phrenic inhibitory reflex in the human fetus near term. *Early Human Development* **22,** 145–9.

Trudinger, B. J. and Boylan, P. (1980). Antepartum fetal heart rate monitoring: value of sound stimulation. *Obstetrics and Gynecology* **55,** 265–8.

Visser, G. H. A., Zeelenberg, H. J., de Vries, J. I. P., and Dawes, G. S. (1983). External physical stimulation of the human fetus during episodes of low heart rate variation. *American Journal of Obstetrics and Gynecology* **145,** 579–84.

Visser, G. H. A., Mulder, H. H., Wit., H. P., Mulder, E. J. H., and Prechtl, H. F. R. (1989). Vibro-acoustic stimulation of the human fetus: effect on behavioural state organization. *Early Human Development* **19,** 285–9.

Walker, D. W., Grimwade, J. C., and Wood, C. (1971). Intrauterine noise: a component of the fetal environment. *American Journal of Obstetrics and Gynecology* **109,** 91–7.

16

Doppler flow measurements

J. VAN EYCK and J. W. WLADIMIROFF

Introduction

With the introduction by Prechtl and Beintema (1964) of a behavioural
state classification in the full-term human neonate, a major breakthrough
was made in developmental neurology. The concept of behavioural states
in the young infant has been used as a descriptive categorization of behaviour and as an explanation of the brain mechanisms that modify the
responsiveness of the infant. Obviously, the next logical study was to
investigate whether behavioural states also exist before birth. It was
Nijhuis *et al.* (1982) who clearly identified four distinct fetal behavioural
states on the basis of fetal eye and body movements and fetal heart-rate
(FHR) pattern as from 36 weeks of gestation.

Based on the marked changes in FHR pattern and the incidence of fetal
body movements between different behavioural states, it is not unlikely
that these changes are associated with alterations in fetal cardiovascular
performance. In fact, from a teleological point of view, it is highly desirable that the fetal central nervous system and cardiovascular regulatory
mechanisms develop simultaneously. With the introduction of combined
real-time and pulsed Doppler systems a non-invasive method became
available for studying fetal haemodynamics in relation to fetal behaviour.

Doppler flow velocity measurements are increasingly performed in obstetric care for monitoring fetal condition and for the early detection and
evaluation of intrauterine growth retardation (IUGR) (Arabin *et al.* 1987).
For a correct interpretation of recorded data it is important to establish the
influence of internal fetal variables, for example fetal breathing movements, FHR, fetal heart rhythm, and fetal behavioural states. So from both
a physiological and clinical point of view it is, therefore, interesting to
evaluate the relationship between fetal behavioural states and BFV waveforms in the human fetus. The objective of this chapter is to report on the
relationship between BFV waveforms obtained from various fetal vessels
and fetal behavioural states 1F and 2F according to the classification of
Nijhuis *et al.* (1982) in the normal-growth and asymmetric growth-retarded
human fetus. Furthermore, haemodynamics at the cardiac level in relation
to behavioural states 1F and 2F are discussed.

Fetal descending aorta

Normal values for the various components of the BFV waveform in the lower thoracic part of the fetal descending aorta in the third trimester of pregnancy have been established by various centres (Jouppila and Kirkinen 1984; Marsal *et al.* 1984; Tonge *et al.* 1984). It has been documented that in the normal-growing human fetus at term, BFV waveforms obtained from this vessel display a clear relationship with fetal behavioural states (van Eyck *et al.* 1985). Under standardized FHR conditions there is a statistically significant reduction in pulsatility index (PI) during behavioural state 2F compared to PI during behavioural state 1F (Fig. 16.1). The marked behavioural state-dependent PI difference is almost entirely determined by changes in end-diastolic BFV and reflects reduced peripheral vascular resistance, suggesting increased perfusion of the fetal skeletal musculature. An inverse relationship was established between PI and FHR in both behavioural states 1F and 2F (van Eyck *et al.* 1985). This inverse relationship is mainly determined by the definition presented by Gosling and King (1975) for PI calculations (i.e. at a lower FHR a more gradual end-diastolic slow-down of the BFV takes place).

In the presence of asymmetric IUGR there is an increased PI, reflecting a raised peripheral vascular resistance. Whereas in the normal growing human fetus PI is behavioural state-dependent, this phenomenon did not occur in the presence of asymmetric IUGR, as demonstrated in Fig. 16.1 (van Eyck *et al.* 1986). This behavioural state-independency may be explained by the fact that chronic hypoxia, probably present in IUGR, stimulates the peripheral chemoreceptors (Dawes 1968; Itskovitz *et al.* 1982), 1982), and subsequent release of vasoconstrictive agents, such as vasopressin and catecholamines (Iwamoto *et al.* 1979; Mott 1985; Oosterbaan 1985). This peripheral vasoconstriction seems to overrule state-dependent PI fluctuations. Again there was an inverse relationship between PI and FHR, which was even more pronounced than in normal growth (see Fig. 16.1).

Since at term, FHR pattern, eye movements, and body movements align with short transition periods from combined presence to combined absence and vice versa, it is not possible to analyse whether one of these state variables is particularly associated with the observed PI changes in the descending aorta in the normal-growing human fetus at term. At 27 to 28 weeks of gestation there are episodes of low and high FHR variability, with and without eye movements and body movements. There is no proper synchronization in the cyclic appearance of these variables. Periods of coincidence often occur by chance and will result in the occurrence of eight combinations of state parameters, providing the opportunity to evaluate the relationship between these single state parameters and PI. Using this

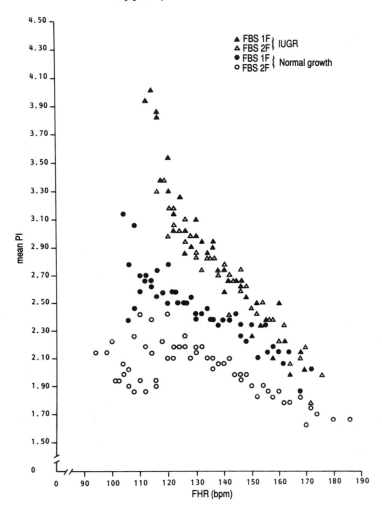

Fig. 16.1. Mean pulsatility index (PI) in the fetal descending aorta in fetal behavioural states 1F and 2F in normal and intrauterine growth-retarded (IUGR) fetuses in relation to fetal heart-rate (FHR). (From Eyck, J. van *et al.* 1986, reproduced by permission of Elsevier Scientific Publishers.)

method for analysis it has been documented that in the normal-growing human fetus at 27 to 28 weeks of gestation, the PI in the lower thoracic part of the fetal descending aorta displays a statistically significant reduction during periods of high FHR variability compared to that during periods of low FHR variability, irrespective of fetal eye or body movements (van Eyck *et al.* 1988a).

Fetal internal carotid artery

Sleep state has been shown to influence cerebral blood flow in animals (Reivich *et al.* 1968), human neonates (Mukhtar *et al.* 1982), and adult man (Townsend *et al.* 1973). These studies have shown an increase in cerebral blood-flow during rapid eye movement sleep (active sleep) compared to that during non-rapid eye movement sleep (quiet sleep).

Comparison of cerebral blood flow measured by microspheres and pulsed Doppler in young piglets (Hansen *et al.* 1983) and newborn lambs (Rosenberg *et al.* 1985) demonstrated that peak systolic and end-diastolic BFV as well as the area under the velocity curve, reflecting the shape of the waveform, closely correlate with cerebral blood flow. Since the PI is determined by all these three variables, the observed reduction of this index, under standardized FHR conditions, suggests an increase in cerebral blood flow during behavioural state 2F.

In 1986 a Doppler ultrasound method was introduced to study BFV waveforms in the internal carotid artery of the human fetus (Wladimiroff *et al.* 1986). In the normal-growing human fetus at term there is, under standardized FHR conditions, a statistically significant reduction in PI during behavioural state 2F, compared to PI during behavioural state 1F, as demonstrated in Fig. 16.2 (van Eyck *et al.* 1987). This decrease suggests a reduced peripheral vascular resistance in the fetal cerebral circulation. In both behavioural states 1F and 2F, PI is inversely related to FHR. During the last four weeks of pregnancy there is a fall in PI in the fetal internal carotid artery with maintenance of behavioural state-dependency (Van den Wijngaard *et al.* 1988*a*), suggesting a haemodynamic redistribution favouring blood supply to the brain during the latter weeks of gestation.

In the presence of asymmetric IUGR, PI showed no behavioural state-dependency in the asymmetric growth-retarded fetus, as demonstrated in Fig. 16.3 (van Eyck *et al.* 1988*b*). In contrast to the marked increase in PI in the fetal descending aorta, state-independency in the fetal internal carotid artery was associated with only a moderate reduction in PI, suggesting the onset of circulatory redistribution with the aim of favouring cerebral blood flow (brain-sparing effect). The degree of PI reduction at this stage seems, however, to be sufficient to overrule behavioural state-dependency. PI is inversely related to FHR, but this was less pronounced than in normal fetal growth.

Umbilical artery

In obstetric care, Doppler measurements are predominantly performed in

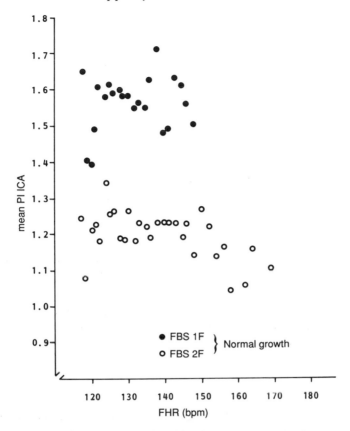

Fig. 16.2. Mean pulsatility index (PI) in the fetal internal carotid artery in fetal behavioural states 1F and 2F in normal fetal growth in relation to fetal heart-rate (FHR). (From Wladimiroff, J. W. and Eyck, J. van 1989, reproduced by permission of Karger Scientific Publishers.)

the umbilical artery, since an increase in PI in this vessel is associated with IUGR and poor fetal outcome. For this reason it is of special importance to investigate whether BFV waveforms in this vessel are also influenced by fetal behavioural states.

Both in the normal-growing (Fig. 16.4) (Mulders *et al.* 1986; van Eyck *et al.* 1987) and asymmetric growth-retarded human fetus at term (van Eyck *et al.* 1988*b*), it was demonstrated that, under standardized FHR conditions, PI in the umbilical artery is fetal behavioural state-independent. These observations are important because it means that Doppler measurements can be performed in the umbilical artery without a prior fetal behavioural state determination. Furthermore, this fetal behavioural state-

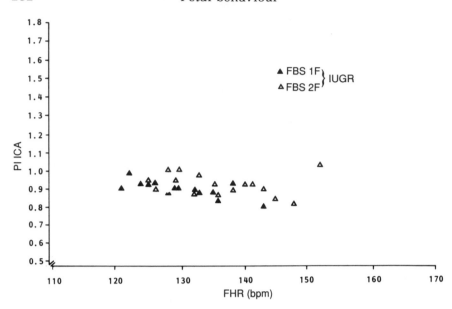

Fig. 16.3. Mean pulsatility index in the fetal internal carotid artery (PIICA) in fetal behavioural states 1F and 2F in intrauterine growth retardation (IUGR) in relation to fetal heart-rate (FHR).

independency suggests a fetal origin of the aforementioned behavioural state-related changes in aortic and carotid BFV. There is an inverse relationship between PI and FHR for both behavioural states 1F and 2F in the umbilical artery (Fig. 16.4).

Blood flow velocity waveforms at cardiac level in relation to behavioural states

Recently, a technique for recording BFV waveforms in the fetal ductus arteriosus (Huhta *et al.* 1987) and foramen ovale (van Eyck *et al.* 1990*a*) became available, which enabled us to investigate the influence of fetal behavioural states on haemodynamics at cardiac level. Ductal peak BFV was significantly reduced during behavioural state 2F compared to that during state 1F (Fig. 16.5); this suggests redistribution in left ventricular and right ventricular output in favour of the left side of the heart (van der Mooren *et al.* 1989). Furthermore, it was demonstrated that ductal peak BFV is FHR-independent (van der Mooren *et al.* 1989) and is modulated by fetal breathing movements (van Eyck *et al.* 1990*b*). BFV waveforms

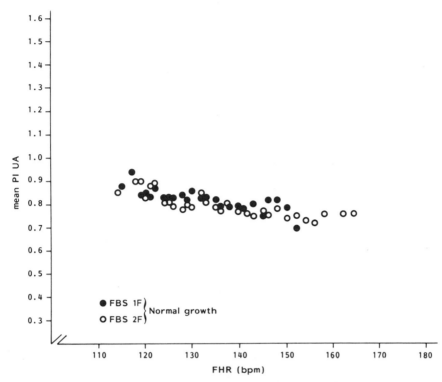

Fig. 16.4. Mean pulsatility index (PI) in the umbilical artery in fetal behavioural states 1F and 2F in normal fetal growth in relation to fetal heart-rate (FHR). (From Eyck, J. van *et al.* 1987, reproduced by permission of Blackwell Scientific Publishers.)

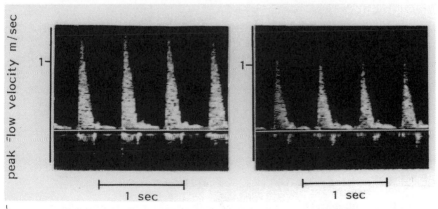

Fig. 16.5. Ductus arteriosus blood flow velocity waveforms in the normal-growing human fetus at term during fetal behavioural states 1F (left panel) and 2F (right panel). (From Mooren, K. van der *et al.* 1989, reproduced by permission of Mosby-Yearbook Scientific Publishers.)

obtained at foramen ovale level are characterized by a typical systolic/diastolic component, as demonstrated in Fig. 16.6 (van Eyck *et al.* 1990*a*). Average BFV was statistically significantly increased in behavioural state 2F compared to that in 1F; this was mainly determined by an increase in BFV during the end-systolic and passive atrial filling phase, as demonstrated in Fig. 16.7 (van Eyck *et al.* 1990*a*). The increase in the average BFV at the foramen ovale level during behavioural state 2F suggests a redistribution of blood flow at cardiac level, resulting in an increased right-to-left shunt, substantiating the behavioural state-related changes observed in the ductus arteriosus.

Discussion

The combined use of real-time and pulsed Doppler systems provides a non-invasive method to study fetal haemodynamics in relation to fetal behavioural states. Table 16.1 summarizes these results. The reduced PI and elevated end-diastolic BFV in the fetal descending aorta and internal carotid artery during behavioural state 2F in normal pregnancy suggest an increased perfusion of the skeletal musculature and brain. Such a response would be necessary to meet increased energy demand resulting from increased muscular and electrocortical activity in this behavioural state. The fetal origin of these changes is suggested by the absence of behavioural state-dependent PI fluctuations in the umbilical artery.

In the normal-growing human fetus at term, haemodynamics at cardiac

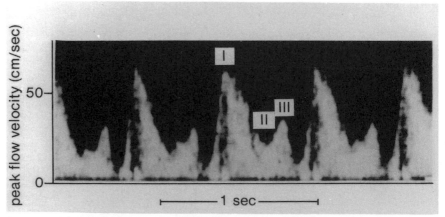

Fig. 16.6. Foramen ovale blood flow velocity waveforms. I = systolic ventricular phase, II = end-diastolic ventricular phase, and III = passive atrial filling phase. (From Eyck, J. van *et al.* 1990*a*, reproduced by permission of Mosby-Yearbook Scientific Publishers.)

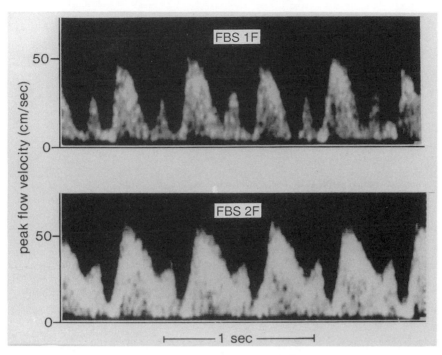

Fig. 16.7. Foramen ovale blood flow velocity waveforms obtained during fetal behavioural state 1F (upper panel) and state 2F (lower panel). (From Eyck, J. van *et al.* 1990*a*, reproduced by permission of Mosby-Yearbook Scientific Publishers.)

level are also clearly modulated by fetal behavioural states. The reduced ductus arteriosus peak BFV during behavioural state 2F suggests a redistribution of ventricular output in favour of the left side of the heart. This redistribution is substantiated by the increased average foramen ovale BFV during behavioural state 2F, reflecting raised right-to-left shunting. The documented increased average foramen ovale BFV is mainly determined by the end-systolic and passive atrial filling phase of the foramen ovale BFV waveform, suggesting increased passive atrial filling during diastole as a result of raised pre-load. Pre-load of the right atrium is the sum of the venous return from the superior vena cava, coronary sinus, and inferior vena cava; the latter is the main determinant of foramen ovale flow. The suggested increased pre-load could be the result of raised inferior vena cava flow, due to preferential streaming in behavioural state 2F of well-oxygenated umbilical venous blood through the ductus venosus into the inferior vena cava to bypass the hepatic microcirculation (Teitel and Rudolph 1985). Since foramen ovale blood-flow is mainly determined by

Table 16.1 Blood flow velocity (BFV) waveform parameters (i.e. pulsatility index (PI), peak BFV, and average BFV in various fetal vessels in relation to fetal behavioural states

Vessel	Normal fetal growth	Intrauterine growth retardation
Aorta	PI in 2F < PI in 1F	PI in 2F = PI in 1F
Internal carotid artery	PI in 2F < PI in 1F	PI in 2F = PI in 1F
Umbilical artery	PI in 2F = PI in 1F	PI in 2F = PI in 1F
Ductus arteriosus	Peak BFV in 2F < Peak BFV in 1F	
Foramen ovale	Average BFV in 2F > Average BFV in 1F	

inferior vena cava blood-flow this mechanism could explain for the behavioural state-related redistribution of blood flow at cardiac level, resulting not only in raised left ventricular output, but also in an increased preferential streaming of well-oxygenated blood directly to the left side of the heart and subsequently to the cerebral circulation and descending aorta. It is suggested that in the normal-growing human fetus at term, fetal behavioural states are related to specific haemodynamic adaptations of pre- and after-load, favouring well-oxygenated blood to perfuse specific vascular beds with increased energy demands.

In asymmetric IUGR, the PI in the fetal descending aorta and internal carotid artery display no fetal behavioural state-dependency. This may be considered as a vascular adaptation that is instrumental in the redistribution of the fetal circulation during IUGR. The rise in PI in the fetal descending aorta and the reduction in PI in the fetal internal carotid artery, which reflect this redistribution (brain-sparing effect), seem to overrule behavioural state-dependent PI fluctuations.

Whereas in the normal-growing human fetus at term fetal behavioural states should be taken into account when Doppler flow studies are performed in the descending aorta, internal carotid artery, ductus arteriosus, and foramen ovale, this does not apply for Doppler flow studies in the umbilical artery. Both in normal growth and asymmetric IUGR, PI in the umbilical artery displays fetal behavioural state-independency, which is of practical importance since in obstetric care Doppler measurements focus on this specific vessel. Furthermore, it was established that in both behavioural states 1F and 2F, PI values obtained from the fetal descending aorta, umbilical artery, and internal carotid artery, were inversely related to FHR (van den Wijngaard *et al.* 1988*b*). The degree of this inverse relationship varies proportionally with the level of peripheral resistance in the vessel studied.

It can be concluded that fetal neurological development expressed by the emergence of fetal behaviour and eventually resulting in well distinguished fetal behavioural states is clearly associated with specific haemodynamic adaptions that can be demonstrated by Doppler flow measurements.

References

Arabin, B., Bergmann, P. L., and Saling, E. (1987). Simultaneous assessment of blood flow velocity waveforms in uteroplacental vessels, the umbilical artery, the fetal aorta and the fetal common carotid artery. *Fetal Therapy* **2**, 17–26.

Dawes, G. S., Lewis, B. V., Milligan, I. E., Roach, M. R., and Talner, N. S. (1968). Vasomotor responses in the hind limbs of foetal and new-born lambs to asphyxia and aortic chemoreceptor stimulation. *Journal of Physiology* **195**, 55–81.

Eyck, J. van, Wladimiroff, J. W., Noordam, M. J., Tonge, H. M., and Prechtl, H.
  F. R. (1985). The blood flow velocity waveform in the fetal descending aorta; its
  relationship to fetal behavioural states in normal pregnancy at 37–38 weeks of
  gestation. *Early Human Development* **14,** 99–107.
Eyck, J. van, Wladimiroff, J. W., Noordam, M. J., Tonge, H. M., and Prechtl, H.
  F. R. (1986). The blood flow velocity waveform in the fetal descending aorta; its
  relationship to fetal behavioural states in the growth retarded fetus at 37–38
  weeks of gestation. *Early Human Development* **14,** 99–107.
Eyck, J. van, Wladimiroff, J. W., Wijngaard, J. A. G. W. van den, Noordam, H.
  M., and Prechtl, H. F. R. (1987). The blood flow velocity waveform in the fetal
  internal carotid and umbilical artery; its relationship to fetal behavioural states in
  normal pregnancy at 37–38 weeks of gestation. *British Journal of Obstetrics and
  Gynaecology* **94,** 736–41.
Eyck, J. van, Wladimiroff, J. W., Noordam, M. J., Cheung, K. L., Wijngaard, J.
  A. G. W. van den, and Prechtl, H. F. R. (1988*a*). The blood flow velocity
  waveform in the fetal descending aorta; its relationship to fetal heart rate pattern, eye and body movements in normal pregnancy at 27–28 weeks of gestation.
  Early Human Development **17,** 187–94.
Eyck, J. van, Wladimiroff, J. W., Noordam, M. J., Wijngaard, J. A. G. W. van
  den, and Prechtl, H. F. R., (1988*b*). The blood flow velocity waveform in the
  fetal internal carotid and umbilical artery; its relationship to fetal behavioural
  states in the growth-retarded fetus at 37–38 weeks of gestation. *British Journal of
  Obstetrics and Gynaecology* **95,** 473–7.
Eyck, J. van, Stewart, P. A., and Wladimiroff, J. W. (1990*a*). Human fetal
  foramen ovale flow velocity waveforms relative to behavioural states in normal
  term pregnancy. *American Journal of Obstetrics and Gynecology* **163,** 1239–
  42.
Eyck, J. van, Mooren, K. van der, and Wladimiroff, J. W. (1990*b*). Ductus
  arteriosus flow velocity modulation by fetal breathing movements as a measure
  of fetal lung development. *American Journal of Obstetrics and Gynecology* **163,**
  558–66.
Gosling, R. G. and King, D. H. (1975). Ultrasound angiology. In: *Arteries and
  veins* (ed. A. W. Marcus and L. Adamson), pp. 61–98. Churchill Livingstone,
  Edinburgh.
Hansen, N. B., Stonestreet, B. C., Rosenkrantz, T. S., and Oh, W. (1983).
  Validity of Doppler measurements of anterior cerebral artery blood flow velocity:
  correlation with brain blood flow in piglets. *Pediatrics* **872,** 526–31.
Huhta, J. C., Moise, K. J., Fisher, D. J., Sharif, D. S., Wasserstrum, N., and
  Martin, C. (1987). Detection and quantitation of constriction of the fetal ductus
  arteriosus by Doppler echocardiography. *Circulation* **75,** 406–12.
Itskovitz, J., Goetzman, B. W., and Rudolph, A. M. (1982). The mechanism of
  late deceleration of heart rate and its relationship to oxygenation in normoxemic
  and chronically hypoxemic fetal lambs. *American Journal of Obstetrics and
  Gynecology* **142,** 66–73.
Iwamoto, H. S., Rudolph, A. M., Keil, L. C., and Heymann, M. A. (1979).
  Haemodynamic responses of the sheep to vasopressin infusion. *Clinical Research*
  44, 430–6.
Jouppila, P. and Kirkinen, P. (1984). Increased vascular resistance in the descend-

ing aorta of the human fetus in hypoxia. *British Journal of Obstetrics and Gynaecology* **91**, 853–6.

Marsal, K., Lindblad, A., Lingman, G., and Eik-Nes, S. H. (1984). Blood flow in the fetal descending aorta; intrinsic factors affecting fetal blood flow, i.e. fetal breathing movements and cardiac arrhythmia. *Ultrasound in Medicine and Biology* **10**, 339–48.

Mooren, K. van der, Eyck, J. van, and Wladimiroff, J. W. (1989). Human fetal ductal flow velocity waveforms relative to behavioural states in normal term pregnancy. *American Journal of Obstetrics and Gynecology* **160**, 371–4.

Mott, J. C. (1985). Humoral control of the fetal circulation. In: *The physiological development of the fetus and newborn* (ed. C. T. Jones and P. W. Nathanielz), pp. 113–21. Academic Press, London.

Mukhtar, A. I., Cowan, F. M., and Stothers, J. K. (1982). Cranial blood flow and blood pressure changes during sleep in the human neonate. *Early Human Development* **6**, 59–64.

Mulders, L. G. M., Muyser, G. J. J. M., Jongsma, H. W., Nijhuis, J. G., and Hein, P. R. (1986). The umbilical artery blood flow velocity waveform in relation to fetal breathing movements, fetal heart rate and fetal behavioural state in normal pregnancy at 37–39 weeks. *Early Human Development* **11**, 283–93.

Nijhuis, J. G., Prechtl, H. F. R., Martin, C. B. Jr, and Bots, R. S. G. M. (1982). Are there behavioural states in the human fetus? *Early Human Development* **6**, 177–95.

Oosterbaan, H. P. (1985). Amniotic oxytocin and vasopressin in the human and the rat. *Thesis*, University of Amsterdam, The Netherlands.

Prechtl, H. F. R. and Beintema, D. J. (1964). The neurological examination of the full-term newborn infant. In: *Clinics in Developmental Medicine*, Vol. 12, p. 74. Heinemann, London.

Reivich, M., Isaacs, G., Evarts, E., and Kety, S. (1968). The effect of slow wave sleep and REM sleep on regional cerebral blood flow in cats. *Journal of Neurochemistry* **15**, 301–6.

Rosenberg, A. A., Narayanan, V., and Douglas Jones, M. Jr. (1985). Comparison of anterior cerebral blood flow velocity and cerebral blood flow during hypoxia. *Pediatric Research* **19**, 67–70.

Teitel, D. and Rudolph, A. M. (1985). Perinatal oxygen delivery and cardiac function. *Advances in Pediatrics* **32**, 321–47.

Tonge, H. M., Struyk, P. C., and Wladimiroff, J. W. (1984). Blood flow measurements in the fetal descending aorta: techniques and clinics. *Clinics in Cardiology* **7**, 323–9.

Townsend, R. E., Prins, P. N., and Obrist, W. D. (1973). Human cerebral blood flow during sleep and waking. *Journal of Applied Physiology* **35**, 620–5.

Wijngaard, J. A. G. W. van den, Eyck, J. van, Noordam, M. J., Wladimiroff, J. W., and Strik, R. van. (1988*a*). The Doppler flow velocity waveform in the fetal internal carotid artery with respect to behavioural states. A longitudinal study. *Biology of the Neonate* **53**, 274–8.

Wijngaard. J. A. G. W. van den, Eyck, J. van, and Wladimiroff, J. W. (1988*b*). The relationship between fetal heart rate and Doppler blood flow velocity waveforms. *Ultrasound in Medicine and Biology* **14**, 593–7.

Wladimiroff, J. W. and Eyck, J. van (1989). Human fetal blood flow and

behavioural states. In: *Achievements in gynecology* (ed. S. Manusco), pp. 17, 63–73. Karger, Basel.
Wladimiroff, J. W., Tonge, H. M., and Stewart, P. A. (1986). Doppler ultrasound assessment of cerebral blood flow in the human fetus. *British Journal of Obstetrics and Gynaecology* **93,** 471–5.

17

Biophysical profile scoring

F. A. MANNING

Introduction

The introduction of high-resolution dynamic ultrasound imaging methods
to the art of obstetrics has resulted in fundamental changes in our understanding of normal fetal activities and responses in health and disease. This
rich new source of fetal information is of major clinical significance since
from it flows a method, fetal biophysical profile (FBP) scoring, that permits
very precise recognition of the normal and uncompromised fetus, and
recognition and classification by severity of disease of the compromised
fetus (Manning *et al.* 1980). The integration of this highly accurate method
of fetal well-being assessment together with the concomitant ultrasound-
derived data on fetal morphometrics, morphology, and functional organ
system assessment yields a very complete picture of fetal condition and
risk. It is the subsequent integration of this set of fetal data within the
contemporary neonatal outcome statistics and obstetric management
schemes that forms the basis for management decisions in modern perinatal medicine. The intention of this chapter is to review the impact of the
existing method for fetal biophysical profile (FBP) scoring on perinatal
mortality and morbidity statistics, and to consider factors that may influence or change the application of the testing method.

Method

Initially four FBP variables are measured concurrently using a dynamic
real-time ultrasound imaging method; these are fetal breathing, fetal tone,
fetal body movements, and fetal heart-rate (FHR) reactivity. Each of these
variables is assessed as normal or abnormal according to fixed criteria and
after an observation period of up to 30 minutes (Table 17.1). The occurrence of cyclical behavioural states in the human fetus has been described
(Nijhuis *et al*). Fetal movements are defined as episodes of movement of
the trunk and limbs either in concert or separately. Fetal tone is described
by extension–flexion movements of the limbs or by the presence of opening and closing of the fetal hand. In recent years we have preferred the

Table 17.1 Biophysical Profile Scoring—technique and interpretation

Biophysical variable	Normal (score = 2)	Abnormal (score = 0)
Fetal breathing movements (FBM)	At least one episode of FBM of at least 30 s duration in 30 min observation	Absent FBM or no episode of at least 30 s in 30 min
Gross body movement	At least three discrete body/limb movements in 30 min (episodes of active continuous movement considered as a single movement)	Two or fewer episodes of body/limb movements in 30 min
Extension or absent fetal movement	At least one episode of active extension with return to flexion of fetal limb(s) or trunk. Opening and closing of hand considered normal tone.	Either slow extension with return to partial flexion or movement of limb in full extension absent fetal movement
Reactive fetal heart-rate (FHR)	At least two episodes of FHR acceleration of more than 15 beats/min and of at least 15 s duration associated with fetal movement in 20 min	Less than two episodes of acceleration of FHR or acceleration of >15 beats/min in 40 min
Qualitative amniotic fluid (AF) volume	At least one pocket of AF that measures at least one cm in two perpendicular planes	Either no AF pockets or a pocket less than one cm in two perpendicular planes

preferred the latter definition of fetal tone since in our experience it is more reproducible (Manning *et al.* 1985). Fetal breathing movements are defined as an episode of chest and abdominal wall movement that lasts for at least 30 seconds. The selection of 30 seconds for this variable is arbitrary on our part and is designed primarily to avoid confusion with general body movements or with the passive effects of maternal respiration. FHR is recorded separately using Doppler ultrasound methods. A reactive FHR trace (normal) is defined by observation of at least two episodes of fetal acceleration of more than 15 beats per minute and lasting longer than 15 seconds associated with fetal movement in a 30 minute period. A non-reactive (abnormal) FHR tracing is defined by the absence of such accelerations in a continuous 30 minute observation of FHR.

The basic premise of FBP scoring is that differentiation of the normal from the compromised fetus is improved by consideration of variables that reflect immediate fetal condition (i.e. fetal breathing, gross body movements, tone, and FHR activity), and a variable that reflects chronic fetal condition (i.e. amniotic fluid volume). In the human fetus at least three acute FBP variables (breathing, movement, and FHR reactivity) are known to exhibit rhythmic variation and expression coincidence with fetal behavioural states (Drogtrop *et al.* 1990; Patrick 1988). The effect of sleep–wake cycles on fetal tone in the human fetus has not been studied systematically. In the animal fetus, hypoxaemia is known to suppress or abolish breathing movements and gross body movements (Boddy and Dawes 1976; Natale *et al.* 1980). In the human fetus hypoxaemia causes similar effects on breathing movements (Manning and Platt 1979). Clinical studies strongly suggest a similar effect on gross body movements, tone, and FHR reactivity (Manning and Platt 1979). Differentiation of behavioural state effects from hypoxaemic effects is achieved by extending the observation time until either the normal variable appears or at least 30 minutes of continued observation have elapsed. The 30-minute observation period works in the majority of cases, but since it is arbitrary it may contribute to a false positive result in a small percentage of cases. Thus, in a very immature fetus for whom delivery carries an exaggerated risk of neonatal complications, an extended testing time of up to 60 minutes or a repeat same-day testing is recommended. This is a technique we use commonly when dealing with a fetus for whom the risks of severe neonatal disease are high. A continued or sustained abnormal test is always an indication for delivery on our part. Amniotic fluid volume assessment by our method is recorded by measurement of the vertical axis of the largest pocket of fluid (Chamberlain *et al.* 1984), although others have employed a four-quadrant recording method (Phelan *et al.* 1987). The presence of umbilical cord loops within fluid pockets is not worrisome provided that the error of confusing a section of umbilical vein for amniotic fluid is avoided. The common association of Doppler ultrasound methods with linear array methods now permits Doppler scanning of amniotic fluid pockets to avoid this error.

A fundamental principle of FBP scoring is that the test is complete whenever all normal variables are observed. In our clinical experience of more than 122 000 tests the average time required to record breathing movement, tone, and amniotic fluid volume has been consistently less than 8 minutes; fewer than 2 per cent of all tests require a full 30-minute observation (Manning *et al*. 1991).

To facilitate recording, the variables are each assigned a score of 2 if normal and 0 if abnormal according to fixed criteria (see Table 17.1). In the initial description of the FBP scoring method it was believed that intermediate values (i.e. a score of 1) would evolve, but accumulating experience to date does not allow definition of such criteria. Therefore the binary concept persists in FBP scoring with each variable being either normal (score of 2) or abnormal (score 0). The test scores that result from this method may, therefore, range from 10 (i.e. all variables normal) to 0 (i.e. all variables abnormal).

As our experience with the testing method has increased two major modifications have been added to the method. First, based on a prospective clinical trial, we now do not routinely perform a non-stress test on all fetuses in whom the four dynamic ultrasound monitor variables are normal (Manning *et al*. 1987*a*). This modification has yielded a new scoring category of 8 (i.e. non-stress test excluded), the predictive accuracy of which equals that of a score of 10. A non-stress test is now routinely performed in all fetuses in whom any of the dynamic ultrasound monitor variables are abnormal. In our experience a non-stress test is required in less than 5 per cent of cases. This modification is of practical clinical advantage because it limits testing time. The second modification is in the definition of oligohydramnios. We have made the definition less stringent such that the largest pocket of fluid of 2 centimetres or less is now used to define decreased amniotic fluid volume. This modification was based on prospective studies of our clinical results (Chamberlain *et al*. 1984; Bastide *et al*. 1986). Despite the observation within our group that subjective assessment of amniotic fluid correlates well with measured pocket size we avoid using subjective impressions of amniotic fluid in the definition of an abnormal score in clinical management. This firm position is taken primarily to ensure uniformity in reporting FBP scores.

Antepartum fetal assessment by FBP scoring is limited at the present to referred patients with recognized maternal or fetal high-risk factors. Our working rule has been to begin the testing scheme when the factors may be reasonably expected to influence clinical management. As a result of this policy the gestational age at initial entry is progressively falling as improvements in neonatal survival increase. At the time of writing patients are accepted from 25 weeks onward. The frequency of repeat testing is also flexible depending on initial and subsequent maternal and fetal condition. In general repeat testing is scheduled on a weekly basis for all but the post-dates and insulin-dependent diabetic patients. Clinical management is based on test score result and obstetric factors (e.g. favourability of the cervix for induction), the extent and progression of maternal disease, and other fetal factors, including the presence or absence of anomalies, and in select cases, confirmation of pulmonary immaturity by amniotic fluid phospholipid profile. Usual management is outlined in Table 17.2.

Clinical outcome

Clinical testing of the concept of FBP scoring began with a prospective blind clinical study in 216 high-risk patients (Manning *et al.* 1980). In these patients FBP scores were obtained within one week of delivery and in most instances (i.e. in 52 per cent) within 2 days of delivery. A relationship between the last FBP score and perinatal mortality was observed. Perinatal mortality increased progressively as the score decreased such that perinatal mortality with a score of 10 was zero and perinatal mortality with a score of 0 was 600 per 1000. The relationship between FBP score and perinatal mortality has been recently reviewed (Baskett 1989). The results of recent published studies on this relationship are given in Table 17.3 (Baskett *et al.* 1987; Golde *et al.* 1984; Manning *et al.* 1981, 1985, 1990*b*; Platt *et al.* 1983; Shifrin *et al.* 1981; Shime *et al.* 1984; Vintzileos *et al.* 1987*a*). The two largest series, which came from Canadian hospitals, were performed in an identical manner and are responsible for most of the reported experience. The corrected perinatal mortality for these two series, involving 16 804 high-risk referred patients, was 2.2 per 1000. These collective data strongly suggest that the application of FBP scoring to the high-risk pregnancy population resulted in a dramatic improvement in perinatal mortality rates.

The false-negative rate of the testing method, defined by fetal death within a week of a last normal test result, is of considerable clinical importance because it may permit conservative management of the high-risk pregnancy and thereby reduce the risk of perinatal immaturity and the maternal risk attendant with expedited delivery. In the two large Canadian studies involving some 24 105 high-risk fetuses there are 17 reported false-negative deaths yielding a false negative rate of 0.7 per 1000 (Baskett *et al.* 1987; Manning *et al.* 1987*b*).

In a recent study of 19 221 referred high-risk fetuses Manning *et al.* (1987*b*) examined the relationship between the last FBP score and perinatal morbidity as well as mortality. Morbidity markers included fetal distress in labour (as defined by the presence of periodic FHR decelerations of

Table 17.2 Fetal biophysical profile (FBP) scores and recommended clinical managements

FBP score	Interpretation	Perinatal mortality within one week without intervention	Management
10 of 10 8 of 10 (normal fluid) 8 of 8 (non-stress test not done)	Risk of fetal asphyxia extremely rare	<1 per 1000	Intervention only for obstetric and maternal factors. No indication for intervention for fetal disease
8 of 10 (abnormal fluid)	Probable chronic fetal compromise	89 per 1000	Determine that there is functioning renal tissue and intact membranes—if so deliver for fetal indications
6 of 10 (normal fluid)	Equivocal test possible fetal asphyxia	Variable	If the fetus is mature—deliver. In the immature fetus repeat test within 24 hours—if <6/10 deliver
6 of 10 (abnormal)	Probable fetal asphyxia	89 per 1000	Deliver for fetal indications
4 of 10	High probability of fetal asphyxia	91 per 1000	Deliver for fetal indications
2 of 10	Fetal asphyxia almost certain	125 per 1000	Deliver for fetal indication
0 of 10	Fetal asphyxia certain	600 per 1000	Deliver for fetal indication

Table 17.3 The relationship of fetal biophysical profile scoring to perinatal death

Author	Number of patients	Number of tests	Total	Perinatal mortality (per 1000)		False-positive rate (per cent)
				Total	Corrected	
Manning et al. (1985)	12,620	26,257	93 (7.4)	24 (1.9)	8 (0.6)	—
Baskett et al. (1987)	4184	9624	45 (8.6)	13 (3.1)	4 (1.0)	71.8
Platt et al. (1983)	286	1112	4 (14.0)	2 (7.0)	2 (7.0)	71.4
Shime et al. (1984)	274	274	0	0	0	100.0
Schifrin et al. (1981)	158	240	7 (44.3)	2 (12.7)	1 (6.3)	42.6
Vintzileos et al. (1987a)	150	342	5 (33.3)	4 (26.6)	0	60.0
Golde et al. (1984)	107	459	2 (18.7)	0	0	75.0
Manning et al. (1987b)**	19,221	42,286	143 (7.95)	38 (1.95)	13	—
Total	23,780	54,337	206 (8)	59 (2.27)	18 (0.77)	42.6–100

* Lethal anomalies excluded
** Includes patients from Manning et al. (1985)

which the patterns, repetitive frequency, and magnitude prompted foreshortening of labour by operative intervention), low 5-minute Apgar score (i.e. less than 7), abnormal umbilical vein pH (less than 7.20 in venous blood), intrauterine growth retardation (i.e. birth-weight less than the third centile for gestational age and sex), and admission to an intensive care nursery for factors other than immaturity (for example, the presence of meconium-stained amniotic fluid or the presence of a major structural anomaly). In addition perinatal mortality, as defined by death of a fetus weighing at least 500 grams and neonatal death of up to 28 days of life, in this population, was examined. Perinatal mortality was further subdivided according to the time of death (stillborn or neonatal) and the presumed aetiology. In this paper a corrected perinatal death was defined as death due to factors other than developmental anomaly. In this study the relationship between the last test score and individual perinatal outcome variables fell into three general categories. For two morbidity variables, the incidence of meconium-staining of amniotic fluid and the incidence of major anomalies, there was no obvious relationship between the last test score and its occurrence (Fig. 17.1). A highly significant inverse linear correlation was observed with last test score. In contrast the morbidity markers of fetal distress, admission to a neonatal intensive care unit, intrauterine growth retardation, a low 5-minute Apgar score, and cord pH less than 7.20 bore a highly significant inverse linear correlation to last test score (Fig. 17.2). In contrast the relationship between last test score and perinatal mortality was inverse and exponential (Fig. 17.3).

The explanation for these observed relationships is intriguing and may offer considerable insight into the nature of fetal compromise and into the characteristics of fetal adaptive responses. The effect of hypoxaemia on the human fetus may be expected to vary according to the characteristics of the hypoxaemia and the fetal responsive mechanisms. From both serendipitous observation of the human fetus and experimental observation in the animal fetus it is known that hypoxaemia abolishes central nervous system-generated acute biophysical activities, and that the duration of the abolition exceeds the duration of hypoxaemia, often by a considerable margin. Variation in sensitivity of discrete central nervous system signal sources to greater hypoxaemia is suspected, but is as yet incompletely characterized (Vintzileos *et al.* 1987*b*). Oligohydramnios is a consequence of hypoxaemia, but is probably due to different mechanisms (Cohn *et al.* 1974) which occur over a long period of time. In the human fetus hypoxaemia is unlikely to be sustained, but is more likely to be intermittent, at least in the evolving stages, the modulation of episodes resulting from superimposed reductions in perfusion of the failing uteroplacental unit induced by spontaneous uterine contractions. According to this hypothesis, changes in the FBP variables, resulting in a change in the FBP score would indicate a

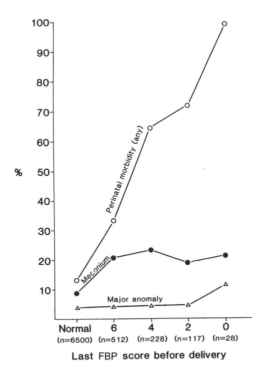

Fig. 17.1. The relationships of all perinatal morbidity, meconium-stained amniotic fluid, and anomalies with the last fetal biophysical profile (FBP) score before delivery, are shown. A highly significant linear relationship with morbidity is noted.

cumulative effect of hypoxaemic episodes. The sequential loss of FBP variables to yield a range of equivocal to abnormal score results reflects the magnitude and repetitive frequency of antepartum episodes of fetal hypoxaemia and therefore serve as an indirect marker of the degree of placental dysfunction. The theory predicts that all markers of adverse perinatal outcome should increase as the test score falls, and the results of this study confirm this prediction. The variation in slope, which was defined by the incremental increase as score falls between select end-points, was predicted by the theory as well. This steepest slope would be expected for fetal distress since this end-point is an almost direct reflection of placental dysfunction which becomes evident in the presence of uterine contractions, and the least slope would be predicted for umbilical vein acidosis since this would reflect the cumulative effects of more severe hypoxaemia. The observations in this study conform to this hypothesis (see Fig. 17.1).

The exponential relationship observed between the last test score and

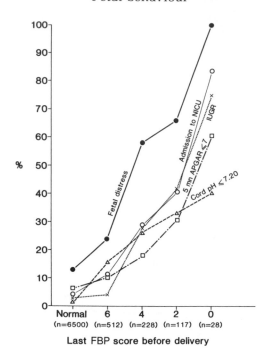

Last FBP score before delivery

Fig. 17.2. The relationships between last fetal biophysical profile (FBP) score and individual markers of perinatal morbidity are shown. All relationships are linear and highly significant.

perinatal mortality is more complex and more difficult to explain. It is likely that there are at least two factors that explain the relationship. Firstly, the degree and nature of fetal adaptor responses, which are not well studied, are likely to be substantial. Accordingly the sharp rise in perinatal mortality with the abnormal and very abnormal scores may suggest a terminal failure of adaptor responses to chronic fetal hypoxaemia. Secondly, the hypothesis predicts that the more severe the degree of hypoxaemia the more abnormal the score should be. Detailed reporting of perinatal outcome in fetuses with the most abnormal FBP score (i.e. 0) conform to this hypothesis (Manning *et al.* 1990c).

Predictive accuracy by variable combination

The FBP score is derived from five variables each of which are graded against fixed criteria and assigned a score of equal value when normal or abnormal. The combinations of normal and abnormal variables that can

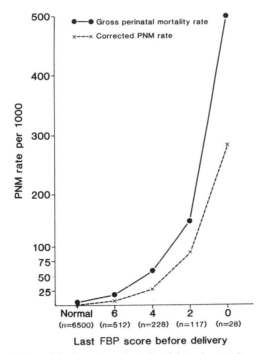

Fig. 17.3. The relationship between last fetal biophysical profile (FBP) score result and perinatal mortality is shown. The relationship is exponential and highly significant.

occur to yield a given score are multiple, for example there are 10 possible combinations to yield a score of 6, 10 possible combinations to yield a score of 4, and five possible combinations to yield a score of 2. Whereas all prospective studies of FBP scoring demonstrate a combination of variables yield superior predictive accuracy to any individual variable it remains uncertain as to whether or not the assigned value to each variable is reasonable. It may be argued for example that amniotic fluid volume is a more important and more powerful predictor of adverse perinatal outcome than fetal tone, for example. The original study on FBP scoring yielded 47 instances of a profile score of 6 or less (Manning *et al*. 1980). A recent study increased this experience by looking at perinatal outcome in relationship to test score composition in 525 fetuses who were delivered or died within 48 hours of a last abnormal FBP score of 6 or less (Manning *et al*. 1990*a*). In this study the relationship of test score composition to perinatal morbidity or mortality was determined. Individual components of the score varied in frequency of occurrence, but not in accuracy parameters. Thus the positive predictive accuracy of a composite of all five variables always exceeded that for any individual variable. This was more easily demonstrated in an analysis of the results of a FBP score of 2, a test combination, which because only a single variable of the composite score remains normal offers unique insight into the relationship between test score and predictive accuracy. When the results of 113 fetuses with a last FBP score of 2 were contrasted with previously reported results of fetuses with normal test results it was noted that while a non-significant variation in the frequency of perinatal outcome end-points was observed, the observed frequency for all abnormal end-points was always many-fold higher than that observed among fetuses with the last score greater than 2. Thus for example a reactive non-stress test in the presence of absent fetal breathing movements, absent fetal movement and fetal tone, and decreased amniotic fluid volume was not reassuring, being associated with as low as a 3.7-fold increase in incidence of low 5-minute Apgar score to as high as a 17-fold increase in perinatal mortality. Further, for all end-points of abnormal outcome, a significant inverse relationship with last test score was observed. This latter relationship was not unexpected since it had been reported previously by our clinical group (Manning *et al*. 1985), by Baskett *et al*. (1987), and by Vintzileos *et al*. (1987).

In the usual description of FBP scoring it was assumed that all variables of a composite FBP contributed to a positive predictive accuracy in an equally proportionate manner. This was the basis for an arbitrary assignment of equal score weights for each variable. The data from the composite assessment of 525 patients with a score of 6 or less casts some doubt on this assumption. It was noted that within sub-groups the distribution of score combinations was not equal, nor was the positive predictive accuracy constant across possible combinations. Thus for example, with a FBP score of 6 the positive predictive accuracy of any abnormal outcome variable was always higher than that reported for a normal score, but the probability of for example, fetal distress or death when the non-stress test for fetal tone was abnormal was significantly higher than when fetal tone and fetal breathing movements were absent, when the probability of fetal distress was lower. Similar significant variations in positive predictive accuracy occurred within the sub-sets of variable combinations yielding a FBP score of 4. These variations disappeared with any FBP score of 2.

The best means of examining these data was by logistic regression analysis. The results of this analysis demonstrated that models that best fit against the spectrum of abnormal outcome end-points varied by both relative variable weight and by variable inclusion. It became evident that the non-stress test, amniotic fluid volume, and fetal breathing movements, emerged as the most powerful variables and were necessary for all end-point equations. Fetal tone played a lesser role and fetal movements were important only in the model for prediction of fetal distress. Of course it remains somewhat unclear as to what extent interdependence of variable assessment contributes to predictive models. An example of variable-independence would be fetal movement in the non-stress test. By the definitions used in FBP scoring a reactive non-stress test implies fetal movements are present. However, we observed examples of a reactive non-stress test in combination with an abnormal movement score. Although it is possible that this paradox arises because the number of fetal movements needed for designation of a normal test is greater than the number of accelerations needed for a reactive non-stress test, it is more likely to be the result of sequential testing method in which fetal movements were recorded initially by a dynamic ultrasound method and then the FHR was recorded later by the Doppler ultrasound method. The interval between recording the two modalities might be sufficient to exceed the usual sleep–wake cycle of the fetus. This problem of course was resolved with the introduction of a simultaneous method for recording both real-time fetal movement and FHR data.

It is clear that these observations are of some technical interest, but their clinical significance is less certain. While the data do demonstrate significant variation and positive predictive accuracy of combinations, they do not diminish the significant relationship between the total abnormal score and abnormal outcome. Thus while a FBP score of 4 in which the non-stress test is reactive and amniotic fluid is normal behaves in a positive predictive accuracy more like a score of 6, the risk of adverse outcome with this combination still remains very much higher than that observed in a fetus with a normal score. This is to say that a score of 6 by this combination is not reassuring, and from our observations is not an indication for conservative management. Thus, the concept that it may be possible to reduce antepartum testing to simple combinations of FHR recording and amniotic fluid assessment is not supported by the data presented in this study. A second problem arising from the data is the concept of predicting a new scoring system based on proportionate weights for different variables. Whereas the data from the prospective study demonstrates that there may be some value in this it will become exceedingly difficult to determine such value in clinical practice because of the very good results achieved to date with the existing method of FBP scoring. Working within a context of a corrected perinatal mortality of around 1 per 1000 it will be exceedingly difficult to collect sufficient numbers to alter the scoring system, at least in the short term.

These data also offer some insight into a concept that has frequently been raised with FBP scoring—that is the concept of sequential loss of variables as the fetus deteriorates (Vintzileos *et al.* 1987*a*). It was our hope in the analysis of these data to determine some sequential pattern of progressive loss, but such a pattern, if it exists, was certainly not apparent.

The spectrum of possible combinations observed yielded the full range of adverse outcome, and the positive predictive accuracy for any of the possible combinations, while varying, was always high. These data suggest that the switching-off of normal FBP variables in the progress to deterioration must depend more on the extent and cadence of the disease than on specific thresholds. Thus while the concept of threshold response to graded hypoxaemia remains attractive it would seem that the complexity of fetal disease is such that the recognition of these patterns will remain exceedingly difficult. It seems evident from this study that future advances in FBP applications will most likely result from the addition of new variables such as Doppler ultrasound assessment of umbilical artery flow than by modification of the criteria of the original variables.

Gestational age

It seems evident that as improvements in neonatal survival continue, the lower limit at which intervention for fetal disease becomes possible will fall. It has been our observed clinical experience over the last 10 years to see this age fall from 32 weeks in the early 1980s down to an age of approximately 25 weeks within our units. As these opportunities for intervention in the compromised fetus become possible at these earlier gestational ages it becomes increasingly important to understand the effect, if any, of fetal age on the positive predictive accuracy and reliability of the antepartum testing methods. This is particularly important because intervention at 25 weeks is associated with a neonatal mortality rate in excess of 40 per cent. There is a paucity of data regarding the positive predictive accuracy of FBP scoring at less than 28 weeks of gestation. Baskett (1988) examined the relationship between gestational age and FBP assessment in 5582 singleton fetuses with a normal perinatal outcome. In this study Baskett demonstrated that the incidence of an abnormal non-stress test rose progressively as gestational age decreased ranging from as high as 31.4 per cent at 26 to 30 weeks compared to 9.2 per cent at 37 to 41 weeks. There is no change between 26 weeks and 44 weeks in the incidence of abnormal test results for fetal breathing movements, fetal movement, fetal tone, or amniotic fluid volume. These data appear to indicate that FBP scoring is effective from a gestational age as early as 26 weeks. In an ongoing study, Manning *et al.* have demonstrated similar relationships (1991). We have examined 1096 fetuses with a gestational age less than 29 weeks serially with FBP scoring. In this population the incidence of an abnormal FBP score (i.e. 4 or less) was 1.8 per cent which is approximately twice the incidence observed in the population at large (0.7 per cent). Interestingly, the positive predictive accuracy in the fetus between 26 and

29 weeks gestation with a profile score of 4 or less was comparable to that observed in a population of older fetuses. More importantly the negative predictive accuracy of a normal score in this younger population remains comparable to that observed in the older fetus (i.e. in the presence of a score of 8 out of 8 the probability of fetal death within a week of the test is less than 1 per 1000). This particular observation is of considerable clinical importance for it means that conservative management is reasonable in the fetus at risk with a normal score. Such management has allowed us to coax several days to weeks out of fetuses with such abnormal findings as intrauterine growth retardation, and in fetuses who had absent end-diastolic flow on Doppler assessment of the umbilical artery. Whereas such conservative management might have little significance at 34 weeks or greater, it is evident that even a few extra days at 25 to 26 weeks of gestation represents a significant improvement of perinatal survival. Ongoing studies of FBP scoring at earlier gestational ages is of great importance.

Conclusion

The introduction of highly accurate methods for observing and recording human fetal biophysical activities has exerted, and continues to exert, profound positive change in the understanding of fetal activities in health and disease. The complexities and organization of fetal response to intrinsic and extrinsic stimuli are quite remarkable. It seems evident that categorization of patterns of response to noxious stimuli such as hypoxaemia must be derived from a framework of understanding behavioural states and gestational age influences. Within such a context it now appears that composite fetal assessment, that is risk determination based on a spectrum of biophysical responses with different time constraints and different controlling mechanisms, will be the most accurate means of differentiating the healthy fetus from the fetus at risk of death or damage *in utero*.

References

Baskett, T. F. (1988). Gestational age and fetal biophysical assessment. *American Journal of Obstetrics and Gynecology* **158,** 332–4.

Baskett, T. F. (1989). The fetal biophysical profile. In: *Progress in obstetrics and gynecology* (ed. J. Studd). 7th Edn, pp. 145–54. Churchill Livingstone, New York.

Baskett, T. F., Allen, A. C., Gray, J. H., Young, D. C., and Young, L. M. (1987). Fetal biophysical profile and perinatal death. *Obstetrics and Gynecology* **70,** 357–60.

Bastide, A., Manning, F. A., Harman, C. R., Lange, I., and Morrison, I. (1986).

Ultrasound evaluation of amniotic fluid. Outcome of pregnancies with severe oligohydramnios. *American Journal of Obstetrics and Gynecology* **154**, 895–900.

Boddy, K. and Dawes, G. S. (1976). Fetal breathing. *British Medical Bulletin* **31**, 3–7.

Chamberlain, P. F., Manning, F. A., Morrison, I., Harman, C. A., and Lange, I. R. (1984). Ultrasound evaluation of amniotic fluid 1. The relationship of marginal and decreased amniotic fluid to perinatal outcome. *American Journal of Obstetrics and Gynecology* **150**, 245–9.

Cohn, H. E., Sacks, E. J., Heyman, M. A., and Rudolph, A. M. (1974). Cardiovascular responses to hypoxemia and acidemia in fetal lambs. *American Journal of Obstetrics and Gynecology* **120**, 817–24.

Drogtrop, A. P., Ubels, R., and Nijhuis, J. G. (1990). The association between fetal body movements, eye movements and heart rate patterns in pregnancies between 25 and 30 weeks of gestation. *Early Human Development* **23**, 67–73.

Golde, S. H., Montoro, M., Good-Anderson, B., Broussard, P., Jacobs, N., Loesser, C., *et al.* (1984). The role of non-stress tests, fetal biophysical profile, and contraction stress tests in the out-patient management of insulin requiring diabetic pregnancies. *American Journal of Obstetrics and Gynecology* **148**, 269–73.

Manning, F. A. and Platt, L. D. (1979). Maternal hypoxemia and fetal breathing movements. *Obstetrics and Gynecology* **53**, 758–60.

Manning, F. A., Platt, L. D., and Sipos, L. (1980). Antepartum fetal evaluation: development of a fetal biophysical profile score. *American Journal of Obstetrics and Gynecology* **136**, 787–95.

Manning, F. A., Baskett, T. F., Morrison, I., and Lange, I. R. (1981). Fetal biophysical profile scoring: a prospective study in 1184 high risk patients. *American Journal of Obstetrics and Gynecology* **140**, 289–94.

Manning, F. A., Morrison, I., Lange, I., Harman, C. R., and Chamberlain, P. F. C. (1985). Fetal assessment based on fetal biophysical profile scoring: experience in 12,620 high risk pregnancies. 1. Perinatal mortality by frequency and etiology. *American Journal of Obstetrics and Gynecology* **151**, 343–50.

Manning, F. A., Morrison, I., Lange, I. R., Harman, C. R., and Chamberlain, P. F. C. (1987*a*). Fetal biophysical profile scoring: selective use of the non-stress test. *American Journal of Obstetrics and Gynecology* **156**, 709–12.

Manning, F. A., Morrison, I., Harman, C. R., Lange, I. R., and Menticoglou, S. (1987*b*). Fetal assessment by fetal biophysical profile scoring in 19221 referred high risk pregnancies. II The false negative rate by frequency and etiology. *American Journal of Obstetrics and Gynecology* **157**, 880–4.

Manning, F. A., Morrison, I., Harman, and Menticoglou, S. M. (1990*a*). The abnormal fetal biophysical profile score. V. Predictive accuracy according to score composition. *American Journal of Obstetrics and Gynecology* **162**, 918–27.

Manning, F. A., Harman, C. R., Morrison, I., Menticoglou, S., Lange, I. R., and Johnson, J. M. (1990*b*). Fetal assessment based upon fetal biophysical profile score: IV Analysis of perinatal morbidity and mortality. *American Journal of Obstetrics and Gynecology* **162**, 703–9.

Manning, F. A., Harman, C. R., Morrison, I., and Menticoglou, S. M. (1990*c*). Fetal assessment based on fetal biophysical profile III. Positive predictive accuracy of the very abnormal test (BPS = 0). *American Journal of Obstetrics and Gynecology* **162**, 398–402.

Manning, F. A., Harman, C. R., Morrison, I., and Menticoglou, S. (1991). Unpublished data.

Natale, R., Clewlow, F., and Dawes, G. S. (1980). Measurement of fetal forelimb movement in the lamb *in utero*. *American Journal of Obstetrics and Gynecology* **140**, 545–51.

Nijhuis, J. G., Prechtl, H. F. R., Martin, C. B., Jr, and Bots, R. S. G. M. (1982). Are there behavioural states in the human fetus? *Early Human Development* **6**, 177–95.

Patrick, J. E. (1988). Fetal breathing movements, gross body movements and rest activity patterns. In: *Maternal and fetal medicine: principles and practice* (ed. R. Creasy and R. Resnik), pp. 239–48. W. B. Saunders, Philadelphia.

Phelan, J. P., Platt, L. D., Sze-Ya, Y., Broussard, P., and Paul, R. H. (1987). The role of ultrasound assessment and amniotic fluid in the postdate pregnancy. *American Journal of Obstetrics and Gynecology* **151**, 304–8.

Platt, L. D., Eglington, G. S., Sipos, L., Broussard, P. M., and Paul, R. H. (1983). Further experience with the fetal biophysical profile. *Obstetrics and Gynecology* **61**, 480–5.

Schifrin, B. S., Guntes, V., Gergely, R. C., Eden, R., Roll, K., and Jacobi, J. (1981). The role of real-time scanning in antenatal survcillance. *American Journal of Obstetrics and Gynecology* **140**, 525 30.

Shime, J., Gare, J. D., Andrews, J., Bertrand, M., Salgado, J., and Whillans, G. (1984). Prolonged pregnancy: surveillance of the fetus and the neonate and the course of labor and delivery. *American Journal of Obstetrics and Gynecology* **148**, 547–52.

Vintzileos, A. M., Campbell, W. A., and Ingardia, C. J. (1987a). The fetal biophysical profile and its predictive value. *American Journal of Obstetrics and Gynecology* **157**, 236–40.

Vintzileos, A. M., Gaffney, S. E., Salinger, L. M., Kontopoulos, V., Campbell, W. A., and Jochimson, D. J. (1987b). The relationship among the fetal biophysical profile, umbilical cord pH, and Apgar scores. *American Journal of Obstetrics and Gynecology* **157**, 627–31.

18

Consequences for fetal monitoring

B. A. P. J. TAS and J. G. NIJHUIS

Introduction

The first section of this book describes the developmental course of fetal motility and fetal behavioural states. It has become very clear that it is important to know what one may expect from a fetus at a certain gestational age. The aim of this chapter is to summarize the consequences of this knowledge for fetal monitoring and fetal surveillance. For example, absence of movements over a prolonged period of time may be physiological at 38 weeks of gestation, but is obviously pathological at 16 weeks. For this reason the above-mentioned consequences for the assessment of fetal condition will be discussed for each trimester.

First trimester

The very first sign of 'fetal activity' that can be observed using a vaginal ultrasound-transducer is fetal heart activity. This is also the very first sign that a pregnancy is viable. Once heart activity has been noted, the chance that the pregnancy will end in a spontaneous abortion is dramatically reduced. Heart activity begins at about 5 weeks of gestation and can be observed from approximately 40 days of menstrual age. From week 6 to week 9 a rapid increase of the mean fetal heart-rate (FHR) from 110 to 167 beats per minute is followed by a slow decrease to 165. A close correlation between crown–rump length and FHR has been established (van Heeswijk *et al.* 1990). Failure of the FHR to show this rapid increase seems to indicate impending embryonic death.

During the following weeks fetal somatic motility begins and has been described by de Vries in Chapter 1. It is clear that the quality of fetal movements may be of greater importance than the quantity at this gestational age (de Vries *et al.* 1982, 1985). This was nicely illustrated by Visser *et al.* (1985) who investigated motor behaviour in anencephalic fetuses. Although the incidence of general movements corresponded to the median values found in normal fetuses of the same gestational age, the quality of the movements was completely different. The body movements and limb movements were forceful and jerky and of large amplitude, in contrast to the fluent appearance and the waxing and waning of movements in normal fetuses. The general movement patterns in eight anencephalic fetuses between 16 and 35 weeks is presented in Fig. 18.1. Although the quantity of fetal movements seems to be of minor importance it is useful to know that absence of movements for longer than about five minutes is certainly abnormal (see de Vries *et al*. in Chapter 1, Table 1.2). From these data it can be concluded that it is worth waiting for the appearance of movements during every ultrasound examination in the first trimester. Absence of movements for a period longer than 10 minutes should be regarded as a warning sign and further evaluation is then indicated.

Second trimester

From 20 to 30 weeks of gestation no new fetal movements emerge. As Visser has already pointed out in Chapter 2, the generalized movements decrease in number per hour (Natale *et al*. 1985; Roodenburg *et al*. 1991) and in percentage of total recording time (de Vries *et al*. 1982). During this gestational period the beginning of the development of a rest–activity cycle can be seen; but the concept of behavioural states is not yet applicable. Compared to the first trimester, this period has the advantage that cardiotocography (CTG) can be used, which adds another tool for evaluating fetal well-being. Unfortunately only a few studies have investigated the use of CTG in this trimester.

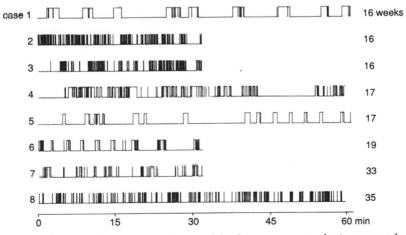

Fig. 18.1. Compiled actogram of general body movements during a one-hour observation of eight anencephalic fetuses. (Reproduced with permission from Visser *et al*. 1985.)

In general a 'silent' FHR pattern (FHR pattern A) is believed to be indicative of fetal distress. This is particularly true at this gestational age as the median duration of FHR pattern A is about 5 minutes (!), and the maximum duration is 30 minutes (Drogtrop *et al.* 1990). Regarding motility, it is clear that the fetus seems to be continually active. The median duration for body movements to be absent is 5 minutes, and the maximum is 16 minutes, while the median duration for eye movements to be absent is 4 minutes, and the maximum is 25 minutes (Drogtrop *et al.* 1990). Breathing movements can be absent for a maximum period of 40 minutes (Natale *et al.* 1985). These durations increase with gestational age (Fig. 18.2). This knowledge has implications for the assessment of fetal condition. For example, if one produces a biophysical profile of a fetus at 28 weeks of gestation according to Manning (see Chapter 17) and body movements are observed only during the last 5 minutes of an observation period of 30 minutes after a period of quiescence of 25 minutes, then the maximum score of 2 points would be justified according to this scoring system (Manning *et al.* 1980, 1990). However, although the fetus makes body

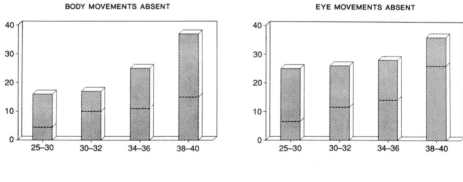

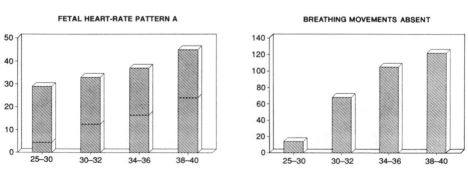

Fig. 18.2. Duration of heart-rate pattern A and body, eye, and breathing movements (in minutes) in different periods of fetal life. Median and maximum durations are indicated.

movements during the last 5 minutes, the period of 25 minutes without body movements is completely abnormal at this gestational age and it is therefore possible that this fetus, or rather its central nervous system (CNS), is abnormal. Rather than concluding that the fetus is in a good condition, it would be more appropriate to perform a further behavioural study.

Third trimester

In the third trimester rest–activity cycles and behavioural states are fully developed. This means that breathing movements, eye movements, and body movements can be absent over long periods and that during the same epoch the CTG will reveal a silent FHR pattern (FHR pattern A) (Chapter 3; Nijhuis *et al.* 1982; van Woerden *et al.* 1988). This has important consequences, especially for the interpretation of CTG recordings.

Before fetal behaviour was understood, the CTG was the only variable used for the assessment of fetal condition. Tracings with good variability indicated a good fetal condition, while a silent pattern was suggestive of a poor condition. While a good condition could usually be predicted (i.e. high specificity), the sensitivity and predictive value of 'fetal distress' was poor. A number of scoring systems for interpreting CTG recordings were proposed (Fischer *et al.* 1976; Visser and Huisjes 1977; Visser 1984), but none has gained universal acceptance, probably because of this problem of insensitivity and low predictive value. What we would like to stress in this section is that knowledge of fetal behaviour has greatly influenced the interpretations of the CTG recordings.

Silent heart-rate pattern

The FHR pattern may be silent during a maximum period of about 45 minutes near term (see Fig. 18.2). If decelerations are absent, extension of the recording time is the first step in evaluating a silent FHR pattern. During this time the use of drugs by the mother must be excluded, because of the well-known fact that some drugs may influence the FHR variability (de Haan *et al.* 1971). Congenital anomalies such as anencephaly should also be excluded.

If the fetus does move while the FHR pattern is still silent then it is most likely that there is a disturbance of the CNS. In Fig. 18.3 an example of such a case is presented. Although fetal distress was suspected when this CTG was recorded, on the base of a behavioural study the presence of hypoxia appeared to be highly unlikely. In the case presented here, an expectant management was advised instead of an emergency caesarean

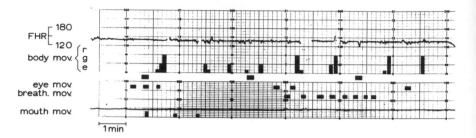

Fig. 18.3. An example of a silent fetal heart-rate (FHR) with several movements present. This child had severe congenital malformations of the brain including hypoplasia of the cerebellum. (r, rotation; g, general movement; e, extremity movement.)

section for fetal distress. After a few weeks a baby was born with congenital anomalies of the CNS including hypoplasia of the cerebellum.

If the fetus does not move, then a contraction stress test can be performed in addition to the behavioural study. If (late) decelerations occur during this test, hypoxia is probably present and a rapid delivery by caesarean section is necessary. If decelerations are absent during this test, hypoxia is most unlikely and a diagnosis of fetal brain death should be considered (Fig. 18.4, Nijhuis *et al.* 1990). At this point a cordocentesis can be performed and if the fetal blood gas analysis excludes hypoxia, further invasive procedures, for example caesarean section, can then be avoided. In all cases of fetal brain death the CTG tracings can be defined as an absolutely silent pattern with a normal or slightly increased base-line without decelerations (Nijhuis *et al.* 1990).

Table 18.1 summarizes the management of a silent FHR pattern.

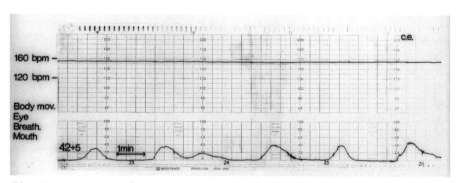

Fig. 18.4. An example of a persistent, absolutely silent fetal heart-rate (FHR) pattern with total absence of fetal movements. Mark the relatively high base-line (i.e. 155 bpm). This recording indicates fetal brain death.

Table 18.1 Differential diagnosis of a silent fetal heart-rate pattern and proposed management (modified from Nijhuis *et al.* 1990)

Differential diagnosis	Management
Behavioural state 1F	Extend the recording time
Effect of drugs	Exclude use of drugs
Tachycardia	Inspect base-line
Anomalies	Ultrasonographic examination Behavioural study
Hypoxia	Contraction stress test (CST)
Brain death	Cordocentesis

Sinusoidal-like patterns

In Chapter 4 it was mentioned that during regular mouthing in state 1F, there are typical oscillations in the FHR, concurrent with clusters of mouthing movements. In 1984 Nijhuis *et al.* showed that fetal sucking movements (probably during state 3F) may simulate a CTG pattern which can be judged as sinusoidal, which can also be seen in severely anaemic fetuses. An example of such a FHR pattern is shown in Fig. 18.5.

Tachycardia

Tachycardia may occur as a sign of fetal heart decompensation, maternal fever, and the use of drugs like beta-mimetics. Normal fetal behaviour may also lead to differential diagnostic problems in fetal tachycardia. Episodes

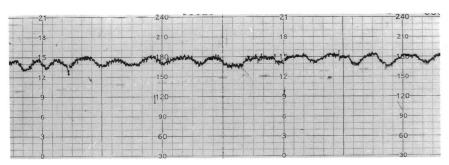

Fig. 18.5. An example of a sinusoidal fetal heart-rate pattern during fetal sucking. Each cluster of sucking movements entrains a short lasting acceleration.

of vigorous fetal movements can evoke large amplitudes and sustained accelerations of the FHR (i.e. FHR pattern D—'the jogging fetus'; Nijhuis 1986). If the observer is not alert to the presence of the motor activity and its effect on FHR, return of the FHR to or toward the resting rate during brief pauses in the activity can lead to a misinterpretation of the pattern as 'tachycardia with decelerations', which is a potentially ominous finding (Fig. 18.6). Such mistakes can usually be avoided if the CTG tracings are examined in the light of the simultaneous fetal activity and/or the recording time is extended when there is a transition to another fetal behavioural state.

Do reactive patterns always indicate a good fetal condition?

In general a reactive FHR pattern reflects a good fetal condition. However, there can be exceptions (Fig. 18.7). In this case, the mother kept complaining that she was unable to perceive any fetal body movement. Nevertheless the CTG recordings were always reactive. This was an indication to perform a fetal behavioural study. The CTG recording stayed reactive, but no movements were seen; it was as if the fetus tried to make movements, but did not succeed. The accelerations, therefore, seemed to be the result of isometric contractions of the fetal muscles. On the base of this fetal behavioural study the diagnosis of arthrogryposis fetalis was proposed and was confirmed after birth.

Conclusions

In this chapter we have emphasized that both quality and quantity of fetal movements are important in the assessment of fetal condition. It is important to know what is normal at a particular gestational age. Furthermore, fetal behaviour can be seen as the output of the CNS activity. If a fetus behaves abnormally, then a CNS anomaly should be excluded, although more peripheral pathology (e.g., some cases of arthrogryposis) may lead to the same phenomenon. Therefore, when discrepancies are present between the recorded CTG pattern and the perception of fetal movements by the mother, a thorough fetal behavioural study is strongly indicated. This is also the case if problems arise when interpreting a certain FHR pattern. Recently Pillai *et al.* presented the case of a fetus with a lethal multiple congenital abnormality syndrome; the CTG and biophysical profile were normal, but detailed analysis of fetal behaviour was grossly abnormal (Pillai *et al.* 1991). In such cases the knowledge and observation of fetal behaviour will lead to the correct diagnosis and avoid unnecessary interventions.

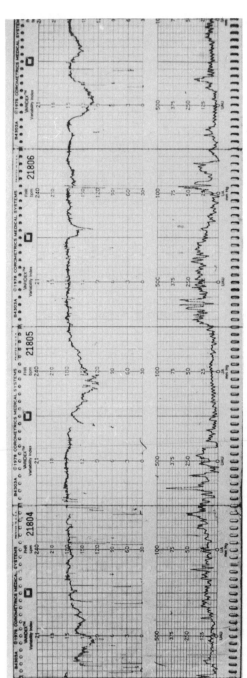

Fig. 18.6. Trace showing sustained accelerations of the fetal heart-rate evoked by vigorous fetal body movements; this was misinterpreted as a 'tachycardia with decelerations'. (Reproduced with permission from Nijhuis 1986.)

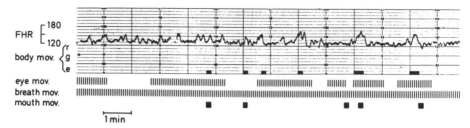

Fig. 18.7. Recording of a reactive fetal heart-rate pattern without real fetal movements. The 'movements' that are indicated with small bars were interpreted as isometric contractions. The diagnosis of arthrogryposis was proposed on the basis of this behavioural study and the diagnosis was confirmed after birth. (r, rotation; g, general movement; e, extremity movement.)

References

Drogtrop, P. A., Ubels, R., and Nijhuis, J. G. (1990). The association between fetal body movements, eye movements and heart rate patterns in pregnancies between 25 and 30 weeks of gestation. *Early Human Development* **23**, 67–73.

Fischer, W. M., Stude, I., and Brandt, H. (1976). Ein Vorschlag zur Beurteilung des antepartualen Kardiotokogramms. *Zeitschrift zur Geburtshilfe und Perinatalogie* **180**, 117–23.

Haan, J. de, Bemmel, J. H. van, and Stolte, L. A. M. (1971). Quantitative evaluation of fetal heart rate patterns. II. The significance of the fixed heart rate during pregnancy and Labour. *European Journal of Obstetrics and Gynecology* **3**, 103–10.

Heeswijk, M. van, Nijhuis, J. G., and Hollanders, H. M. G. (1990). Fetal heart rate in early pregnancy. *Early Human Development* **22**, 151–6.

Manning, F. A., Platt, L. D., and Sipos, L. (1980). Antepartum fetal evaluation: development of a fetal biophysical profile score. *American Journal of Obstetrics and Gynecology* **136**, 787.

Manning, F. A., Morisson, I., Harman, C. R., and Menticoglou, S. M. (1990). The abnormal fetal biophysical profile score. Predictive accuracy according to score composition. *American Journal of Obstetrics and Gynecology* **162**, 918–27.

Natale, R., Nassello-Peterson, C., and Turlink, R. (1985). Longitudinal measurements of fetal breathing, body movements, and heart rate accelerations and decelerations at 24 to 32 weeks of gestation. *American Journal of Obstetrics and Gynecology* **151**, 256–63.

Nijhuis, J. G. (1986). Behavioural states: concomitants, clinical implications and the assessment of the condition of the nervous system. *European Journal of Obstetrics and Gynecology and Reproductive Biology* **21**, 301–8.

Nijhuis, J. G., Prechtl, H. F. R., Martin, Jr. C. B., and Bots, R. S. G. M. (1982). Are there behavioural states in the human fetus? *Early Human Development* **6**, 177–95.

Nijhuis, J. G., Staisch, K. J., Martin, Jr. C. B., and Prechtl, H. F. R. (1984). A sinusoidal-like fetal heart rate pattern in association with fetal sucking—report of two cases. *European Journal of Obstetrics and Gynecology and Reproductive Biology* **21,** 353.

Nijhuis, J. G., Crevels, A. J., and Van Dongen, P. W. J. (1990). Fetal brain death: the definition of a fetal heart rate pattern and its clinical consequences. *Obstetrical and Gynecological Survey* **46,** 229–32.

Pillai, M., Garrett, C., and James, D. (1991). Bizarre fetal behaviour associated with lethal congenital anomalies: a case report. *European Journal of Obstetrics and Gynecology and Reproductive Biology* **39,** 215–18.

Roodenburg, F. J., Wladimiroff, J. W., Es, A. van, and Prechtl, H. F. R. (1991). Classification and quantitative aspects of fetal movements during the second half of normal pregnancy. *Early Human Development* **15,** 19–36.

Visser, G. H. A. (1984). Antenatal cardiotocography in the evaluation of fetal well-being. *Australian and New Zealand Journal of Obstetrics and Gynaecology* **24,** 80–5.

Visser, G. H. A. and Huisjes, H. J. (1977). Diagnostic value of the unstressed antepartum cardiotocogram. *British Journal of Obstetrics and Gynaecology* **84,** 321–6.

Visser, G. H. A., Laurini, R. N., Vries, J. I. P. de, Bekedam, D. J., and Prechtl, H. F. R. (1985). Abnormal motor behaviour in anencephalic fetuses. *Early Human Development* **12,** 173–82.

Vries, J. I. P. de, Visser, G. H. A., and Prechtl, H. F. R. (1982). The emergence of fetal behaviour. I. Qualitative aspects. *Early Human Development* **7,** 301–22.

Vries, J. I. P. de, Visser, G. H. A., and Prechtl, H. F. R. (1985). The emergence of fetal behaviour. II. Quantitative aspects. *Early Human Development* **12,** 99–120.

Vries, J. I. P. de, Visser, G. H. A., and Prechtl, H. F. R. (1988). The emergence of fetal behaviour. III. Individual differences and consistencies. *Early Human Development* **16,** 85–103.

Woerden, E. E. van, Geijn, H. P. van, Swartjes, J. M., Caron, F. J. M., Brons, J. T. J., and Arts, N. F. Th. (1988). Fetal heart rhythms during behavioural state 1F. *European Journal of Obstetrics and Gynecology and Reproductive Biology* **28,** 29–38.

Epilogue: Do we really need the concept of fetal behavioural states?

CHESTER B. MARTIN JR

My answer to the question posed in the title is (predictably from the context in which it appears) an emphatic yes. Every physician responsible for the care and assessment of fetuses, and every researcher studying fetal physiology must be aware of behavioural states, for these certainly affect the interpretation of both clinical and laboratory observations. In the two decades that have passed since Dawes and associates (1970) described the association of breathing movements, eye movements, and electrocortical activity patterns in fetal sheep, and since the demonstration 12 years later of the existence of behavioural states prior to birth in the human fetus (Nijhuis *et al*. 1982), it has become very clear that the fetal state is not a 'steady state'. The alternation of activity states is accompanied by significant changes not only in fetal motility, but also in fetal physiology, metabolism, and response to stimulation. The investigator who does not take this state into account may be faced with explaining inconsistencies in data and come to erroneous conclusions. The clinician who ignores behavioural states risks committing errors in patient management.

While in one context states are a descriptive categorization of behaviour, they are also 'distinct conditions, each having its specific properties and reflecting a particular mode of nervous function' (Prechtl 1974). The differing incidence and character of somatic, eye, and breathing movements in each state are readily understood as expressions of differing modes of neural function. Regional differences in brain blood-flow and uptake of substrates between states, as described in Chapters 8 and 9, are predictable consequences of different patterns of brain activity. Since fetal heart-rate (FHR) and FHR variability are greatly influenced by control mechanisms involving the central nervous system, an association between these variables and the mode of brain function is also to be expected. Indeed, the pattern of base-line FHR variability is one of the variables used to define the behavioural states of the human fetus.

With the refinement of non-invasive ultrasound methods to study blood-flow and the application of these to the human fetus, it has become apparent that there are substantial changes in the fetal circulation associated with the behavioural states. These are described by Van Eyck and Wladimiroff in Chapter 16. State-related alterations in the fetal circulation involve not only cerebral and peripheral vascular beds, but also include changes in central shunting through the foramen ovale and ductus arteriosus. Moreover, Rizzo and associates (1990) have demonstrated an increase in left ventricular output and a decrease in right ventricular output in state 2F in comparison to state 1F. Combined ventricular output did not change between these two states. Although the ultrasound measurements suggest that umbilical vascular resistance does not differ with state in the human fetus, there is evidence that umbilical blood-flow differs not only between states, but changes over time within the same state in the fetal sheep (Slotten *et al.* 1989). Circulating catecholamine levels also differ between electrocorticographic states in fetal sheep (Reid *et al.* 1990). It seems certain that future research will continue to demonstrate circulatory, metabolic, and endocrine changes in association with behavioural states. It is imperative, therefore, that behavioural state is taken into account in experimental design and data interpretation in studies of human or laboratory animal fetuses.

An appreciation of behavioural states is as important for the clinician, who deals with pregnant women and their fetuses, as it is for the fetal physiologist. State-related changes in fetal motility and FHR have obvious implications for the assessment of fetal well-being by any biophysical method. The clinician must be aware of the normal spectrum of human fetal behaviour in order to distinguish the abnormal with greater certainty.

The influence of the fetal rest–activity cycle on the antepartum cardiotocogram (CTG) was recognized early by the developers of this technique, indeed well before fetal behavioural states were identified. However, real-time ultrasound observation of fetal motility simultaneously with the CTG has improved our ability to interpret many of the FHR patterns seen in the antepartum CTG, as van Woerden and van Geijn, and Tas and Nijhuis point out in Chapters 4 and 18, respectively. Behavioural states are present in the mature fetus during labour, and cycles of activity and rest continue during labour in the preterm fetus. These cycles in motility and behaviour affect the intrapartum CTG, as noted by Spencer in Chapter 5. Clinicians must be as aware of the FHR patterns associated with normal behavioural phenomena during labour as they are with antepartum tracings. For example, I have reviewed two cases in which a caesarean section was performed for 'fetal tachycardia with decelerations, and inability to do a scalp sample', where the FHR pattern strongly suggested a state 4F epoch, but no assessment of fetal movements was done! Both infants were vigorous at delivery, as could have been predicted from the FHR tracing had the pattern been recognized (see Fig. 18.6). Most clinicians recognize that episodes of fetal quiescence and low FHR variability often last longer during labour than antepartum, and do not confuse these with fetal distress. Changes in the FHR response to uterine contractions in the different behavioural states warrants further study, as does the effect of analgesics given to the mother on fetal behavioural states and motility cycles (see also Chapter 18).

One of the intriguing findings that has emerged from the study of fetal motility at different stages of development is the increased duration of epochs of absent movements as the fetus matures. In first trimester fetuses de Vries (see Chapter 1) found median durations of epochs of absent fetal movements ranging from 2 to 6 minutes, with a maximum of 13 minutes. This does not change through the second and early third trimesters, for Drogtrop *et al.* (1990) observed a median duration of absent body movements of 4.4 minutes in 25 to 30 week fetuses, with a maximum of 16.5 minutes. After this time, however, there is an increase in the median duration of somatic quiescence to 10 minutes at 32 weeks, and a further increase to 16.5 minutes at 40 weeks (see Chapter 3). The corresponding maximum epochs of absent body movements were 15.5 and 37 minutes, respectively. A similar pattern was found for epochs of absent fetal eye movements (Drogtrop *et al.* 1990). The criteria for interpretation of biophysical tests for fetal well-being do not take this developmental trend in motility into account; however, the test durations for both the non-stressed CTG and the biophysical profile substantially exceed the longest epochs of absent movements to be expected at 32 weeks of gestation and earlier. Perhaps this is at least a partial explanation for the relative lack of correlation between the score for the body movement component of the biophysical profile and adverse fetal outcomes (except for fetal distress) described by Manning in Chapter 17.

On the other hand, a marked decrease in the number of fetal movements may be a relatively late occurrence during the development of fetal distress. Although Arduini *et al.* (see Chapter 13) describe a significant decrease in the number of and proportion of recording time occupied by gross fetal movements in growth-retarded fetuses, they also found a substantial overlap between the affected fetuses and normal controls. Bekedam *et al.* (1987) had noted earlier that a decrease in fetal movements only became evident after the occurrence of late decelerations in the FHR. Experiments have shown that although body movements are suppressed by acute hypoxaemia in fetal sheep, movements subsequently return to normal levels when the hypoxaemia is prolonged at moderate, sub-lethal levels (Bocking *et al.* 1988). Further quantitative investigations of movement patterns in pregnancies with complications other than fetal growth retardation which threaten fetal well-being are needed to resolve the role of fetal body movements in identifying subacute fetal distress.

Qualitative aspects of fetal movements may be more predictive of neural dysfunction than the quantity of movements (Prechtl 1990). As noted by Arduini *et al.* (see Chapter 13), several investigators have described the movements of growth-retarded fetuses as weak, slow, or monotonous. Although qualitative analysis of fetal movements is subjective, Prechtl (1990) found a high degree of inter-observer agreement in the assessment of movement quality from videotapes of preterm infants. If the same can be demonstrated for ultrasound recordings of fetal movements, the quality of fetal movements may become a powerful tool in the prenatal detection of fetal compromise.

The development of behavioural states has been studied in two categories of abnormal pregnancies: pregnancies complicated by fetal growth retardation (see Chapter 13) and pregnancies of women with type 1 diabetes mellitus (see Chapter 14). Despite the fact that one of these complications results from chronic fetal hypoxaemia and/or undernutrition, and the other is often accompanied by fetal overnutrition, the differences from normal pregnancies in fetal behaviour were rather similar. In both groups, states appeared late, and in a high proportion of near-term fetuses states could not be identified. The reasons for the absence of states in both groups were prolonged transitions between periods of coincidence of the state variables, and interruption of epochs of coincident association of the state variables by episodes of no coincidence. Since these two disparate disorders produced similar effects on the development of behavioural states, the disturbances observed seem to represent non-specific effects of sub-optimal fetal metabolic conditions rather than specific behavioural pathologies.

Lastly, the importance of the rapid eye movement (REM) state (state 2F) for development of the fetal and neonatal brain deserves emphasis. As pointed out by Swaab, Honnebier, and Mirmiran in Chapter 7, growth and maintenance of neural tissue are promoted by stimulation. REM is a mechanism by which this stimulation can be self-generated during the fetal period when the individual is relatively cut off from environmental stimuli. Experimental suppression of REM during early development in laboratory animals has been shown to lead to permanent structural brain differences as well as physiological and behavioural defects. A number of commonly used drugs can affect the synthesis and action of brain neurotransmitters, and thereby suppress REM. The potential hazards of these drugs for the developing fetal brain are reviewed by Mirmiran and Swaab in Chapter 10. Physicians should be as cautious in prescribing potential behavioural teratogens for pregnant women as they are with possible structural teratogens.

References

Bekedam, D. J., Visser, G. H. A., Mulder, E. J. H., and Poelmann-Weesjes, G. (1987). Heart rate variation and movement incidence in growth-retarded fetuses: the significance of antenatal late heart rate decelerations. *American Journal of Obstetrics and Gynecology* **157**, 126–33.

Bocking, A. D., Gagnon, R., Milne, R. M., and White, S. E. (1988). Behavioural activity during prolonged hypoxemia in fetal sheep. *Journal of Applied Physiology* **65**, 2420–6.

Dawes, G. S., Fox, H. E., Leduc, B. M., Liggins, G. C., and Richards, R. T. (1970). Respiratory movements and paradoxical sleep in foetal lambs. *Journal of Physiology* **210**, 47–8.

Drogtrop, A. P., Ubels, R., and Nijhuis, J. G. (1990). The association between fetal body movements, eye movements and heart rate patterns in pregnancies between 25 and 30 weeks of gestation. *Early Human Development* **23**, 67–73.

Nijhuis, J. G., Prechtl, H. F. R., Martin, C. B., Jr, and Bots, R. S. G. M. (1982). Are there behavioural states in the human fetus? *Early Human Development* **6**, 177–95.

Prechtl, H. F. R. (1974). The behavioural states of the newborn infant (a review). *Brain Research* **76**, 185–212.

Prechtl, H. F. R. (1990). Qualitative changes of spontaneous movements in fetus and preterm infant are a marker of neurological dysfunction. *Early Human Development* **23**, 151–8.

Reid, D. L., Jensen, A., Phernetton, T. M., and Rankin, J. H. G. (1990). Relationship between plasma catecholamine levels and electrocortical state in the mature fetal lamb. *Journal of Developmental Physiology* **13**, 75–9.

Rizzo, G., Arduini, D., Valensise, H., and Romanini, C. (1990). Effects of behavioural state on cardiac output in the healthy human fetus at 36–38 weeks of gestation. *Early Human Development* **23**, 109–15.

Slotten, P., Phernetton, T., and Rankin, J. H. G. (1989). Relationship between fetal electrocorticographic changes and umbilical blood flow in the near term sheep fetus. *Journal of Developmental Physiology* **11**, 19–23.

Index

acetylcholine 113
acetyl salicylate 95
acidaemia 93, 185
acidosis xvi, 222, 249
acids in amniotic fluid 57, 108, 133, 137–
    42, **212–18**, 221–2
active sleep (state 2F)
    in animals 92, 105
    and apnoea 219, 220
    and blood flow velocity 227, 230, 233–7
    and brain development 78–80, 272
    in diabetic pregnancy 198–200
    fetal 30, 42, **49–52**, 91, 114, 209
    and movement 22
    REM 78–80, 91–2, 105, 114, 230, 272
    and stimulation 215
    transitions 188–90
    see also behavioural states
activity, see hyperactivity; movement; rest-
    activity cycles
adenosine 94
adrenaline 161, 168–72
adrenocorticotrophic hormone 170, 172
alcohol 96, 109, 166
almitrine 94, 105, 109
alpha-melanocyte-stimulating hormone 202
alpha-methyldopamine 79, 80, 113–17
amino acids 113, 136
amniotic fluid xviii, 136, 242–4, 251–4
amphetamines 114, 116
anaemia 49, 263
analgesics 271
anencephaly 148, 258–9, 261
animal research xv, vii, 100-11
    applicability to humans 101, 118–20, 69
    behavioural states 37
    circadian rhythms 139
    conspecific preferences 147
    drug effects 109, 115–18
    fetal psychology 129
    growth retardation 217–18
    hypoxaemia/hypoxia 97, 184, 243, 248
    psychological stress 169, 170, 171
    sleep states 79, 92, 105, 230, 272
    spinal cord transection 14
    stimulation 108, 138, 148–9, 217–18
    see also rats; sheep
antidepressants 113, 114, 115, 118
antiepileptics 115
antihypertensives 114, 118

anxiety 158–69, 172
aorta 182, 228–9, 234–7
Apgar score 220, 221, 248, 252
apnoea 219–20
arginine-vasopressin 81–4
arm/leg movements 6, 49, 50, 163
artery
    fetal internal carotid 230-7
    umbilical 230-4, 237, 254
arthrogryposis fetalis 264, 266
asphyxia xvi, xvii, xix
assessment of well-being 3, 66–7, **70**, 164–
    6, **179–267**, 270
atropine 95, 96, 104, 109
audition 131–3, 137–9, 143–6, 211, 217
autonomic nervous system 168–70

Babinski reflex 210
barbiturates 116, 118
Bayley Scales of Infant Development 159,
    164, 166, 203
behavioural states
    1F, see quiet sleep
    2F, see active sleep
    3F (quiet awake) 30, 41–2, 114, 263
    4F (active awake) 30, 41–2, 114, 215
    or activity cycles 101, 108, 109
    assessment of 27–8
    and biophysical profile 243
    and blood flow velocity 227–37
    and circadian rhythms 80
    coincidences **31–2**, 68, 103, 186–8, 198–
        9, 201
    concept of vii, 66, 100-1, 227, **269–73**
    definition of 26–7, 30-1
    and diabetic pregnancy 35, 37, 193–4,
        198–203, 272
    disturbance of 79, 108–9
    drug effects **35**, 109, **114–17**, 271
    duration of 35, 67, 103
    and epileptic pregnancy 35
    functional significance 109
    and growth retardation 35, 37, **186–8**,
        272
    and heart rate 21, 27–31, 37, **41–57**,
        270-1
    incidence of 35
    and interpretation of tests 269

behavioural states (*cont.*)
  in labour 59, **61**, 62, 91
  and maternal emotions 161–5, 171
  neonatal and fetal 26–31, 36, **65–9**, 91,
    109, 129
  and nervous system 37, 109
  second trimester 23
  in sheep 36–7, 103–9
  and state concomitants 33–5, 37, 67, 102
  and stimulation 133, 209–11, 215–16
  third trimester 182, 261
  transitions 32, 37, 67–8, 187–90, 200
  variables 21, 32, 41–2, 102–3, 187, 190
  see also fetal behaviour; movement;
    neonates; rest-activity cycles
beta-mimetics 263
biological clock, see circadian rhythms
biophysical profile xviii–xix, 35, 185, **241–
    57**, 260-1, 271
birth, *see* labour; stillbirth
blood flow 181–2, 187, 190, 230, 269, 270
  end-diastolic flow 182, 228, 230, 234
  peak systolic flow 230, 232, 235, 236
  in sheep 92, 106–7, 270
  velocity waveforms 227–40, 254
blood pressure 159, 170
body movements
  and biophysical profile scoring 242–3
  in diabetic pregnancy 195, 201
  first trimester 5, 258–9
  and heart-rate 41, 53, 228–9
  and maternal emotions 163
  and neurological assessment 70
  second trimester 17–23, 259
  sheep 105–6, 183
  third trimester 30, 32, 188
borborygmi 138
brain
  and active sleep 78–80, 272
  and auditory pathways 217
  and behaviour 76, 227, 272
  blood flow 106, 234, 269
  and circadian rhythms 75, 78–84
  damage 181
  death 262
  delayed maturation 202, 204
  drug effects 79–80, 112–25, 271–2
  glucose level effects 200
  hormone effects 170
  and sensory information 132, 145
  stem transection 92–4, 96
  see also central nervous system; neural
    mechanisms
brain-sparing effect 181, 188, 189, 230,
    237
Brazelton Neonatal Behaviour Assessment
    Scale 159, 202

breast-feeding 116, 119, 146–7, 163, 164,
    166
breathing movements xviii–xix, 269
  and biophysical profile 241–4, 252, 254
  and circadian rhythms 76, 84, 107, 171
  and Doppler flow measurements 227,
    232
  and drug action 96
  first trimester 6, 199
  and glucose levels 19, 107, 196–9, 201
  and growth retardation 185–6, 188
  and hypercapnia/hypocapnia 218
  and hyperoxia 218–19
  in labour 57, 61, 62
  and lung tissue 14
  and maternal emotions 163, 169
  and meals 19, 20, 23, 196
  paradoxical 219
  periodic 202, 204
  in quiet sleep 27, 45, 47, 92, 93
  second trimester 18–20, 23, 260
  in sheep 92–6, **104–5**, 185, 220, 243, 269
  and sound/vibration 160, 214–15
  third trimester 27, 28, 33–4, 37, 261

caesarean section 261–2, 270
caffeine 166
cardiography 162
cardiotocography 163
  in fetal monitoring xvi, 28–9, 52–3, 271
  neonates 67
  pathological 190
  and rest–activity cycles 270
  second trimester 259
  third trimester 261–4
  see also heart-rate
cardiovascular mechanisms 227, 232–5
carotid artery, internal 230-7
catecholamines 168, 170, 228, 270
central nervous system xviii, 70, 75–99,
    227, 269
  and behaviour 37, 100, 109, 187, 261,
    264
  in diabetic pregnancy 193, 194, 198, 203
  and growth retardation 181
  and movement 13, 14, 23, 54, 106, 194
  and sensory information 132, 145
  see also brain; neural mechanisms
cerebral palsy xvii
chemosensation 136–7, 139
chlorpromazine 116
circadian rhythms 18, 20, 35, **75–84**, 107–
    8, 139, 171
circulation xv, 35, 237, 269–70
citric acids 136

cleft lip/palate 159
clomipramine 113, 114, 115, 117
clonidine 79, 97, 113–19
cocaine 35
coincidences **31–2**, 68, 103, 186–8, 198–201
communication 146
concomitants, *see* state concomitants
conditioning 141–2
contractions 169, 271
cordocentesis viii, 181, 188, 262
corticosteroids 170
cortisol 82, 161, 171, 172
crying 31, 159, 166
cutaneous senses 134–5, 139, 145

depression 119, 161
descending aorta 182, 228–9, 234–7
dexamethasone 118
diabetic pregnancy 19–20, 35, 37, **193–208**, 272
diazepam 115, 116, 118
distress viii, xvii
  and biophysical profile scoring 245, 248, 249, 252
  and growth retardation 181, 183, 186
  and heart patterns 49, 59, 260, 261
  in labour 59, 221, 222, 245, 270
  see also fetal condition
diurnal rhythms, see circadian rhythms
dopamine 112–13, 171
Doppler methods 43, 244, 253, 254
  flow measurements 181, 182, 187, 190, 227–40
Down's syndrome 148, 159
drugs 109, 119
  effects on developing brain 79–80, **112–25**, 271–2
  in pregnancy 35, 117–19, 148, 261
  site of action 95–6
Duchenne muscular dystrophy 53
ductus arteriosus 232–7, 270
ductus venosus 235

ear 210
echography 162
electrical stimulation 109
electrocardiography 43
electrocortical activity 101, 103, 234
  in sheep 91–6, **104**, 217, 220, 269
electroencephalogram 67, 202, 204
electromyogram 67
electronic artificial larynx 212, 214, 215, 217, 221, 222

electro-oculogram 67
emotional influences 130, 157–78
  on behavioural outcome 159
  on obstetric outcome 158–9
  underlying mechanisms 167–72
end-diastolic flow 182, 228, 230, 234
endocrinology 167–71, 270
  see also hormonal influences
endorphins 171
epileptic pregnancy 35, 118, 119
eye movements xviii, 163, 271
  and behavioural states 28, 49, 62, 67, 269
  first trimester 7
  and glucose levels 195
  and growth retardation 184–5, 189
  and heart rate patterns 184–5, 228–9
  second trimester 20-23, 260
  in sheep **105**, 184, 220, 269
  and sound stimulation 137
  third trimester 28–31, 261
  see also REM sleep

fatty acids 136
fetal behaviour xvii–xviii, vii, 270
  and central nervous control xviii, 76, **91–2**, 264
  circadian rhythms 18, 20, 35, **75–84**, 107–8, 139, 171
  in diabetic pregnancy 19–20, 35, **193–208**, 272
  Doppler flow measurements 181, 182, 227–40
  and fetal psychology vii, 127–78
  first trimester 3–16
  and gestational age vii, 26, 187, 258
  and growth retardation 35, 181–92, 216–18
  in labour 57–64, 221–22
  and maternal emotions 157–78
  monitoring 28–30, 220-22, 258–67
  in normal pregnancy 3–72, 194
  quantitative analysis 8–10, 31–3, 258–9, 264, 271
  research 73–125
  second trimester 17–25
  and stimulation 58, 101, 108–9, 133, **209–26**
  third trimester 26–40
  and well-being 179–267, 270
  see also animal research; behavioural states; biophysical profile; breathing movements; central nervous system; distress; drugs; eye movements; heart-rate; mother's emotions; micturition; movement; neonates; physiology; psychology; sheep; stimulation; stress; tone

fetal condition 3, 100
  and behavioural states 35, 209
  and biophysical profile 241, 243
  and blood flow velocity 227
  and breathing movements 105
  and heart-rate patterns 264
  and learning 147
  and stimulation 212, 214, 220, 221
  see also distress
fetus
  compromised 243, 248, 254, 272
  'jogging' 264
  malformations 193
  psychological health of 130, 149
  research techniques xv–xvi, 131–2
finger movements 6
foramen ovale 232, 234, 235, 237, 270

gamma-aminobutyric acid 115
gastrointestinal problems 159, 166
gestational age vii, 26, 187, **254–5**, 258
  and drug teratogenicity 119
  and response to stimulation 214, 220,
    221
glucocorticoids 118
glucose 19, 107, **193–6**, 198–204, 217
growth retardation 181–92, 271–2
  and behavioural states 35, 37, **186–8**,
    272
  and biophysical profile 248
  in diabetic pregnancy 201
  Doppler flow measurements 227–32,
    236–7
  and oxygen therapy 218, 221
  and stimulation 216–18

habituation 140-1, 148
haemodynamics 181, 227, 230, 232, 234,
  237
hand–face contact 7, 20, 23, 28
handicaps xvi, 159
head movements 6, 20, 23, 28, 49–50, 163,
  165
hearing, *see* audition
heart accelerations 41, 97, 264, 265
  and behavioural states 42, 49–54
  and circadian rhythms 76
  in diabetic pregnancy 195, 196
  in labour 57, 58, 61
  and maternal emotions 160, 169
  and stimulation 209, 214–18, 222
heart-beat of mother 138, 143, 159
heart decelerations 41, 52, 261, 271

  and circadian rhythms 76
  and growth retardation 184, 188–90
  in labour 245
  and maternal emotions 161, 168
  and tachycardia 264–5, 270
heart patterns/rhythms 41–56
  and blood flow velocity 227
  in diabetic pregnancy 198, 200
  and fetal distress 49, 59, 260, 261
  and growth retardation 182–3
  and maternal emotions 161
  and micturition 34
  and movement 184, 228–9, 264, 270
  normal/reactive 41, 42, 264
  silent 260-2
  and stimulation 212
heart-rate xviii–xix
  base-line frequency 41, 52
  and behavioural states 21, 27–31, 37,
    41–57, 270–1
  and biophysical profile 241–3, 253
  and central nervous system 54, 96–7,
    269
  circadian rhythms 76, 84, 108, 171
  and Doppler flow measurements 227–9,
    232, 237
  drug influences 261
  and eye movements 184–5
  and fetal movements 22–3, 41–57, 97,
    102, 209, 228–9, 262–5
  and gestational age 214, 221, 258
  and glucose levels 194–6, 198, 200
  and growth retardation 181–3, 184–90,
    217
  and hypercapnia/hypocapnia 218
  implications for monitoring 28–9, 52–4,
    258–67
  in labour 57–62, 168, 222
  and maternal hyperoxia 218
  monitoring 52–4
  oscillations 49, 53, 263
  pulsatility index 228, 229
  in sheep 96–7, 106
  sinusoidal 45, 49, 263
  and stimulation 133–7, 160-1, **212–15**,
    221, 222
  and sucking 45, 48–9, 53, 263
  tachycardia 160, 166, 214–15, 263–5,
    270
  see also cardiotocography; heart
accelerations; heart decelerations; heart
patterns/rhythms; heart variability
heart variability xvii, xviii, 261, 269, 270
  and blood flow velocity 228–9
  and circadian rhythms 76
  in diabetic pregnancy 196
  and growth retardation 182–3, 188

in labour 58–62
and movement 41, 52
in sheep 96–7, 106
and stimulation 215–18
hiccups 6, 20, 23, 50-2
homeostasis 167
hormonal influences 76, 84, 107, 161, 166–72, 202, 270
'hot-housing' 148
hyoscine 95, 104
hyperactivity 79, 148, 159, 160, 166
hypercapnia 218, 220
hyperglycaemia 195, 196, 198, 201, 204
hyperkinesia 160
hyperoxygenation 188–90, 218–21
hypertensive pregnancy 119
hypocapnia 218, 220
hypoglycaemia 195, 196, 202
hypothalamo-pituitary-adrenocortical
    system 168, 170, 171, 172
hypotonia 202
hypoxaemia xix
    and biophysical profile scoring 248–50, 254
    in sheep 93–7, 106, 183, 185, 220, 243, 271
    hypoxia xvi, xix, 262
    and cortical function 220
    and endorphins 171
    and growth retardation 228
    in sheep 93–6, 105–6

imipramine 113, 115, 116, 117
imprindole 115
indomethacin 95, 109
infants, see neonates
insulin 172
    see also diabetic pregnancy
intercostal-to-phrenic inhibitory reflex 219–20
internal carotid artery 230-7
intrauterine growth retardation, see growth retardation

jaw movements 6, 20, 23, 67
'jogging fetus' 264

kinesthetic sense 135

L-5–hydroxytryptophan 109

labour 57–64, 91, 168
    and circadian rhythms 77–8, 84
    endorphins 171
    fetal distress 59, 221, 222, 245, 270-1
lactation 116, 119, 146–7, 163, 164, 166
lactic acid 136
lambs, see sheep
language 146
learning and sensation 129–31, 139–49
leg/arm movements 6, 49, 50, 163

maternal, see mothers
meclofenamate 95
melatonin 81, 107, 108, 139
memory 144
metabolism 69, 269–70
methadone 35
methodological problems 157, 160-1
mianserin 115
micturition 34, 37
monitoring
    fetal behaviour 28–30, 220-22, 258–67
    fetal heart-rate 52–4
    first trimester 258–9
    intrapartum 221–2
    second trimester 259–61
    third trimester 261–4
    see also cardiotocography
monoamines 80, 112–13, 115
morphine 95–6
mortality
    intrauterine 183, 221, 252
    maternal xv
    neonatal 78, 248
    perinatal xv, 241, 245, 247–52
mothers
    anxiety 158–69, 172
    blood pressure 159, 170
    circadian rhythms 80-1, 84
    depression 119, 161
    diet 107, 146
    emotions 130, 157–78
    fatigue 167
    glucose levels 19, 107, **193–6**, 198–201, 204, 217
    heartbeat 138, 143, 159
    homeostasis 167
    hostility 161
    hypercapnia/hypocapnia 218
    mortality xv
    odour 147
    oxygen 148, 188–90, 218–19, 221
    panic 160
    physical activity 167
    psychophysiological functioning 167

mothers (*cont.*)
  smoking 148, 166
  stress 158–60
  ultrasound feedback 161
  voice 138, 142–3, 145–7
  see also pregnancy
motility, *see* movement
motor activity, *see* movement
mouthing
  and behavioural states 43–6, 49–53, 67, 263
  and maternal emotions 163
  third trimester 28, 35, 37
movement xvii, xviii, xix
  absent 9, 184, 259, 271
  and active sleep 22
  amplitude 8, 11, 12
  and analgesics 271
  and anatomy 13
  arm/leg 6, 49, 50, 163
  and behavioural states 28, 49, 101, 270
  and biophysical profile 241, 252–4
  classification of 4
  clustering 17, 21, 45, 49, 220
  and distress 271
  diurnal variations 18, 20, 35, 76, 171
  duration of 9, 53, 103, 166, 271
  finger 6
  first trimester **3–16**, 66, 194, 197–8, 203, 258–9, 271
  force of 8, 11, 12
  functional significance 13–14
  generalized, *see* body movements
  and glucose levels 107, 194–6, 198, 201, 203
  and growth retardation 183–4, 188–90, 217
  hand/face contact 7, 20, 23, 28
  head 6, 20, 23, 28, 49–50, 163, 165
  hereditary influences 167
  hiccups 6, 20, 23, 50-2
  and hypercapnia/hypocapnia 218
  incidence/occurrence 9, 12, 17–23, 166, 201, 269
  individual differences 10–11, 23
  jaw 6, 20, 23, 67
  just-discernible 4
  in labour **57**, 58, 61, 63
  and maternal emotions 162–6, 168–71
  and maternal hyperoxia 218
  maternal perception of 91, 264
  and meals 195
  mouth, *see* mouthing; sucking
  muscular structures 13, 234
  neural mechanisms of 3, 13, **65–6**, 269
  normal 12
  patterns **3–12**, **17–20**, 23, 201, 203, 259

quality of 70, 258, 264, 271–2
quantitative aspects 8–10, **31–3**, 258–9, 264, 271
quiescence 10, 30, 57, 270
rotation 7, 31
second trimester 17–25, 259–61
sex differences 11
  in sheep 105–6, 183–4, 220, 269
speed of 8, 11, 12
startles 4–5, 20, 23, 30
and stimulation 133–9, 160, 210, **214–16**, 221
stretches 5, 20, 23, 30, 66
swallowing, *see* sucking
third trimester 28–9, 261–4
tongue 7
and ultrasound feedback 161
yawn 7, 20, 66
see also body movements; breathing movements; central nervous system; eye movements; heart patterns; heart-rate; heart variability; mouthing; rest-activity cycles; sucking
muscular dystrophy 53
music 144, 160
myometrium 76, 77, 79, 80, 169

N-acetyltransferase 81–2
naloxone 115
narcotics 35
neonates 65–72
  behaviour of xvii–xviii, 26–31, 57, 129, 131
  Brazelton Neonatal Behaviour Assessment Scale 159, 202
  breast-feeding 116, 119, 146–7, 163, 164, 166
  breathing 219
  circadian rhythms 80-1
  conditioning 142
  of diabetic mothers 193, 202–3
  and fetal behavioural states 26–31, 36, **65–9**, 91, 109, 129
  irritability 159, 170
  and maternal emotions 157–78
  mortality 78, 248
  neural mechanisms 68–70
  premature 80-1, 84, 131, 140, 270
  psychology 130-32
  research techniques 131
  responses to stimulation 142–4, 209–10
  sleep 66–8, 84, 159, 163, 202, 230
  sucking 68, 142–3, 146–7
  temperament 160, 163, 166

neural mechanisms
  of fetal movement 3, 13, 65–6, 269
  of neonates 68–70
  and sensory experience 132, 145
  and stimulation 133–4, 148–9
  see also autonomic nervous system;
      brain; central nervous system
  neural tube defects 193
  neuroleptics 166
  neurological assessment 3, 66–7, 70,
      164–6, 203, 209
neuroteratology 112–14, 118–20
neurotransmitters 95, 171, 172
  effect of drugs 79, 112–14, 115, 272
noise, *see* sound
nomifensine 115
non-stress test 244, 252–4
noradrenaline 112–13, 115, 161, 170–2

olfaction 131, 132, 136
oligohydramnios 244, 248
opiates 114, 115
oxygen 148, 188–90, 218–21
oxytocin levels 77

pain 135, 171, 210
panic 160
parturition, *see* labour
peak systolic flow 230, 232, 235, 236
pentobarbitone 95
peptides 113
perceptions 91, 131, 132, 135, 167, 264
perinatal morbidity 241, 245, 250, 251
perinatal mortality xv, 241, 245, 247–52
physiology xv, 269
placental dysfunction 249
pons 92–6
pregnancy
  depression in 119, 161
  diabetic 19–20, 35, 37, **193–208**, 272
  drug use during 35, 117–19, 148, 261
  duration of 68–9
  epileptic 35, 118, 119
  hypertensive 119
  maternal emotions during 157–78
  normal 3–72, 194
  pathological 35
  see also mothers
premature infants 80-1, 84, 131, 140, 270
prolactin 107, 108, 172
propranolol 96, 113, 115, 116, 117
proprioception 135–6, 139, 210-11
prostaglandins 95, 107

psychobiology vii
psychology vii, 127–78
pulsatility indices 35, 228–37
pyloric stenosis 159

quality of movements 70, 258, 264, 271– 2
quantitative aspects of movement 8–10,
      31–3, 258–9, 264, 271
quiescence 10, 30, 57, 270
  see also rest-activity cycles; sleep
quiet sleep (state1F)
  and blood flow velocity 227, 230, 233,
      236–7
  and breathing movements 27, 45, 47, 92,
      93
  in diabetic pregnancy 198–201
  effects of drugs 114
  and electrocortical activity 92–3
  and growth retardation 188–90
  and heart-rate 42, **43–9**, 53, 263
  second trimester 22
  and stimulation 215, 220
  third trimester 27, 30
  see also behavioural states

rapid eye movement sleep, *see* REM sleep
rats 113–19
real-time ultrasound 28, 131, 162–3, 227,
      234, 241, 270
reflexes 3, 92, 106, 211
  Babinski 210
  intercostal-to-phrenic inhibitory 219–20
  More 210
  righting 135
  rooting 134
  vibratory 210
REM sleep 78–80, 91–2, 105, 114, 230,
      272
  see also active sleep
research 73–125
  and clinical practice xvi
  methodological problems 157, 160-1
  techniques xv–xvi, 131, 132
  see also animal research
reserpine 113, 116
rest-activity cycles 182, 209, 243, 270
  or behavioural states 101, 108, 109
  and circadian rhythms 81, 82, 84
  and drug influence 115
  first trimester 10
  and heart-rate 57, 61–2
  second trimester 17, 20-3, 259
  third trimester 261

rhythmicity, *see* circadian rhythms
ritodrine 117, 119
rotation 7, 31

schizophrenia 148
sensation
 chemosensation 136–7, 139
 cutaneous 134–5, 139, 145
 kinesthetic 135
 and learning 129–31, 139–49
 maturation of receptors 210-12
 and neural mechanisms 132, 145
 sensory environment 130-9, 147–9
serotonin 81, 112–13, 115, 171
sex differences in movements 11
sheep
 auditory structures 217
 behavioural states 36–7, 103–9
 blood flow 92, 106–7, 270
 body and limb movements 105–6, 183
 brain stem transection 92–4, 96
 breathing activity 92–6, **104–5**, 185, 220,
  243, 269
 circadian rhythms 107–8
 electrocortical activity 91–6, **104**, 217,
  220, 269
 eye movements **105**, 184, 220, 269
 heart rate variation 96–7, 106
 hypoxaemia/hypoxia 93–7, 105–6, 183,
  185, 220, 243, 271
sigmoid blip 161
silent heart-rate pattern 260-2
sinusoidal heart-rate 45, 49, 263
sleep xviii
 neonatal 66–8, 84, 159, 163, 202, 230
 problems 79–80
 REM 78–80, 91–2, 105, 114, 230, 272
 see also active sleep, quiet sleep, rest-
  activity cycles
smell, *see* olfaction
smoking 148, 166
social development 147
sound
 environment 138
 responses to 108, 133, 137–9, 142, **212–
  16**, 220
 see also vibro-acoustic stimulation
startles 4–5, 20, 23, 30
state concomitants 33–5, 37, 67, 102
State Trait Anxiety Inventory 162–5
stillbirth 78, 248
stimulation 209–26
 auditory 137, 145, 146
 clinical significance 220-22
 electrical 109

of exteriorized fetuses 65
 fetal responses to 101, 108, 133–9, 142–
  4, 160–1, **209–26**, 269
 and gestational age 214, 220, 221
 habituation 140-1, 148
 in labour 58
 neonatal responses to 142–4, 209–10
 neural mechanisms 133–4, 148–9
 prenatal courses 148–9
 stressful 172
 tactile 133, 134, 139
 temperature 135
 vibro-acoustic 57, 108, 137–9, 141–2,
  212–18, 221–2
 visual 136, 211
stress xvi–xvii, 158–60, 169–72
 non-stress test 244, 252–4
 see also distress
stretches 5, 20, 23, 30, 66
sucking
 first trimester 6
 and heart-rate 45, 48–9, 53, 263
 neonatal 68, 142–3, 146–7
 second trimester 20
suprachiasmatic nucleus 75, 76, 81–4, 139
surveillance, *see* monitoring
sympatho-adrenomedullar system 168, 172

tachycardia 160, 166, 214–15, 263–5, 270
taste 136, 146–7
temperament 160, 163, 166
temperature 81, 84, 135
teratogenicity 112–14, 118–20, 272
testosterone 172
thyroxine 172
tone xviii–xix, 241–2, 244, 251–2, 254
tongue movements 7
touch 133, 134, 139
transitions 32, 37, 67–8, 187–90, 200
triamcinolone 171
trimesters
 first 3–16, 66, 194, 197–8, 203, 258–9, 271
 second 17–25, 259–61
 third 26–40, 182, 188, 198–201, 261–4
trisomy 21, 148

ultrasound xvi, xvii, 3, 269
 and classification of movement 4
 feedback to mothers 161
 and growth retardation 181
 real-time scanners 28, 131, 162–3, 227,
  234, 241, 270
 see also Doppler methods

umbilical artery 230-4, 237, 254
umbilical vein 248, 249
uric acid 136
uterine contractions 169, 271
utero-placental insufficiency 181, 190

valium 117
vasopressin 81–4, 228
vestibular system 69, 135, 136, 211
vibro-acoustic stimulation 57, 108, 137–42,
    160, **210–18**, 220-2
    see also sound
vision 131, 132, 136, 211
voices 138, 142–3, 145–7

wakefulness 30-1, 57, 82, 84, 104,
    114
    see also behavioural states; rest–activity
    cycles; sleep
well-being 179–267, 270

yawning 7, 20, 66

zimelidine 115